The International Library of Sociology

ADOLESCENT GIRLS
IN APPROVED SCHOOLS

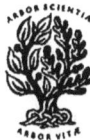

Founded by KARL MANNHEIM

The International Library of Sociology

THE SOCIOLOGY OF EDUCATION
In 28 Volumes

ADOLESCENT GIRLS IN APPROVED SCHOOLS

by

HELEN J. RICHARDSON

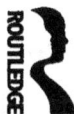

ROUTLEDGE

First published in 1969 by
Routledge

Reprinted in 1998, 1999 by
Routledge

2 Park Square, Milton Park, Abingdon, Oxfordshire OX14 4RN
711 Third Avenue, New York, NY 10017
First issued in paperback 2014
Routledge is an imprint of the Taylor and Francis Group,
an informa business

Transferred to Digital Printing 2007

The publishers have made every effort to contact authors/copyright holders
of the works reprinted in *The International Library of Sociology*.
This has not been possible in every case, however, and we would
welcome correspondence from those individuals/companies
we have been unable to trace.

British Library Cataloguing in Publication Data
A CIP catalogue record for this book
is available from the British Library

Adolescent Girls in Approved Schools
ISBN 978-0-415-17748-1 (hbk)
ISBN 978-0-415-86394-0 (pbk)
The Sociology of Education: 28 Volumes
ISBN 978-0-415-17833-4
The International Library of Sociology: 274 Volumes
ISBN 978-0-415-17838-9

Publisher's Note
The publisher has gone to great lengths to ensure the quality of this reprint
but points out that some imperfections in the original may be apparent

'What people do not understand, M. le Juge, is that more is owing to these children than to others . . .'
'Yes, I know . . . (A silence) And they always have less . . .'
'Always! Whatever one does, whatever one gives them, they will always have less . . .'

Trans. from Michel Cournot's
Enfants de la Justice, Editions Gallimard, 1959

Lancaster University refectory committee has started a special watch on crockery and cutlery, after thefts by students estimated to cost £350 . . .
The University bookshop has reported loss by theft of 300 books since it was opened a year ago.

The Guardian, 18.2.66

She broke into a shop and stole a lipstick and a packet of pellets, total value 7/9d . . . She was brought before Halifax Juvenile Court charged with breaking and entering and larceny and was committed to an Approved School.

From a Classifying Approved School report, 1957

ACKNOWLEDGMENTS

I am grateful firstly to Dr Gordon Rose, who encouraged me to write this book, and gave much time to advice and criticism. A generous financial grant from the Calouste Gulbenkian Foundation made the task possible.

Miss I. Wannop, who was Headmistress of The Shaw in the main three-year period of the research, not only read the manuscript, but was the spirit guiding the writer and most of the other workers into the deeper channels of classification. Hers was the calm amid turmoil.

Thanks are due besides to my long-suffering husband, to a vast number of supportive or goading friends, and to various academic advisers, also to unexpected benefactors less soulless than their reputation—computing experts.

I owe a debt to the Home Office for permission to extract data from files of the former Shaw Classifying School, and to the H.O. Archives Department which gave me access to the files.

Lastly a few individual helpers or suppliers of information whom I wish to thank: Mr Ainsworth, Mr and Mrs Goode, Mr Curr, Mrs Thomas, Mr Moore, Miss Francis, Miss Redfarn (author of one pen picture quoted), the Managers of the two Training Schools described in Chapter Two, and of course the Managers of the former Shaw Classifying School who appointed me and tolerated some of my less 'normal' ideas.

The conclusions drawn and opinions expressed in the book do not, of course, represent the views of any of the above, nor of my colleagues and our charges, from whose stories I have freely borrowed for the text without their permission.

CONTENTS

Contents

Contents

TABLES

Chapter One

INTRODUCTION

When the subject of delinquency hits the headlines, the discussion rarely has much reference to women and girls. When it does the usual commentators remain uneasily silent.

This happens too in the lecture hall, whether the audience is academic, professional or lay. Reticence and even avoidance of the subject of female delinquency extend to police, to male magistrates, and even to many psychiatric clinics, except where women are in charge. A seam of something we might vaguely call chivalry runs through our society, and while women in the main are realistic about their own sex, most men are afraid of their mixed guilt and anger at the worst demonstrations of women or girls 'going wrong'. Deeper emotions apart, crime is a man's world, and female delinquency tends all too often to be shrugged off or avoided.

The subject is more easily avoided, for far fewer girls come before the Courts than do boys, and they appear initially at a later stage. The number of boys aged 14 to 17 found guilty of indictable offences in 1962 (when figures for this research were first being compiled) was 30,569; the number of girls of the same age was 3,764. The number of boys found guilty of indictable offences in 1954 was 13,387; the number of girls of the same age was 1,577. For non-indictable offences we also see large discrepancies. Going back to 1851, to Mary Carpenter's famous book on Reformatory Schools,[1] we find approximately the same ratios; proportions vary from one in five to one in eight. When we look at the number of boys and girls reported by local authorities as committed to Approved Schools by order of Court in each year from 1952 to 1957 (the period covered by this study) we find a consistent ratio of one girl to six boys. As the Boys' Approved Schools were normally larger institutions, the proportion of Girls' Approved Schools was thirty-nine, to eighty-eight for boys, at the end of 1954.[2] The average size of the Girls' Schools was only thirty-three at the end of the same year.

Another marked difference between the sexes is that, for those years, the peak age range of committal for boys was (except in 1954) 13 to 15 years; for girls it was always 15 to 17 years. Again we have Mary Carpenter noting in 1851[1] a comparable time lag.

A third outstanding difference is that about 64 per cent of the girls

1

are committed to Approved School as being in need of care or protection, being in moral danger, or being beyond parental control,
whereas much the largest group (95 per cent) of the boys sent to
Approved School are committed as offenders.

The fourth difference, quoted annually in Home Office statistics,
but one more open to question and criticism—and one which will be
dealt with at length in this study—is that between the success rates
after Approved School training. The 'satisfactory' figures quoted in
the Eighth and subsequent reports on the work of the Children's
Department of the Home Office[2] for boys and girls placed out between the years 1953 and 1959 are:

	1953	1954	1955	1956	1957	1958	1959
Boys	62%	61%	56%	51%	50%	43%	43%
Girls	83%	85%	88%	84%	85%	86%	82%

'Satisfactory' denotes not having been found guilty of an offence
during the three years following placing out. This criterion will be
discussed fully in relation to girls; the spectacular differences in the
success rates appearing above are, to say the least, questionable.

It would be surprising, then, if boys and girls in Approved Schools
did not present different types of problems, yet much more emotion
than cool common-sense has been expressed on the subject. Indeed
little has been written, either by people engaged on the work, or by
the skilled lay observer.

Of what has been said most is negative. Social science lecturers,
students and ex-students tend to comment in two ways:

(a) that most of the residential staff working with delinquent girls
are middle-aged spinsters and therefore cannot understand the sexual
problems of the girls; one obvious answer is, that women who, for
various reasons, have to deny their natural instincts, may be better
able to understand the girls' temporary deprivations; another answer
is that married women, as unmarried women, have varying depths of
experience, some grandmothers being noticeably adolescent. In any
case the more deprived delinquent girls are extremely demanding of
attention, and single-mindedness on the part of staff often means
more to her than the awareness that staff lead 'normal' married lives.

(b) The second oft-repeated comment is that girls in Approved
Schools have to do domestic work, which they hate. They will, however, be doing some kind of domestic work for the rest of their lives.
They may as well come to grips with their femininity at a stage when
they can be taught to do domestic work more efficiently and less
arduously than their mothers, so as to leave time for some of the
leisure pursuits and hobbies that, in fact, take up more time in the

Approved Schools—and which the same girls in the outside world would rarely pursue.

Occasional allusions to maladjusted or delinquent girls appear elsewhere; in the Report of the Committee on Maladjusted Children[3] (Par. 297) we read: 'The experience at one school (i.e. a mixed school for maladjusted) has been that girls make much greater affective demands on the staff, female as well as male.' This is repeated by David Wills in *Throw away thy Rod*;[4] 'In any case, all maladjusted children need the personal attention and affection of adults; girls seem to need it much more than boys, seem to be more conscious of their need, and more deliberate in attempts to secure it.' The writer would add that by the time they are dealt with as maladjusted adolescents they have behind their excessive demands for attention an increased sophistication of experience; this is a particular problem with the girls in Intermediate and Senior Approved Schools.

In another allusion, from the mid-nineteenth century, Mary Carpenter[1] suggests that young girls 'are generally much less prone to crime than boys of the same age', but that their tendency to it rapidly increases with their age, and that 'when they have once embarked on a criminal career, they become more thoroughly hardened than the other sex'. To confirm this she quotes from the Bishop of Tasmania, a witness to the condition of female convicts in the colonies:[1] 'Female felons are so bad, because, before a woman can become a felon at all, she must have fallen much lower, have unlearnt much more, have become much more lost and depraved than a man. Her difficulty of regaining her self-respect is proportionately greater.'

Sophisticated sexual experience is a main feature of the Girls' Approved School population, as we shall see. It is therefore relevant to quote from Michael Schofield's still recent report on the *Sexual Behaviour of Young People*[5] (p. 229): 'It is clear that experienced girls have gone much farther than experienced boys in rejecting family influences. Relations with both parents were often strained.' He assumes that, because a girl is more influenced by her family, she must go farther in overcoming these pressures and 'derogate her family loyalty' before she can kick over the traces. Such extreme reactions by the Classifying School girls (carried over from family derogation often to derogation of the new community) will be demonstrated in a statistical analysis on projective testing carried out in the school.

To generalize and talk of *the* delinquent girl, who does not exist, is difficult. Rose Giallombardo,[6] a sociologist studying a 'Society of Women' in an American Women's Prison, can write with academic detachment of the responses of individual women to a setting, contrasted with the responses of men prisoners to their different setting

—each having been cut off from meaningful relationships outside, and having brought their cultural roles with them. Amid the incessant strivings to form meaningful relationships within a Girls' Classifying Approved School, and to interpret for the girls their failures in relationships outside, it was inevitable that we tended to have a blurred picture of the degree to which they succeeded in running their institution lives independently of us. And so there will be gaps—serious to some—in what follows.

It is not therefore without anxiety that the writer sets out to chart some of this relatively uncharted territory, using experience as well as recorded material. In doing so the story may become more personal and intimate than was intended at the outset of the research. A description of one of the two Classifying Approved Schools for Girls in the two decades which have passed must inevitably bring in the other group of characters in the story—those who were privileged to have unusual experience of a deviant population at a peculiarly personal level. We, the workers, learned from the girls as they learned from us; in the process we sometimes gained more insight into ourselves, which we needed for the next day's challenges.

Chapter Two

HISTORICAL SUMMARY

Scolds and harlots are older phenomena than pick-pockets and car-thieves. Much of what passes for female delinquency in the 14 to 17 age-group (the group to be studied in this research) is off-beat in a very primitive way. Studies of penal reform make little mention of the minority group of women and girls. They are 'covered' by numerous Acts of Parliament just as the men are covered, but not much historical research is devoted to them as a distinctive group from men, nor as to how far the legislation of the past century has catered for their differing emotional and social needs. 'Covered' is indeed the right word, for it is often difficult to find a mention of female delinquency.

Dr Gordon Rose[1] has given an excellent account of the Approved School system in *Schools for Young Offenders*. For an objective account of the system as a whole and its past and current administration, this is the best source of information. Historically it does not offer a comparative basis for this present study of 14 to 17-year-old Approved School Girls, for 40 per cent of the research sample (the 16-year-olds) would not have been in the Reformatories of the nineteenth and earlier twentieth centuries, but in prisons (later on in Borstals), if guilty of offences punishable in these days. Otherwise a good many might have been camp-followers or on the streets.

The account in this chapter is, in contrast to most, not a background to the study of delinquency in general, but a skeleton built up from a few historical remains of female wrongdoers—a skeleton into which it is hoped to breathe something of the spirit of the 600 delinquent girls studied in this research, and known personally to the writer. Because the skeleton is a female one, it may seem oddly disproportionate to those accustomed to male views of long-term delinquency studies.

Prior to the mid-sixteenth century, which saw the founding in England of the first Bridewell for 'the vagabond and ydle strumpet',[2] the punishment of women, as of men who were felons or vagabonds, was mainly physical and public, and the more permanent removal from the sight of their more law-abiding fellows was through imprisonment, death, banishment, or later, from the early sixteenth century, through compulsory transportation.

Among the public and physical punishments of women were branking, branding, ducking, whipping and the pillory.[3] While most victims of these devices would be older than the group being studied, the descriptions of scolds, harlots and petty thieves of the middle ages fits a proportion of our more rebellious, more unseemly 14 to 17-year-olds of the mid-twentieth century, and doubtless some of those we shall be studying might have had such peremptory 'treatment' a few centuries ago.

In the sixteenth century a number of Bridewells were built, to reform and deter the idle and the erring. On admission the wrongdoers were to be severely whipped, and 'have putt uppon hym, her, or them, some clogge, chaine, collars of irons, single, or manacle'[2] before the corrective routine of prayer, work and good behaviour began. The women were to live separately, and work at spinning or mending. A reference to 'fourteen yeares old' as a lower age limit suggests an early comparative group for the present research group of 14 to 17-year-old girls in the mid-twentieth century.

Perhaps the Bridewell system seemed the right one for the times, and contemporary evidence pointed to a reduction in vagrancy and petty crime. Possibly because the system was carried on later by people who no longer believed in it (as has happened to our reformative system to some extent) the Houses of Correction (their other name) deteriorated into places of mass incarceration.

By the later eighteenth century we learn of John Howard, of Bedfordshire, on his inspection of local prisons, finding women as well as men confined in irons. Herded in groups without heat or sanitation, sometimes with their children, the women were sickly and filthy. That the age group for the present study (14 to 17) would not have been exempt, is shown from John Howard's finding of a girl locked up all day in a work room with two soldiers, and a boy and a girl imprisoned in the same room.[4]

By degrees of reform, we find some segregation of the sexes, but no age limit to female imprisonment (as there was none to male). We find occasional witnesses to the peculiar difficulties of women prisoners. A batch of thirty-six arriving at the new Millbank prison in the early nineteenth century were 'liable to fits until the threat of shaving and blistering their heads produced a miraculous cure'[5] (Griffiths, 1884, and Ann Smith, 1962). When some of the prisoners were removed for the good of their health to hulks in the Thames, they were hard to discipline. When a draft of men prisoners passed, 'the whole of the women commenced to shout and yell and to wave their handkerchieves. They abused the deputy matron with choice invectives and appeared quite beyond control.' These behavioural descriptions are still true of inherent possibilities with most female delinquents *en masse*, though in the past hundred years we have not needed to witness the physical degradation which accompanied the moral in the earlier nineteenth-century prison.

That these women could be controlled was the lesson taught by Elizabeth Fry in her work at Newgate Prison, which, as everyone knows, had been a hive of degradation and vice. She took a direct hand in the reorganization of the women for work and education, while devoting much additional time to outside pressure for prison reform, and the needs of the juvenile offenders who too had been liable to imprisonment and the gallows.

Reporting before a Committee of the House of Commons in 1818, Elizabeth Fry said, 'I think I may say we have full power among them, though we use nothing but kindness, I have never proposed a punishment, and yet I think it is impossible, in a well-regulated house, to have rules more strictly attended to than they are.'[6]

In Yarmouth Gaol about the same time Sarah Martin was treating the women with charity, and providing them with work, and proving again that these were the first needs.

Most of the reforms suggested by Elizabeth Fry came long after her death, but the second half of the century brought Mary Carpenter to the fore. We shall come soon to her work for children, which will overlap into our category of girls, but we also find her much concerned with the treatment of women prisoners, whom, with vision unusual in the reformers, she saw to have different needs from men. Within her era of reform the women (like the men) became subject, in some prisons, to solitary confinement for months on end, and this she saw as totally wrong for her sex, especially after their life of unrestrained excitement outside.

In 1848 came an Act whereby the age of 16, and not 14, delineated children from young persons. It is with this section of our present 14 to 17 year group—the 14 to 16's—that Mary Carpenter's name is most closely linked, for the stimulus she gave to the Reformatory Schools movement from 1851 onwards.

Whether classed as children or young persons, few institutions existed then solely to benefit the delinquent or needy child of tender years, though Ragged Schools, some Industrial Schools and a few Reformatories served as guides and inspirations to what might be. Even as early as 1758 the Magdalen Hospital was founded in Whitechapel under Sir John Fielding's *Plan for Preserving Deserted Girls*, most of whom were young prostitutes. The Magdalen was until recently still in existence, having evolved, since its removal to Streatham in 1869, into a Home Office Approved School, and finally a Classifying School. In 1788 the Philanthropic Society was founded to protect the young, and reform children, and extended its work to training 'pauper girls' as well. In the main the delinquent and deprived child was treated as harshly as the adult. A quotation given by Mary Carpenter[7] from evidence presented to the House of Lords, speaks of a girl of 9 under sentence of transportation for house-breaking (p. 16); elsewhere in the book (p. 218) we hear of a Liverpool Magistrate who had been compelled, for want of other provision, to send to gaol a little girl—'a child of whose beautiful appearance any mother might be proud'—for begging on the streets, at her mother's instigation. The same child went to prison at least twice subsequently. The chaplain of Liverpool Borough gaol is later quoted (p. 267) as visiting a class held for girls numbering fifty-four to sixty, who were housed in twelve cells. Quotations (p. 263) about the lack of segregation of juveniles in Newgate Prison, while referring to males, leave little doubt that the same was true of girls, though the number of females was smaller. We read in Elizabeth Fry's Memoirs[6] of her concern for the young women, as well as for the children of prisoners. Mary Carpenter quotes an extract (p. 304) giving the number of convicts at one prison as 600, 'a third of them being at the age of 16 and under. In March 1847, there were ten under 8 years of age, 36 at the ages of 8, 9 and 10; *one third of the whole throughout the year being females, but not so young as the males.*'

Figures for prisoners 'up to 16 years inclusive, committed for trial at the Middlesex Sessions during the year 1846', show trends in the proportions of the sexes much as we might find them today. About one in eight of the young offenders (16 and under) was female, but varied from one in fourteen for those under 14 years old, to about one in six for those aged 14, 15 and 16. One would wish to include some of the descriptions given by Mary Carpenter of the horrors of transportation, and the futility and starkness of the prisons—though children were quoted as preferring them to the depravity and squalor of their own homes. Girls seemed, proportionately, to be treated slightly more leniently, representing only one out of the thirteen (mostly aged 16) sentenced to ten years transportation.

Finally we have the staggering national figures of 10,703 children and young persons under 17 sent to prison or transported in 1849, often for trivial offences.[8]

Against such a background we see the campaign waged by Mary Carpenter as the fight of a visionary, and the evangelical language of her plea must have melted many hearts in her time. Her zeal about methods makes fine reading even today—her plea that 'love must be the ruling sentiment of all who attempt to influence and guide these children'; that 'no severity on his (i.e. the teacher's) part shall alienate them from him'; 'no punishments of a degrading or revenge-

8

ful nature will ever be employed'.[7] Corporal punishment 'not only inflicts a disgrace most sensitively felt by all high-spirited children, but usually excites a vindictive spirit'. Yet just as forcefully she says, 'Energy, faith, and love, though indispensable, are not sufficient for such a work'. The master only so equipped could 'break up the fallow ground', but he needed to learn 'good modes of sowing and watering'.[7] Training in teaching methods and in organization of the group were necessary, or more harm than good might be done.

As the Reformatory School Movement grew after the Youthful Offenders' Act of 1854 (which provided a statutory basis for these schools) most of the girls from 14 to 16 who were seriously recalcitrant or immoral would presumably be sent by the Courts to these institutions, though only after an initial taste of prison life for two weeks. (This condition, retained hitherto despite Mary Carpenter's hatred of it, became optional in 1893, and was abolished in 1899.) The girls were at first often in the same reformatories as boys; this soon led to objections by reformers.

In some reformatories a hard régime of work was set for the children, to diminish expenses. School work only gradually took its rightful place. We can still see what were regarded as suitable buildings, for some of the early schools, adapted and with annexes, are still in use. At a time when leniency (such as the substitution of whipping for imprisonment of young offenders) was suspect in the highest quarters, these Victorian buildings, with unplastered dormitories their full length under the rafters, must have seemed as madly luxurious as would the best purpose-built modern building seem to the more punitive anti-reformers today.

Over this same period there grew up a system of Industrial Schools for lesser offenders and needy boys and girls under 14 years of age. Because of the age range these are not of interest for comparative purposes in this research, except that their approach to the teaching of the poor and needy merged with the doctrines behind the Reformatory School methods. For eventually, after many years of agitation by Penal Reformers, an Act of Parliament was passed in 1932 (consolidated in 1933) merging these Industrial Schools with Reformatory Schools, and creating more neutrally named 'Approved Schools'. By this Act the upper age was extended to 17. This brings in the largest age-group of the research reported in this book—the 16 to 17-year-olds, who previously, as we have noted, were in adult women's prisons, or (at a later period) in borstals, if guilty of offences. Those who subsequently were subject to Court appearances as in moral danger, in need of care or protection, or beyond parental control, would be more difficult to trace back over the years.

Before 1919 the Reformatories were financed by the voluntary societies or other bodies initiating the schools, and partially by the state, which in return had set standards and had inspected the schools. Since 1919 the financial arrangement has been as at present, with a *per capita* contribution rate to cover total needs. Of this half is paid by the Treasury, and an account is sent by the schools to the relevant local authority for the remaining half of the contribution per child, part of which may be a sum collected by the Local Authority from the parents.

The actual setting up and administration of Girls' Approved Schools does not differ from those for boys, except that, as noted in the Introduction, they are (or were) generally smaller. To illustrate what has been written above, the beginnings and continuity, and in one case the ending, of three different, and not necessarily typical girls' Approved Schools are outlined. The last of the three is the Shaw Classifying Approved School, where the 600 girls studied in this project were assessed and observed from 1952 to 1954, and in 1957.

The first, was a purpose-built institution. Its history has been most adequately traced for the writer by the Correspondent to the Managers in 1962 as follows:

The School was built about 1870 out of monies raised partly by a Bazaar and partly by Subscription. It was originally used as a Home for Discharged Female Prisoners from the Gaol and it was run by a Committee of Magistrates and depended on private subscriptions. There was a laundry which helped to reduce part of the cost.

After the Great War women prisoners ceased to be sent to gaol so the original need for the Home ceased and the Committee asked the then Bishop if the Diocese would be willing to take it over together with various properties adjoining for use as a Rescue Home. This was done and the Committee, consisting of members from the Diocese with the Archdeacon as Chairman, was appointed and took in cases from the Preventive and Rescue Council and also certain cases from the Guardians. Owing to increasing costs of maintenance the Committee found difficulty in making the income balance the expenditure, and in 1937 the Home Office were asked if the premises could be converted into an Approved School under the Children and Young Persons Act, 1933. This was agreed to and the girls who were then in the School were gradually transferred to other Schools or discharged, and the School then became wholly an Approved School, which it has remained up to date. It is run by a Committee with representatives from the various organizations in the Diocese and the Archdeacon is the present Chairman.

It needs little imagination to see that a late nineteenth-century building, built for its specific purpose, with a laundry to 'wash the sins away', hardly speaks of the present day. A conscientious body of Managers, and energetic Headmistresses had contrived to keep the interior remarkably bright still in the mid-1950s, but the exterior was forbidding, and few girls were overjoyed as their escort from the Classifying School brought them on to the doorstep.

The form of the building, however, gave it a guaranteed place as the 'tough' school of the Northern half of England—a designation which was neither accurate nor desirable, but was hard to eradicate. As we shall see, 'disturbed' or 'amoral' would have been wiser epithets for the difficult girls who were admitted there.

The second illustrative example again has its setting in a Yorkshire mill town—indeed what is now a Girls' Approved School was built as the private house of a nearby mill-owner. A later owner converted it to more luxurious standards, at a cost of £20,000. In the 1940s the building was taken over by the Salvation Army, to be opened in 1945 as an Approved School with the Headmistress and some of her staff trained and selected by that organization. The dark oak panelling (and perhaps the dark uniforms of staff) gave a calm and sobering effect, and the orderly régime and carefully trained personnel seemed particularly helpful to the girl from a deprived social background needing control to her emotions and some stimulus to her intellect.

It can be said, briefly, that nearly all the Approved Schools for girls in the North were large or largish houses of a bygone age—cheap, because too large for 'family' houses. They ranged from the gracious to the plain ugly—red brick anachronisms on industrial fringes, with grounds not spacious enough for the activities so much favoured latterly in the rehabilitative process.

Our third example, the setting for the present research, was a Victorian mansion, Appleton Hall, leased by the Ministry of Labour in the 1930s as a Training Centre for unemployed women and girls. When in the latter part of that decade the Hall became redundant, negotiations took place between the Ministry of Labour and the Home Office for the transfer of the property for use by the Approved School service.

The School, re-named The Shaw, received its certificate of approval from 1 August 1937, 'for the education and training of girls to be sent there in pursuance of the Children and Young Persons Act, 1933'. The total number of girls resident in the school at any one time was not to exceed forty.

The Victorian mansion and eleven acres of land, leased from an estate which had belonged to a County family (said to have royal connections) was set amid green Cheshire fields, with surrounding parks and very handsome trees. The situation was most pleasant, and being on the fringe of a densely inhabited industrial area had quicker access to the busy outside world than had some rural Approved Schools for girls.

11

Historical Summary

From 1937 to 1942 a Committee of Local Managers formed under the Chairmanship (initially) of the Chief Education Officer of the Borough, managed it as a training School for senior girls, allocated by Magistrates of the committing courts as being suitable for a short training, and providing a domestic training on the level of the Ministry of Labour Training Centres, some of the staff being seconded for this purpose. Selection for a shorter term (9 to 12 months) of training for girls who had aptitude and desire for domestic work by courts up and down the country, inevitably brought in misfits. In this more privileged training a fair degree of freedom was inherent, and girls unready for this were frowned on by middle-class neighbours, proud of their past proximity to 'The Hall'. By 1942 the number of girls suited to this training had dropped, and a more adaptable house was found in a quiet market town, to which Headmistress, Staff and girls were transferred. This new school achieved marked success with suitably classified girls, until it closed in the later 1950s.

Classification for Approved Schools was inaugurated in 1942 at Aycliffe (for boys) and a little later at the Magdalen (already mentioned) for girls. The Shaw was ear-marked as a suitable establishment for classifying non-Roman Catholic senior girls (15 to 17 years) in the Northern half of England and Wales, and the Managers were asked by the Secretary of State to re-staff and re-establish it for this purpose. Later the School also received 14-year-old girls (intermediates) but, though the matter was explored in some detail, and outline plans for dividing the building suitably were much discussed, girls under 14 (juniors) were never admitted except as 'special cases', by permission of the Secretary of State.

The Shaw was the centre for classification of senior and intermediate Approved School girls from the northern half of England (down to, but not including, Birmingham) until 1960, when, because of administrative difficulties, mainly connected with the cost of maintaining and improving the building, the Managers relinquished the Certificate of Approval. The Hall itself has now been demolished.

Chapter Three

CLASSIFICATION

We have seen in the historical section that for many years scant thought was given to classification of offenders, even by sex and age. With the growth of the Reformatory system, a ceiling age of 16 was set, up to which limit ages were mixed, and girls, though fewer in number than boys, shared the institutions. By 1860 classification by sex was the rule.

Classification by religion had been inherent in the setting up of the Reformatory Schools by religious and philanthropic bodies; there were separate schools for Roman Catholic children, and this separation has remained.

Some classification by age was inherent in the type of training set up by the various voluntary bodies. In the case of girls, the hospital type of establishment for the treatment of girls with venereal disease would usually receive the older delinquent; Cottage Homes would tend to receive the younger, less contaminated case. Apart from schoolroom facilities, there was less classification inherent in the actual training facilities for girls than in the case of boys—no parallel, for instance, to the tough discipline of the training ship. Laundries for older girls sometimes went—symbolically—with the cleansing services of the medical treatment institution.

The 1933 Children and Young Persons Act, with the combining of Reformatory and Industrial Schools into Approved Schools, raised, as we have seen, the admission age to 16-plus, and further classified the girls' schools for age, into Senior Schools for those aged 15 or 16 on admission, and Junior Schools for those under 15 on admission. From 1948 they followed the pattern of the Boys' Schools in having Intermediate Approved Schools for girls, but the ages on admission were 14 or 15, and for Juniors the admission age was up to the fifteenth birthday. (For boys the ages are 13 and 14 for admission to Intermediate Schools.)

In order to streamline training facilities further, reforming bodies had been urging the setting up of Observation Centres for more careful observation and assessment of delinquent children than could be achieved in the Remand Homes. The first Classifying School, fulfilling a rather different function, in that only children first committed to Approved Schools came into its net, was set up experimentally at

13

Aycliffe in 1942. John Gittins,[1] the Principal, says: 'Despite the previous discussions the actual beginning of the scheme was probably due more to administrative problems than anything else.' Although the Home Office had in 1942 set up a central department for allocating children to Approved Schools, rather than leaving the placement to the courts, there was, especially with a wartime upsurge of delinquency, seen to be room for further system in both the administrative procedure of allocation, and in the filing of careful scientific studies of the individual child. Shortly two other Classifying Schools opened for boys; another followed some years later.

Eventually, in 1942 and 1943 two Classifying Schools were opened for girls, the Magdalen School, at Streatham, for girls from the southern half of England and Wales, and the Shaw School, near Warrington (the site of the present research findings) for girls from the northern half of the country.

At first the Girls' Classifying Schools made their assessments and observations, compiled a 'classifying report' on a girl and sent the papers, usually with a recommendation for placement, to the Children's Branch of the Home Office, whose responsibility it was to decide the selection of a Training School. By the period covered in this research it had become the Classifying School's responsibility to allocate the girl, except in particularly difficult cases, when the Home Office Children's Department's ready advice was sought.

By the 1952 Children and Young Persons (Amendment) Act, the Classifying Schools were given statutory recognition, and the relevant Classifying School (if one was available for a child of the age and description) was named on the Committal Order. The transfer of the child to a suitable Training School, after classification, remained the Secretary of State's responsibility, as for other occasional transfers from one Training School to another, and an order had to be signed accordingly; this was a mere legal formality.

In November 1957 the Association of Headmasters, Headmistresses and Matrons of Approved Schools, reporting its evidence for presentation to the Ingleby Committee, summarize their approval of classification procedure to date in the following terms:

It was, in our view, an excellent idea to begin classification in the Approved Schools service, after the committal order had been made. This gave an opportunity for trying out the various possible techniques in a relatively homogeneous service, where personal relations—between schools, with other interested agencies, with the Home Office—are close. This has had the effect of very considerably reducing the various possible number of variables in the situation and enabling attention to be concentrated on the most important factor of all—the personal relationships involved.

This statement presupposes that the committal of the child to Approved School (quite a difficult measure to retract) was the right decision, based on sufficient good evidence at an earlier stage. Whether the findings from this research will always be consistent with this belief, or whether earlier classification might have influenced the use of other modes of treatment for some female delinquents, this is not the place to discuss. We may even want later to argue (on evidence) that the circle of Schools and Home Office was too circumscribed for a broad view of present situations, and a continued clear view of surrounding fields of activity and thought.

That further differentiation in treatment was necessary for girls, was proved by the marked success of allocation of most girls of very dull intelligence to one particular school attuned to them; by the more careful differentiation of the stabler girl for short-term training, the one school of this type, set up in pre-classification days could become more specialized. Occasionally courts continued to make recommendations on placement, sometimes singularly unenlightened ones for short-term training, as in one instance where a girl of violent inclinations was clearly in need of longer training than most. Their other recurrent recommendation (often guided by a psychiatric report) was for treatment at Duncroft School, where girls could have fairly intensive psychiatric treatment. Again this recommendation was not always realistic, considered in the fuller knowledge available to the Classifying School, whose recommendations were indeed later subject to careful scrutiny by the Duncroft establishment.

Mainly the practical training for girls was less differentiated than between boys' schools, and the value came to be in the presentation of a more comprehensive picture of the girl to the Training School prior to her admission. With corresponding study of what each Training School had to offer on the emotional and practical planes, discussion could revolve round all sorts of aspects at the biennial review meetings held in conjunction with the Home Office, with the possibility of a growth of self-knowledge in all parties. Personalities at the head of girls' schools seemed the vital point to consider, and here it may be permissible to say these seemed more colourful and diverse than their opposite numbers, the Headmasters of boys' Approved Schools.

Chapter Four

SAMPLING

In the three years 1952, 1953 and 1954, admissions to the Shaw Classifying School were as follows:

Year	Number
1952	216
1953	182
1954	164
Total	562 girls

Three of these represent girls admitted from licence for re-classification, and therefore not new cases. A fourth, re-committed within that time, was also not a new case.

Two parents successfully appealed and the girls concerned went home after a few days in the Classifying School. A further re-committal was invalid, and the girl, though her stay was less short, has not been included in the study.

In three cases too many of the relevant documents were missing, and in three more the files, apart from test material, were completely missing.

The 562 cases were thus reduced to 550.

REDUCED SAMPLE OF 500

Study of the main sample of 550 showed that it contained certain non-representative groups, some being selected special cases proved at an early stage to have been unsuitable for Approved School committal, and therefore falling out of the ranks at this point.

There were six sub-groups of these:

(i) Twenty-three girls were admitted below the prescribed age of 14. These twenty-three are not considered representative of the girls of their age-groups, since the latter were normally sent direct to Junior Approved Schools by the Courts. Special permission of the Secretary of State had to be given for admission to the Classifying School, usually on grounds of being very

16

difficult. Also some of these younger girls were from the southern half of the country.

(ii) Nine older girls (from the southern half of England and Wales) were not fitting into the Training Schools where they had been allocated by the other Girls' Classifying School, and were judged as needing a completely new assessment, or were Roman Catholic girls, not previously in a Classifying School. Seven of the under-14's on committal in section (i) were also in category (ii).

(iii) Three girls, were committed to Borstal, two from the Classifying School, and one within a month of going to a Training School.

(iv) The stay of five girls in the Classifying School was much shortened by reason of serious mental instability, and they were in Mental Hospital for long or short periods. Only one of these five was in a Training School, and that after a long period in hospital, and briefly.

(v) Eight girls were certified under the Mental Deficiency Act soon after their committal, five while at the Classifying School, and three within a few months of admission to a Training School.

(vi) Two were among those girls who were pregnant at the Classifying School; one evaded training by absconding from the Mother and Baby Home, the other eventually reached a Training School, but was certified quickly as mentally defective.

Though these fifty non-representative cases may be referred to, either in their sub-groups, or as special individual problems for the Classifying School, they will not be part of the main sample of 500, where the effects of Approved School training and after-care will be of such importance. The reader should note that some of the most difficult problems were in the excluded 50, so that the study of the 500 is far from exaggerating our difficulties.

FURTHER SAMPLE OF 100

In the year 1957, when the writer was visiting Educational Psycho-logist at the Shaw Classifying School, 167 girls were admitted. The Rorschach and the Porteus Mazes had been added to the test battery, and the diagnostic and predictive values of these tests with this population seemed due for testing. It was found that for exactly 100 girls who had done them, follow-up reports were also available for at least two years.

This later sample, despite the disadvantages of the short follow-up period, seemed likely also to be valuable for comparison with a group born earlier in relation to the war years and the welfare state, as well as supplying an interesting check on more subjective data.

17

Sampling

For most purposes there are two main samples in this study:

(a) the more comprehensive sample of 500 girls, almost entirely from the northern half of England and Wales, who were classified between 1952 and 1954, and allocated to Training Schools, from which, and after which, reports came back to the Classifying School, so that their progress can be followed for at least five years from committal.

(b) The later sample of 100 girls who did certain additional psychological tests at the Classifying School in 1957, and whose progress was followed for about two years after allocation to a training school.

The remaining fifty cases, belonging originally to the main sample, were extracted for various reasons as being atypical, but will be referred to, as their impact on the life of the Classifying School was often out of all proportion to their number.

THE WRITER IN RELATION TO THE SAMPLES

The writer, then a graduate, a trained teacher with fully seven years' experience, was appointed as a Remedial Teacher at the Classifying School in January 1950. About November that year she was promoted to the post of Deputy Headmistress (see chapter on Staffing). Apart from an absence for University post-graduate studies in Education and Psychology, she was in this position until 1955, when she was appointed Headmistress. Soon after her marriage in 1956 she returned as an outside worker, in the role of part-time Educational Psychologist, until 1958. Thus the 1952 to 1954 sample of 500 girls were known closely and personally to the writer, as fellow-residents, and the few who had been forgotten were easily brought back to memory by reading their files when the research was begun in 1962. The 1957 sample of 100 girls were not remembered, as they were seen for two-, three- or four-hour sessions only. For details of how the samples came in and went out, the reader must see the next few chapters.

18

Chapter Five

THE SETTING FOR THE RESEARCH

In 1948 the lease of Appleton Hall (later the Shaw Classifying School) expired and nine Managers were appointed joint Trustees of the building and land, 'purchased with the approval of the Secretary of State with moneys provided by Parliament and paid from the Exchequer to the Managers under Section 104 of the Children and Young Persons Act 1933'.

Unfortunately the house and land, as described by a Home Office Inspector at a Managers' Meeting in 1948, were 'an island', for the long main drive, used throughout the era concerned, was merely a right of way, shared with other property owners for most of its length, and was in a deplorable state. There were two other rights of way; one was grassed over, and the other was muddied, but providing a quick, though nerve-wracking, unlit path for staff to bus journeys, or for the girls on absconsion sprees.

Scarcely a Managers' Meeting in all the months from 1946 to 1960 was not taken up in part by the problem of 'the Drive'. Home Office assistance was sought, or the Home Office urged the Managers to act, according to which side was progressive and which was economizing. A new Manager was appointed to the Committee in 1949 for the specific purpose of making a firm move; in 1960 the drive was in a sorrier state than ever. Not only was isolation of staff and girls thereby increased, but it was one of the ways in which a sense of helplessness could grow.

The house itself, which, by reason of the 'closed' life of the Classifying School, was almost the only part of the property that mattered, was, from two views but not from the drive, a fairly gracious Victorian mansion of grey brick on two floors; there were a few attic rooms, but much of the roof space was occupied by enormous reservoirs of soft water from the gutterings; this once overflowed into a dormitory in the early hours, when a mains pipe running through the largest reservoir sprang a leak, and Jean thought she'd wet the bed. This is a minor example of the unscheduled challenges of residential work, which could draw the community together, or prove the breaking point when staff were already over-taxed.

Most of the main rooms were well lit, yet only two of the public rooms (one the schoolroom, the other unused at the time of this

19

account) had a sunlit look, and a few important rooms, including the Headmistress's study, saw only a glimmer of mid-summer sunlight. While this could be conducive to hard work, and a defence against unsettledness in staff and girls, those whose work lay entirely indoors and had the longest hours could suffer the effects of light and air starvation. (Windows were blocked so as to open only a few inches top and bottom.) Staff bedrooms were generally spacious and airy, however, and often more sunny than the reception rooms, though a few opened on to the yard, or peculiar corners and were neither handsome nor salubrious. In winter they were heated by fires in ancient grates—if the occupant was long enough off duty to have time to light a fire. The girls' dormitories enjoyed large windows and adequate space; only a girl's individual feelings about communal sleeping needed to make or mar her pleasure in that part of her surroundings, if she was aware of them in the habitual home-sickness of bedtime. Sometimes she was mainly aware of the large windows and the measures needed to gain exit from them (for example a filched table-knife to undo blocks, and a few counterpanes as rope-ladders).

The main school entrance was by a handsome door into a lobby, then by double swing doors into a spacious hall with a large fireplace. It was usually possible (at the research period) to leave this main entrance unlocked, and so the greeting of a new girl could be effected without a jangling of keys.

The Hall, which had the schoolroom, the staff dining-room and the Head's study opening off it, and the fine carpeted staircase, were polished with zeal each day by a girl who had aspired to this status task. Above these rooms were the chapel, kept immaculately, two staff bedrooms (with verandahs) a dormitory for eight girls and adjoining toilets, a staff bathroom, and the Headmistress's bedroom and bathroom; these last, part of the Head's 'suite', were quite separate from the remainder, her study, which, as mentioned, was downstairs and had to do double service as her official working quarters, rendering it unsuitable for private reception of personal friends.

These downstairs rooms were locked at bedtime, for obvious reasons. Dormitory doors were not locked and there were no night patrols, apart from the readiness of each member of staff to be disturbed.

The side outside-door gave on to the main downstairs corridors leading to the girls' dining-room and to their recreation room, a large, square, oak-panelled and noisy place, the old billiard room of the Hall. Nearby were the main clothing stores, the 'testing room', many bleak toilets, beside one set of which was a useful, but odorous stance for the member of staff on 'corridor duty'. From here the 'back stairs' (uncovered and very creaky) led to the dormitories (there were, all told, four, accommodating a total of thirty-six girls) and to the girls' bathrooms and toilets, interspersed, at intervals suited to supervision, with five more staff bedrooms, some too large, some too small. Also along the two long, creaky corridors lay a staff bathroom and an odd toilet—so that one was guaranteed many kinds of 'Good mornings' on one's first emergence of the day. A stair to the second floor led to two staff bedrooms, a toilet, and a third room whose role changed from extra dormitory to empty space.

A further corridor led to Sick Wing—a bathroom, two small double-bedded sick rooms, and the resident Nurse's small bedroom sandwiched between. Above, by a steep, narrow stair, was a water tower, then two small bare rooms which officially (in fact, rarely) were 'detention rooms', and then a secluded staff bedroom. On the ground floor, in a rather shoddy wing of this later part of the mansion house (it had held the servants' quarters) were the surgery and 'treatment' room.

There were, besides a large kitchen, many store rooms, and the corridors, upstairs and down, contained various odd dark cubby-holes and pantries and sluices—all fine hiding places for mischievous or rebellious individuals or little gangs. The large well-lit 'butler's pantry', lined with cupboards and drawers, became the Deputy Head's office; the butler's silver safe accommodated stage props.

Below were large expanses of cellars, with the boilers and the coke, sometimes inhabited by rats, at one period by half wild cats, and dreamed of by the girls as an escape route, but their uncharted depths were feared too much for them to be exploited.

The whole school, and the outside access points, were inadequately lit, for the electric wiring (until 1956) was unfit for new lighting points (or for any power points) and fuses frequently blew. Electric light bulbs were known to drop from their decayed moorings, but no girl or member of staff was electrocuted. Returning to the school late at night, one negotiated a dark field and a dark lane to a dark building, and walked the length of a corridor before reaching a light switch. Then one extinguished that and climbed the stairs in darkness to another, and so to bed.

The central heating system, where it existed, was fierce, but uneven, for unheated spaces, and thresholds hollowed by generations of feet, brought freezing draughts. In the evening, with the furnace banked down, one often basked in fumes.

Outside, round the yard, were the old stables, with a clock tower, and a clock which worked. The problem whether to repair and convert these attractive, but very decrepit old buildings—coach houses, coachman's rooms, and the stables and sheds—into further school buildings or staff rest rooms was debated almost as often at Managers' Meetings as the subject of the drive—and never solved.

A little further from the house than these others, and regarded as a special little world, was an old-fashioned laundry with a few pieces of modern equipment, where a small group of girls under an Instructress worked more cheerfully and noisily than those in the dignified mansion. Here many minor emotional problems were solved, away from it all.

On the south of the house were terraced lawns and flower beds. These were beautifully kept, and did service for the very rare opportunities for the girls to work or relax outdoors. (It was too overlooked for staff relaxation.) One part was in daily use, a sweep of sloping grass—as fine a setting for outdoor games as was ever known. Beyond that cows grazed in a lovely sweep of Cheshire fields among some very fine trees. Opposite the recreation room windows, on the school boundary, was a particularly fine old beech which the sex-starved girls named Charlie. Deprived or not, their exclusion from life was not emphasized by walls or barbed wire, only by outside doors being mainly locked and by spoken and unspoken prohibitions.

In a Girls' Approved School, as in a woman's own home, the surroundings are embedded in her existence. As well as being the environment which she absorbed, or which she resisted, it was often her work setting; her scrubbing or polishing of the corridors, her washing of the walls, her cleaning of the baths and toilets, or her hard work in the schoolroom, were a measuring rod of her keenness or her unwillingness to conform and show progress.

The Shaw School was blessed in its surroundings, and in some of its amenities, but its deficiencies from the domestic angle became latterly more and more marked. It is amusing now to read in a 1938 description of short-term schools, that the 'Shaw School was fully equipped as a domestic training centre', (*Young Offenders* by Geraldine Cadbury, p. 95). As the stringencies of the War years receded, one could no longer feel ennobled by the sacrifice of physical comforts. Surprisingly enough, the staff slowest to grumble at discomfort and decay in the building were those who had no home apart from the School; partly they were not reminded so much of the contrast from normality, and partly they tended to be the staff with the most comfortable bed-sitting-rooms. All shared the responsibility and inconvenience of dormitory supervision—from bedtime till the rising bell. And superficially at least most duties, scheduled and otherwise, were done serenely, often with gaiety.

22

Chapter Six

STAFFING, ROUTINE, AND
WORK CONDITIONS

The staffing in Girls' Approved Schools at the time of this research project was very different from that of the Boys' Schools, where the few women employed were in traditional female roles of looking after the cleanliness of boys and building, and the nourishment of boys and of unmarried male staff. Most men were married, living with their own family group in separate houses in the grounds, and the wives sometimes played parts in the female programme, with the Headmaster's wife traditionally cast as Matron. Cleaning was generally done by outside employees.

At the Shaw Classifying School, as was usual in the Girls' Training Schools, the only male regularly about the place, but generally non-resident, was the gardener. The remainder of the fifteen who formed the establishment in the period dealt with were all female. Except for perhaps the kitchen instructress, all were of the 'career woman' level, either because they were young, unattached and fairly ambitious, or because they were widowed or divorced, and required a post with residence and of suitable status. While past training varied, or was non-existent, the socio-cultural level was fairly constant; few were of working-class backgrounds, and if they were they concealed the fact carefully. Generally their norms of conduct and thought were good middle class. Manners were gracious, and bickering was usually taboo. An indication of the cultural level was that the school was never, in the research period, without three good pianists, and interest in the arts was considerable, even if outlets were few.

The establishment was for

1 Headmistress
1 Deputy Headmistress
1 Housemistress
2 House Instructresses
1 Laundry Instructress
1 Kitchen Instructress (or Cook)
1 Sewing Instructress
2 Relief Instructresses

23

1 Nurse
1 Secretary
1 Gardener–Handyman
2 Teachers

In fact there was much over-lapping, and only one teacher (who usually was non-resident) had cut-and-dried hours and duties. The Classifying School remained in full swing for seven days of the week and for fifty-two weeks of the year, except in times of serious epidemics. Leave rotas had to be covered by staff on duty, and sick leave had similarly to be covered. A brief description of the normal duties, and of those sometimes covered, follows.

The Headmistress, who was normally very fully occupied for at least twelve hours of the day, by administrative and 'hostess' duties (such as receiving escorts, and official visitors, who came from as far as India and Canada) plus much counselling and intermediary work with girls, and the supervision of one meal per day with the girls and the others with her staff, had in the eight (theoretical) weeks of her deputy's leave, to cover some of the latter's report-writing duties, and sometimes do routine intelligence or scholastic testing. Then she would probably work a 15-hour day, possibly a 7-day week. If her journeys for her own (uncertain) leave and day off or one-in-three (theoretical) free weekends lay in the required direction, she would possibly escort a girl to her Training School to maintain knowledge of the establishment, visit a particularly complicated home, or attend the Home Office for discussion of a problem. If she remained in the school for any odd hours off duty, or for a day off, it had to be in her bedroom, as her sitting-room was also her office.

The Deputy Headmistress, whose main duties were report-writing, and who, because of previous academic background and interest in this period, covered the routine intelligence, scholastic and personality tests, shared individual counselling and intermediary work with the Headmistress, and had to deputize totally for the Head's (theoretical) eight weeks' annual leave, day-off per week and her one-in-three weekends off. Likewise she did an escort duty within part of her day or longer-term leave journeys, if this was helpful to the school. Total work hours were not far from being as limitless and leaves as uncertain, as the Headmistress's.

The Housemistress's role was to care for much of the girls' leisure time and more free individually occupied time. As one person was unlikely to have either the elasticity or nervous resources to fulfil this in her $5\frac{1}{2}$-day week, she tended to be occupied for part of her time with the work of an absent instructress, while instructresses, in turn, used their varied talents in organized leisure time. The

24

Housemistress did a share of escort duties, mainly in duty, sometimes in free time.

House Instructresses were responsible for the large Hall, with all its dormitories, bed-sitting-rooms and public rooms, being maintained in a highly polished state, both in the interests of hygiene, and to satisfy the Managers and many interested visitors from home and abroad. Nine or ten girls were allocated each day to the household tasks, and as far as possible orderly succession was adhered to, so that a girl learned jobs of graded difficulty (from corridor scrubbing to dormitory cleaning, to turning out staff-bedrooms, and finally serving meals or tea and coffee to staff). As the capable learners were outnumbered by the (usually) willing but sloppy worker, the Instructresses (one upstairs, one down), had, as well as teaching and demonstrating and handing out materials, to supplement with a good share of her own elbow-grease. As this was all happening during the intense preoccupations of testing, report-writing and receiving of strangers and conducted tours, the tact and ruses of these excellent staff were further exercised to maintain quiet smoothness. Strike action was minimized, and an offer from the intermediary (the Head or her Deputy) to do the abandoned job, usually saw the girl scurrying (or dragging) back to her task. This relative smoothness was amazing when seen against the work records of most of the girls, with frequent changes and often serious recalcitrance, but it was not achieved without expertise and nervous strain. Some girls if not from the start, at least learned to set an example to others. From the figures tabulated for this research, 60 per cent of the girls listened to instructions and usually followed them, even one who 'could hardly hold a duster at first', but at most, less than half the girls were satisfactory workers, even with maximum tact. The greatest difficulty was in concentration, and in capacity to work without supervision; 12 per cent were recorded as having 'weak' concentration and persistence, and a further 40 per cent as being only 'fair' in this respect. Only about one third could be left to work unsupervised, while one-in-five needed unbroken supervision.

If mothers who doubt their daughters' potential in such circumstances reject these figures as irrelevant, it can be said that work records before committal will be found to differ significantly from that of the average teenager, and these pre-committal work records correlated significantly in this research with concentration and persistence at the Classifying School (p. 283, Table XV).

Perhaps it was as well that most House Instructresses appointed had some specific talents which they could use with relief for an evening session (unless they were spending the afternoon on general supervision, or on escort). In the research period this varied from musical appreciation classes (by an L.R.A.M.), to being accompanist to hymns or bee-bop or parlour games, and to conducting crafts classes.

Laundry Instructress. All the institution's laundry was at this stage done on the premises, in the laundry equipped for the Ministry of Labour training scheme in the 1930s, and with few refinements since. Generally four girls worked under instruction here (or rather with the Instructress), away from the main building. It was a happy and more settled department mostly, partly because singing at work, and a lapse into horse-play and merriment could not disturb the intensity of classification. One girl's letter back from her Training School said: 'I do miss having Miss —— chasing me round the laundry with a broom.' The same Miss —— released a great deal of tension by her weekly evening duty of conducting parlour games, sometimes competitive, and often with costumes. She could just as successfully arrange programmes for religious festivals, and a Sunday evening programme of hymns.

The Kitchen Instructress (or Cook) worked a normal day, without evening sessions, being relieved then by one of the others. Four girls assisted (or hindered), two preparing vegetables in a back kitchen, and two taking varying degrees of responsibility in the main kitchen. Here a good worker often proved herself, but a failure caused much irritation, and the dim became more bewildered, putting floor sweepings into the bread bin instead of the dust bin, and eleven tablespoons of salt in the potato pan instead of a level one. Yet all fared well, the girls on fairly equal terms with staff, if with less refinement and more starch.

Sewing Instructress. This was a misnomer, as the only instruction given in plain sewing was when the weekly 'bundle' was darned on Friday evening, ready for donning after the Saturday bi-weekly bath. It was an unnecessarily disheartening session, when girls who had usually discarded their outworn flimsy underwear were required to repair navy interlock knickers, and darn white or navy socks. They used their irritation to accuse the Instructress of 'taking it out on them' by giving them the worst garments, and generally the mood blackened. Otherwise the Sewing Instructress spent at least fifteen hours a week sorting out clothing, repairing clothing and 'bundling' clothing, and fitting up new girls, helped usually by a reliable girl who responded to the individual notice and pungent advice she could gain in this small department. The Instructress relieved in other departments, did escort duties, and contributed to classification from her fund of memories of old girls and shrewd assessments of the current group.

The Relief Instructresses relieved on any, or all of these duties, for

26

the six weeks' annual leave of others, on day and weekend leaves, and for the many occasions of sick leave or staff not replaced.

The Nurse had a mainly full-time job of attending to major and minor ills, consulting on girls with the School Medical Officer, and escorting girls to hospitals and clinics for specialist help. She supervised the bi-weekly baths, and in times of shortage might be required to cover a vacant department, according to other interests. Perhaps it was a pointer to some distortion of emphasis, that while the Home Office Inspectorate was emphatic that the nurse employed should, if at all possible, be State Registered, their approval was given for advertising for a Headmistress as *'preferably* a graduate', while Instructress staff could be of all diversities of training or none . . . (In fact a Headmistress with one or more degrees came our way, and everyone seemed duly surprised, while Instructresses occasionally had a degree or a diploma, but not often with reference to the work of their department.)

The Secretary. Even the Secretary was not immune from calls on her other faculties, if only to harbour a difficult or upset girl in her office while her work continued. For part of the time of which we are writing, the Secretary (though non-resident) spent an occasional evening on duty with the girls, and in bed-time supervision and sympathetic listening.

The Gardener–Handyman was also the stoker of four boilers, and the overseer of workmen doing repairs on the premises. In theory he was assisted by a 'garden girl' or girls, but at the Classifying School in the time described it was only for occasional periods that we had a girl with genuine and more than passing interest in outdoor work, and at the same time the ability to resist the easy opportunity of running away; the ready-made outdoor worker tended to be the tough Borstal candidate. There were plenty of girls without either the drive to abscond, or the drive to work without perpetual prodding, who were surprised not to be given the propagating of seeds which would sprout and blossom by tea-time. Occasionally a reliable girl also enjoyed the work, and was prepared to send off the butcher's boy, who found her in the wood-shed and thought he was in clover. But it was sad that assistance was not readily available to an excellent male gardener who was tactful and patient with the grossly maladjusted girls, while seeming impervious to their femininity.

The Teachers. One of the two teachers worked normal school hours, and (relatively to the criss-crossing of most duties) on normal schoolroom activities. The work was challenging, not because of large numbers, low standards or high standards, but because of the mobile population, the very mixed educational standards and

27

attitudes, mixed ages, and sudden swings of group mood in and out of the schoolroom.

The schoolroom itself was a large sunny room. Equipment was adequate or not according to the teaching interests of the person in charge. Into morning school came all new girls, usually for about their first fortnight in the Classifying School, and 14-year-olds throughout their stay, as well as a few older girls whose stabilization was clearly helped by more schoolroom time (plus a few whose gross instability or practical ineptitude made life even more intolerable elsewhere). These girls had come, with an interval at different Remand Homes, from schools all over the northern half of England, mainly Secondary Modern (mixed or girls') but also many still from all-age schools, and a few from Grammar Schools and from Special Schools. To some school had spelt encouragement and even success; to some it had spelt discouragement, with consequent resistance or apathy or persistent truancy. Now and then a 'school attendance' case retreated into illness or rebellion before she could at last be eased into our schoolroom.

The best source of cheer to the discouraged was to tell them that they would mostly work on their own, show just what they could do, and be helped over the things that had worried them before. Not all the teachers, however, could escape from their own rigid training in class-teaching, and for a girl to be allowed to choose her work was then regarded as weakness. In fact, with a good remedial teacher unobtrusively guiding her choice, and sometimes insisting on an imposed piece, a girl who had felt a failure could work her way into a state of enthusiasm which carried into the remainder of the community life. However, finding a teacher interested enough in this backwater of education was so difficult that she was usually left to find her own compromise between teaching a very heterogeneous group as a group, or being prepared to unbend to the individual whims within the group. Then a 14-year-old girl might be reading to the teacher from an infants' primer in one corner, while a 16-year-old ex-Grammar School girl might be doing pre-School Certificate English in another.

Part of the 1957 group, which comes less directly into this research, were involved in an experiment in activity methods, adapted by an ex-teacher of city primary schools with an advanced degree in Education. The emphasis was away from paper-and-pen, to painting, modelling, free drama, and free verbal expression, written and oral. There is, of course nothing very revolutionary in this, even with Secondary children in Special Schools, but the disapproval of some of the resident staff, imbued mainly with Grammar School outlook, and aghast at the occasional violence when a girl felt insecure in this schoolroom milieu, was such that much unhappiness ensued. The medical departments impinging on the institution's routine could be borne unquestioningly as a sacrosanct, specialist field, but the educationist's policy was assailed on every side.

In the patterned life more favoured in the schoolroom there could be contentment and personality growth, and the inevitable jealousies and frustrations built up in the competitiveness for love and for success during most of the morning, could be solved in the painting sessions, which were free under most of our teachers. The schoolroom walls were papered with a collection of gloomy skies, sensual hills, belligerent or lost males and females; under the influence of one charming teacher, wearing an engagement ring, there were many lovers in the park. Fashion-plates in remote, untouchable glory, were always favoured subjects, as were rigid, sometimes lurid, designs.

Afternoon school, attended by all but a very few girls, was divided between an hour of outdoor games—rounders or netball—and an hour of needlework, usually cross-stitch embroidery, which appeared to answer a need in most for periods of controlled movement and concentration.

In two of the three years of the main part of the research, schoolroom was relieved during the other teacher's total of eight weeks' leaves by the second teacher, who habitually shared the afternoon by conducting outdoor games, and managing to encourage a team spirit through team prizes when earned; this was not achieved without much tact and cajoling, partly by the team-members themselves. As this teacher (for most of the research period) had a degree in Psychology, her other contribution was the major one of assisting with group and individual cognitive testing, and with extracting social data for the classifying reports.

Total devotion was called for in this Classifying School Staff; meals in the staff dining-room, which was also the board-room, and was very austere, were rather formal occasions. General conversation, mainly directed to the head of the table, tended to the trivial, for controversial and distasteful topics were avoided and talk became animated only when girls present, past or future were discussed, for then no subject was taboo at table, even venereal diseases. Jokes about the girls—usually kindly jokes—evoked restrained mirth. In the Headmistress's absence total loyalty was preserved in the communal talk, and contradiction in her presence was rare; fortunately there was little to contradict, for the quality of leadership was exceptional, but over the years this was not particularly healthy. The atmosphere, despite all this formality, was rarely sour, or disgruntled, but was mainly benign, and was elevated in its sentiments

29

about people. Only in the absence of several of the liberal-minded did the talk of girls or parents savour of a 'them-and-us' outlook.

While there was not actual tension, neither was there release of tension. No one could do the work well without a keen sense of humour, and this burbled through just now and then with hilarity. What was missing was loud fun, mockery and ribaldry.

The staff endeavoured, where congeniality existed, to have a closer social life at the end of the day, when, by 9.30 p.m., all was reasonably settled. Not all staff enjoyed gathering in twos and threes in staff bed-sitting-rooms, and, from the supervision angle it was well it was not so, for some ears had to be attuned to corridor noises, there being no separate night duty staff. But, even where there was slightly more jollity in these gatherings, it had still to be restrained so as not to penetrate to dormitories, which were never more than a few feet away. No radio could be played loudly, and of course no gramophone. Smokers must keep the tempting cigarette odour from permeating the corridors, just as no one smoked in the presence of the girls.

Behind all this almost superhuman sacrifice there was not the soullessness of regulations, but generally a sincere belief that they could not expect more self-control in the girls than they perceived in themselves, and indeed the assumption of quietly dignified manners, low-pitched voices, pronounced stillness of bearing, and a calm smiling face and gently teasing humour in times of difficulty, had an impressive effect. The most rumbustious girls, if at all suggestible, learned, without the necessity of rebuke, to be outwardly controlled for much of the time. Others needed verbal reminders of what helped people to live in such close proximity. Reward (in the way of two inches of red ribbon to sew on a tunic) helped most girls to remember. Unfortunately the occasional true psychopath was neither able nor willing to respond to suggestions of this kind, and the pity was that, while staff frequently discussed the unsuitability of such girls for the régime (or rather for approved school) they seldom saw that the régime was too lacking in means of self-expression. True they gave more rope to the psychopathic girl away from the group, through individual therapy, than most similar institutions proffer, a good deal of 'letting-off' being possible then, but the permissiveness necessary for her to regress to infancy, and the warmth missing in her childhood, could not be incorporated into the group atmosphere which stabilized the larger groups of socially retarded girls, the very dull and backward girls, and the neurotic girls. William and Joan McCord,[1] in their study of the psychopath note (p. 152) that of the children handled in the permissively therapeutic milieu of Wiltwyck, the neurotic and borderline psychotic children improved less than the behaviour-disordered and the psychopaths. Since the Shaw was first and foremost a Classifying School, and was only by the necessity of living without too much hazard (and—confessedly—by the direction of the Staff's interests) a therapeutic institution, there was more constraint towards catering for the greater proportion of manageable problems and finding training schools for the others at record speed. Yet it can be said that, however far staff failed to provide the group milieu, through their handling of the psychopath as an individual, they did as well as most of the receiving schools did subsequently, and with one or two succeeded to the extent of retaining them until they were more ready for training. It will also be clear from some histories to follow that we had girls who had failed in the most progressive institutions in the country.

The present-day response to this summary of their problems would be to group the girls suitably, and set up a 'house' system with some sort of imagined similarity to a family. The writer would have to be convinced by experience. Certainly one or two less pacific, rather masculine staff, succeeded better with a few girls, and cultivated a one-sided loyalty. This could surely have been disastrous if such a feeling were built up in one House, under a liberal régime. In the larger group, while more girls were exposed to the disruptive behaviour of a few contemporaries, there were also more girls and staff to share the trials, and to act as buffers. Insecure girls gravitated to their favourite 'teacher', and mature staff were able to tolerate and utilize the playing-off of one adult against another which sometimes ensued. Again, of course, one thinks in terms of ideal staff, and for *part* of the period studied in this research they were not far short of the writer's ideal.

Daily Routine

Before seven o'clock—sometimes earlier for a special escort's breakfast—one of the relieving instructresses was in the kitchen, followed by her four girls. At 7.15 the two House Instructresses on duty roused their girls, their usual nine, plus the girls who would spend the later morning in the schoolroom, but would share the early morning tasks. Offices had to be ready for occupation, this involving at that time open coal fires. The girls' five dining tables and the staff dining table had to be laid, and at 8.15 all had to stop work to be ready for breakfast at 8.30.

Habitually the Headmistress had breakfast (at a separate small table) with the girls, after serving their hot dish, and while they ate their extra bread (on request) with butter and marmalade, she had time to plan some lines of action for their day.

About 9 o'clock the girls were conducted to the school Chapel, where the Headmistress conducted a short, simple service and one of the Staff was organist. A particularly high standard of decorum was asked at this time, and only acute rebels showed their paces in or to and from Chapel. An emotional outlet was sometimes supplied by an expressive hymn, especially if selected as someone's favourite hymn, as when a girl was due to leave that day.

This was followed by morning assembly in the Hall, with talks on matters concerning the group, and individual matters like birthday greetings. Girls were allocated to the work departments, and applications for changes of job were received. Once a week this was the time for 'ribbon' awards for conduct (red), work (green) and prefect (yellow), following Staff verdicts the previous evening. These awards were taken very seriously, and tears and exultation were the order during bed-making, which the girls did very carefully, under supervision; a weekly award for a dormitory of particular merit, for tidiness or good behaviour, fostered team work under a dormitory prefect.

The morning routine of concurrent house, laundry, kitchen and schoolwork began in earnest about 9.30, and, with a break for drinks, continued until 12.45, when manual workers changed out of blue cotton working dresses into their school tunics.

The afternoon programme of outdoor games and needlework lasted, with a short break, from 2 to 4.45. Apart from arrivals of new girls, or a rebel or two who might resist the activities prescribed, the afternoon was a time when concentrated paper work in the respective offices had a better chance of being done in peace.

After tea (5 to 5.30) preparations were on for the evening recreational class, or for the bath rota on two evenings, when the girls not in the bath embroidered gifts for sending home, or read books, magazines and comics, played quiet games, or just huddled and moped. But a hot bath often tempered a storm.

Then there was a light supper, with letters from home, after which a queue formed for attention by nurse at the surgery, and other applicants had interviews with the Head or her Deputy about special problems (real or magnified); frequently it was 'When am I going to my school, miss? I don't really want to go, but the sooner I go the sooner I'll get home'. One extreme form of this request was: 'Can you tell me when I'm going, miss, for I've smashed up every place I've been to, and I don't really want to smash this place for I've got to like it.' The reply to the ultimatum was as calm and non-committal as to other requests of a challenging nature: 'We're doing our best . . .' Sometimes the request for an interview arose from a letter from home, or the lack of a letter. Ultimately power and influence were minimal compared with attentiveness from home, while a letter announcing a visit, or the impossibility of visiting could revolutionize a girl's mood. On these issues, associated with so much insecurity and rejection in the past, hung the majority of abscondings, though this might be inverted, and a girl abscond on the eve of a parental visit, to annoy.

During these all too limited doses of individual physical and emotional bolstering in the surgery, and emotional bolstering in the Headmistress's office, the remainder chatted or read or hung around. The one or two members of staff on general supervision, then as at other such intervals of the day, had the most difficult job, for they had to be friendly, cheerful and outwardly relaxed, and yet miss nothing of what was going on in the little knots of conspirators, or studiedly casual loiterings near possible and impossible exits. Absconding was infectious, and there were spells of sublime contentment, but even one girl feeling seriously unsettled and managing to escape could shake the composure of all but the most bovine of the group. Those who say absconding is not serious seem rarely to think of this aspect. If staff allowed a girl or girls to elude them, it was not because they believed it did not matter, but either because (as in most cases) the staff ratio was too small to cover all contingencies, or because the member of staff was too new, too naïve, or not observant enough. The school was rarely without a few loyal girls who, at some personal risk, told of 'plans', and an excuse had to be found to probe the reasons behind the plans. This was not called 'snitching' but regarded as a sign of girls indentifying with the adult role of preserving the community. Sometimes a nosey-parker or a trouble-maker—after perhaps inviting the girls concerned to abscond with her—came, and her information had to be evaluated, but the informer was granted scant approval.

Further occasions for absconding at the tired, restless end of the day were to evade the line going to or from the evening Chapel service, or after lights-out, when all Staff seemed to have gone to sleep. Those near to dormitories were alert for unusual noises; it was always easier to nip trouble in the bud than to be roused from a first sleep by a smashed window-pane. No staffing allowance covered such emergencies, which might mean three or four people losing several hours of sleep, with one or two—a driver alone or with a companion —going miles in the school car to collect the girls if apprehended quickly by the police. With several specially difficult girls, this could happen two or three nights in a week, and successful absconders might need to be collected from as far as London or Glasgow. The Headmistress or her Deputy would be roused, would make the necessary telephone calls, and later receive not only police telephone calls, but one from the Press if information had leaked. Yet the following day every demand had to be met as if no sleep had been stolen. Not only abscondings, but serious or feigned illness, or attempted suicides, or rainwater leaks, or any nocturnal happenings, like nightmares and sleep-walkings, or refusals to settle down in a dormitory, could sap the energies in adults already tight-strung by longer than normal duty-hours and the effort of being a still centre in a storm. Not surprisingly Staff sometimes handled girls with diminished tact on these occasions, though mainly only after break-outs, and then suffered the aftermath of their own guilt and of the girls' rancour. Absconders collected and returned at 4 a.m. were likewise not at their sweetest and most reasonable, and were less so if stripped of ill-gotten gains, such as money from male associates (with which we bought classical records for school).

Staff often were most vulnerable if a longish spell of contentment and relative comfort had preceded a very unsettled phase. Conditioning to unrest, and ability to take turbulence and abscondings without rancour were essential to the way of life the Classifying School represented.

While it is true that problems in the work tend to be exaggerated, and the 'good girls' passed over, it is also true that little idea can be given to the lay reader of the crises that arose; indeed to the other residential workers with delinquents a reminder may be necessary that this difficult age-group of girls in the Classifying School were themselves unclassified, and sometimes a Juvenile Court committed a girl subsequently found to be totally unsuited to Approved School training. A few quotations from the Headmistress's report to the School Managers' monthly meetings during the latter part of the research period may highlight departures from routine, and the impossibility of watertight timetabling. These are taken mostly from consecutive reports.

Our numbers have risen slightly . . . thirty-nine being the peak number on our register. We have admitted some very difficult cases during the last few weeks and have maintained stability by a narrow margin. Yesterday was a day of crisis. A small group played up deliberately at intervals during the day. We averted absconding until last thing in the evening when five girls got away. Two of these gave themselves up at 11 p.m. and were in school again before midnight. The other three . . . are still at large.

The difficulty experienced immediately prior to the last meeting recurred a week later and we had a serious crisis on Sunday . . . involving four of the girls who had been difficult the previous Sunday. . . . On the evening of Saturday, during the bath period, they congregated in a small room on the second floor, barricaded themselves in and did considerable damage to walls and furniture before they allowed entry to the room on the morning of Sunday.... [One of these girls had become a national figure through earlier violence before admission and reputed mishandling of her case.]

We have made no progress in the matter of J's transfer (from mental hospital to a training school). Miss ——, the Headmistress of ——, consulted with her managers and they agreed to give J a trial there. Miss —— came over . . . and went with me to the hospital to visit J. She made excellent personal contact with her, but was unable to interest J in her school. J suggested that she might commit suicide if she went there! [This was not one of the above cases.]

In the same monthly report:

We had a particularly difficult girl in the school over Christmas. She was not only provocative, threatening and at times violent with other girls, but also turned her attention to members of staff, behaving quite dangerously on occasions. She was a girl who had spent all her life in institutions.... Great patience and tact were required in handling her and staff are to be congratulated that they managed it so well. She behaved almost normally during her last week in the school....

The Christmas and New Year festivities pass off remarkably happily in view of this, and other minor problems . . . Then [separately in report] we had the unfortunate experience at about 10 p.m. on Christmas Eve of discovering a serious burst in a water pipe in our boiler house....

We have had more anxiety than usual over individual cases, both inside and outside school. J, who had absconded from the mental hospital, where she was still a voluntary patient, at first refused to return [i.e. to hospital].

On —— we admitted a girl . . . with a record of difficult behaviour in —— Remand Home. A week later we admitted another difficult case . . . straight from hospital where she had been receiving treatment after swallowing needles. Unfortunately these two girls immediately became friends and a few days later there were rumours that both of them had swallowed needles. [One had two needles, and the other four needles and a hairpin inside her.] . . .

I am pleased to be able to report that Dr —— has been able to arrange for the admission of M to (mental) hospital as a voluntary patient. M is the 15-year-old epileptic girl who is pregnant....

Further excerpts show that the difficult girls were also difficult elsewhere.

(The above epileptic girl, who was pregnant) was removed from the mental hospital to a general hospital for the birth. She was difficult and unsettled and it was thought she should return to the Mental Hospital. She refused to go voluntarily, became violent, putting her hand through a window and sustaining a serious cut on her wrist, and eventually had to be taken back on a three-day order....

35

The two girls who were operated on in the —— Infirmary after swallowing needles made a satisfactory recovery. . . . Both were seen by a psychiatrist while still in hospital, and it was considered that —— should go into a mental hospital for a period of observation. . . . The two girls had been in the same ward and became very hysterical when they knew they were to be parted. —— swallowed a ring and a brooch-pin before being removed to mental hospital. —— had to be brought back to school by ambulance and was still hysterical on arrival ——.

Three of the twenty-eight girls admitted (since last report) were transferred from training schools where they had previously proved difficult. Some recent admissions are also troublesome cases . . . consequently it is not easy at present to maintain stability. . . .

Twenty-two girls have been admitted and twenty-two transferred since the last meeting. . . . It has been a difficult period. X, before her transfer here, had been bound over by the Court to be of good behaviour for twelve months. She was never able to conform for long to school routine and absconded from here—along with two other girls after stealing a key. There was a second incident on Saturday, when she threatened a member of staff with a fire extinguisher and afterwards smashed a glass panel in a fire-escape door. Her behaviour was by this time causing unrest and dissension in the school so that it seemed time to take action. The Home Office gave approval for a charge of absconding. . . .*

These were a few selected episodes, usually the more serious ones. Whilst they represented atypical behaviour in the school group, the time taken in dealing with it was out of all proportion to the number of girls involved.

The Approved School Rules stated that: 'Every effort shall be made to enforce discipline without resort to corporal punishment.' Corporal punishment of girls must be 'on the hands with a cane of a type approved by the Secretary of State—but only girls under fifteen shall be so punished'. In the research period covered about 130 girls under 15 passed through the Classifying School. As far as the writer knows no cane existed in the school, and the use of such an instrument, or other instrument of punishment was never discussed. This kind of disciplinary treatment was far removed from the school's methods, which would not, however, have excluded a smack on the bottom (to about one girl in a hundred) to quell dangerous hysteria; mainly Staff used verbal challenge or soothing in such cases, but in the rare case of a physical method it would probably not have occurred to them to enter it in the regulation punishment book, because they did not regard such a measure as

---

* This girl was diagnosed as pre-psychotic, and there was a history of withdrawal behaviour since before puberty, yet no other avenue of disposal was open but seeking for Borstal training.

punitive, but as remedial, and if it was done in such a way as to produce rancour (or devotion) in the girl they would have deplored its use. Advice was strongly against physical handling, because, however slight, it roused retaliatory actions, and danger existed of misinterpretation by any girls who had had sordid sexual experiences. Restraint during a rage, even by taking an arm, was avoided if at all possible. If a girl seemed likely to harm herself or others, two or three Staff, with or without some stable and helpful girls, stood by, as relaxedly as possible, and used all their powers of persuasion and suggestion, interlaced with humour. The writer recalls one occasion when she stood for about ten minutes alone between a very powerful girl in a frenzy of rage, and her 'enemy', until the former collapsed in tears. On another occasion the writer and a colleague stood for twenty minutes between a girl and her quarry—all four of us in stillness until the statue-like aggressor fell in a faint. To be without compassion at such times could only have led to brutality—by someone.

There was no formula of punishment, and often girls, needing something to blame, blamed the lack of punishment for their misconduct. Staff did not say what they thought—that the girls had mostly been punished enough by life, nor that punishment would do little good (for someone might at a later stage apply it) but, with a degree of truthfulness, that the Classifying School wanted to plan their future by seeing how they behaved; if they behaved well from fear of punishment we had learned very little.

The Home Office rules for punishment by separation from others were as follows (for 'boys' one reads 'girls'):

   (i) No boys under the age of 12 shall be kept in separation.

  (ii) The room used for the purpose shall be light and airy and kept lighted after dark.

 (iii) Some form of occupation shall be given.

 (iv) Means of communication with a member of the staff shall be provided.

  (v) If the separation is to be continued for more than twenty-four hours the written consent of one of the Managers shall be obtained and the circumstances shall be reported immediately to the Chief Inspector.

During the period of this research the two small detention rooms were very rarely used, and inevitably with a sickening sense of defeat, before and after. If a girl was so bent on absconding that this means had eventually to be used in order to retain her for psychiatric interview and mental and physical tests, then she still could resort to abnormal ruses to find a way out; one damsel, with flowing tresses and wearing bra and pyjama trousers was found two-thirds out through an unbelievably small window aperture; an earlier case had widened such an aperture and fractured her spine—but walked several miles before giving herself up. When a girl was so anti-social and frenzied that she had to be forcibly removed into a room away from the others, she became even more frenzied, and the night-light, bell and everything were put out of action in a trice, and eventually the lock and even the reinforced door. So the natural policy of treating a girl to every persuasive and therapeutic tactic, within the group, or individually, though, in its own way, harder, remained in force except in a small proportion of cases, and detention as a rule of thumb after absconding was likewise contrary to Staff's belief in trying to amend the cause behind the absconding—faulty relationships in the past.

Punishment was tried, with doubtful success, by another permitted method—'Forfeiture of rewards or privileges', but as the girls received no pocket money while at the School, and most awards in lieu (such as soap and toothpaste) were readily enough stolen without staff taking them, there remained the weekly ration of sweets and chocolate; fortunately other girls shared theirs with the absconder so she was rewarded with love as well as deprived of it!

Rule 33 said: 'The discipline of the School shall be maintained by the personal influence of the Headmaster and staff and shall be promoted by a system of rewards and privileges.' There may have been a tendency in recent years to diminish the role of the personalities of those in control, and belief in rather vague principles of child care may to some extent have taken their place. Indeed under the old emphasis there could grow up in a few girls' institutions such a nucleus of personal force as to overwhelm the growth, not only of evil but of good; junior staff could not develop their influence fully, and many girls ceased to question anything. In recent years what science of delinquency there is has filtered among the personnel in Approved Schools for girls. But the role of strong, good adult personality (preferably with stillness at the centre) cannot be underestimated; nor can the role of scientific knowledge. A father wrote to the Headmistress of the research period: 'It takes a person like you with very high qualities to bring the best out of people.'

Not surprisingly some members of staff tired of the long, arduous duties, and the continued self-restraint within the building, and little outlet in what was a strange neighbourhood to most, for staff came from as wide a geographical field as the Orkneys and the Isle of Wight. Lengthy sick leave was probably more common than in ordinary boarding schools. In the middle year of the research period, one key member of staff was absent for a year, and another for recurrent long periods. Replacements were hard to find, and much doubling of duty was necessary. It is probably safe to say that the required establishment was never complete in these three years, quite apart from absences for leave, longer and shorter. Generally staff (other than the Head and her Deputy) had full leave of six weeks (in instalments) or eight weeks for teachers.

Final departure of staff at this time in the school's history was less common than later. During these years, a pattern was set of devoted staff deciding their strength could not hold, resigning for another post, and later returning when a vacancy occurred at The Shaw. No fewer than *four* staff left and returned in this way between 1952 and 1954. Another on leave of absence for further study returned with no hesitation. The intellectual stimulus of the classification itself was added to the challenge of residential work, to the sense of being necessary, and all compounded in a régime built on loyalty and affection, made it possible to renew one's strength in a way that is barely credible in retrospect.

There were six final departures in the three-year period, but only one of these had failed to settle and stayed but briefly. One left for further study and a new branch of social work; two (a relief and a kitchen instructress) for other similar fields.

Neither pay nor prestige were binding factors in holding staff; few can have been 'in it for the money'. The basic salary of Instructresses at the beginning of this research period was £270 per annum,* and extraneous duty allowance was paid up to ten hours weekly, at the rate of a maximum of £3 per week. Residential emoluments of £108 per annum were charged out of this. Vocal complaints were few: a rueful smile when reports came back of educationally sub-normal girls now out in the world earning higher pay than the Approved School Instructress, or some difficulty in relating calmly the remark of a girl, whose mother had written to say she was once a maid at the Hall in its palmy days—'She was doing the same job as you, miss.' Mainly, however, the girls did lend equal prestige by calling all staff 'teachers'.

The other staff paid on a scale other than national was the Housemistress, who merited £400 per annum† at that time, if qualified by training, or awaiting the verdict of a Board if untrained. She was not, however, paid for extraneous duties, being expected, presumably, to do her many additional stints for love. Yet the Deputy Headmistress, on Burnham Scale, could be paid extraneous duty up to fifteen hours a week, as well as a responsibility allowance, and increments for

* Unqualified instructresses at girls' schools were paid on a scale of £650 to £760 in 1967.

† Qualified Housemistresses in 1967 were paid on the scale £860 to £1,510. Emoluments varied for single quarters from £145 to £195.

Approved School work. Fortunately habitual restraint extended to discussion of respective earnings.

In their Evidence for Presentation to the Ingleby Committee (1957) the Technical Sub-Committee of the Association of Headmasters, Headmistresses and Matrons of Approved Schools wrote (p. 23),

> Approved Schools require teachers, instructors, housemasters, housemistresses and so on but the over-riding requirement is that while technical or other proficiency is an advantage, certain personal qualities are essential. These are not easy to define and it has long been recognized that they are often possessed by people lacking in academic or technical training. It seems to us that candidates for work in an Approved School must essentially be chosen on the basis of these personal qualities and that specific training should follow the selection ... Certain professional requirements are, and should be, laid down for teachers and instructors but these, too, will profit from specific training probably after some Approved School experience.

By the time this was written (1957) a pilot training scheme was under way for four house-masters and two housemistresses, working initially in an Approved School, eventually studying almost full-time in a University Department of Education.

The Ingleby Report (1960)[2] regarded 'Matters relating to the staffing of Approved Schools as falling largely outside our terms of reference' (par. 506). However the report had, in paragraph 463, stressed the difficulties of staffing girls' Approved Schools adequately, in order to cover a wide range of activities for a small number of girls, quite apart from the shortage of senior staff of quality. Pre- and in-service training of staff was encouraged. Moves have been made in recent years towards both kinds of training, so that the writer's concern may well seem out-dated. At the time of this research little encouragement came from employers about the need for further training of instructresses, and indeed *all* grades of staff. Such training would have stimulated intellectual interest, encouraged a healthier degree of detachment, given time for renewing interest in the world outside, and confidence for seeking ultimate promotion. Only one of the staff in the three-year research period is still directly in the Approved School service (with promotion), but at least eight are in situations of considerably more status, but possibly less personally satisfying, in allied fields. Settling elsewhere is initially difficult. The continual running in high gear, the over-dose of excitement, the close personal demands, and the insight gained from them; the subsequent lack of understanding outside of the depth and quality of experience gained inside, together with the adjustment needed to a life without the community's props—all gradually give way, and a return to the circumscribed, defensive life would be harder to contemplate.

Chapter Seven

THE GIRLS 1

Was there anything about these girls to look at, to listen to, to live with, that makes them worth writing about?

We have heard comments by one writer on maladjusted children about the restlessness of the girls as against the boys, about their failure to lose themselves as easily in group activities. But this is largely true of all adolescent girls. Sex rears its head earlier than with boys, but not only in delinquent girls in Approved Schools. Most segregated girls, in day or boarding schools, will look and sigh when a male crosses the playground. They assert their femininity and remind the poor schoolmistress of whatever age that she is 'past it'. It is doubtful whether the private conversations of the average adolescent girl are less knowledgeable or cleaner than the average Approved School girls'. At one extreme of both is the girl who knows the crude aspects of sex, while at the other is the girl who is too immature socially for her to do more than gape and imitate the talk and postures of others. The range of emotional immaturity in the delinquent girl is the thing that distinguishes them most from the normal so that the more sophisticated in knowledge is driven more to experiment than would be the average adolescent girl—to satisfy her infantile sensual needs for tactile comfort; to demonstrate to her superior contemporaries that she could win love; to pay a parent off for neglecting her. The experimental love life of the least mature of the delinquents differed mainly in its unselfconsciousness, like the pre-school child in its experimental sexual phase.

While the danger of over-generalization is still present, this difference in emotional maturity is perhaps the key to most of the apparently bizarre, or just off-the-beam, behaviour of the adolescent girl in Approved School.

This is well illustrated in an article in the *Approved Schools Gazette* of June 1962, which was a reproduction of a paper given to the Scottish Approved Schools Staffs Association by their President, Mr T. S. Jack.

Mr Jack had been placed as Acting Headmaster for a short time, as an experiment, in a Girls' Approved School, where the rest of the staff were the established female contingent. He had previously heard what he regarded as 'unlikely tales of girlish misdemeanours', and came therefore not forearmed against what he found a 'most alarming' difference in dealing with the mentally or emotionally disturbed girl, as against delinquent boys. He notes they are 'much more emotional, much more irrational and as a result much more insolent and difficult to handle than boys'. With the robust, infectious humour one finds in most of the extraverted Headmasters of Boys' Approved Schools, Mr Jack recounts how one girl ate floor polish, or food from the pig swill; another refused to get out of her bath; the impasse when a violently hysterical girl would neither conform in the group or go quietly into isolation. 'With the really difficult girl, there always had to be a fight. . . .'

Any Head or member of the Staff of a Girls' Approved School may tend to envy the candour with which this 'experimental' Headmaster can talk of his experiences. Most women (perhaps because they tend to take things more personally than men) are reticent about difficulties with their charges. This is in many ways a good thing, because they have quietly evolved ways of meeting difficult situations which Mr Jack had not yet dreamt of—ways of side-stepping to avoid the ugliness of physical struggle; to make insolence and defiance less likely, even from the most aggressive. But when the hard-to-define measures have been taken and trouble still ensues, the defeat to an exhausted staff is more sore.

The lurid behaviour of a few cases can take attention away from the wistful and the woebegone. Sometimes the two could blend into an incident. One Sunday morning at the Classifying School a rather sad but poised 16-year-old was doing her before-breakfast stint, sweeping a corridor. An unbalanced youngster came past, muttering, 'They're all thieves here, and you're one too.' A terrible fight started, of course, just outside the writer's bedroom door. Separated, but not calm, the unbalanced one proceeded downstairs, grabbed a large knife from the kitchen hatch and careered along the corridor. A little colourless dullard, all nervous twitches and grins, calmly put her hand out and said, 'Thank you, I'll have that!'—and neatly retrieved the knife.

It is easy to go on to recall the same berserk girl absconding the same evening and biting about twelve policemen on their hands or arms and the Inspector on the ankle.

This was 'over the border' behaviour. Somewhere on the border-line one recalls a finely built, intelligent, 16-year-old lying screaming and kicking on a toilet floor, in a typical toddler tantrum. A neurotic ex-Grammar School girl showed her rebellion in a more ladylike way—in a simulated faint on the same toilet floor. A mentally defective Black Country girl gave a casual glance, and asked tonelessly, 'Is 'er dead, Miss?'

Sometimes the dopey appearance of the dull girl was belied, as when a diplomatic Senior member of staff said sadly to a returned absconder, 'I *was* disappointed when I heard you'd gone.' 'You'll get over it, Miss,' was the sympathetic reply.

The robust behaviour problem could be a relief after purely neurotic and regressive strains. A stalwart who worked hard in the garden one winter's day and left on the gardener's bicycle, typified more the delinquent boy, and the change was relished. When she later played the prostitute in a U.S. camp, she had reduced her stature in staff eyes.

The extremes in hysteria were usually drinking disinfectant or swallowing foreign bodies. Certain girls specialized in this, another might do it once by imitation; others might claim they had needles or brooches inside them, but a diet of cotton wool sandwiches made them more truthful.

These are, indeed, among the lurid episodes which tend to be retold wherever two or three former staff are gathered together. Tragedy and comedy were mixed, and had to be, so that callousness and mawkishness could be avoided.

More difficult, in some ways, than the dramas, which often culminated in the exit to a more suitable stage of the leading player, were the day-to-day petty rebellions, and even more than the 'day' ones, the evening and overnight clashes with authority, for tired nerves on both sides made the end of the day hardest—as any overwrought mother of toddlers would confirm. A girl stumping about, muttering, or dragging her feet more noticeably than usual; a girl saying 'Aw, Miss!' to every polite request; a girl spending twenty minutes in a toilet to evade work, or smoothing down her hair with water at the mirror for an extra five minutes to keep everyone waiting for a meal; a girl prodding the girl beside her, or giving a vacuous grin across the room during serious discussions; a girl refusing to have a bath, or refusing to take off her brassiere at bedtime—all these were the everyday little goads which, except in a raw mood, staff either ignored or turned into positive behaviour by a change of subject or a funny remark, in the best tradition of family management. Thus the days passed, without too many serious crises, and with only the very rare 'show-down'.

Inexpert staff, or the expert in a 'raw' mood could prolong a very minor rebellion into a major crisis. But when one considers how major some of the minor rebellions would seem in the normal girls' school, it should not be necessary to make excuses. We shall see later that over 30 per cent of the main group had been 'definitely unacceptable, unreliable, uncooperative' at school, and a further 42 per cent had been less than reliable. This leaves 28 per cent who had not been much trouble, or even had been very good, and at the Classifying School such a nucleus also existed.

Standardized differences between the sexes which would substantiate, and partially explain, the difficulties noted so far, either with maladjusted children elsewhere, or with Classifying School girls, might be summarized as follows:

(1) *Vital Capacity.* In a chapter by Lewis M. Terman and others in *Manual of Child Psychology*[1] we read, 'the superiority of boys in vital capacity is about 7 per cent by age 6, and rises to about 12 per cent at age 10, and to about 35 per cent at age 20. 'It may be one of the factors underlying sex differences in play interests, drive for achievement, and liking for activity and adventure.' Against this, the same chapter stresses the more rapid *physical maturation of girls.*

(2) *Stability of Bodily Function.* Most types of glandular imbalance are quoted in the same chapter as being much more common in females. Also, 'The male shows less fluctuation than the female in body temperature, basal metabolism, acid–base balance of the blood and level of blood sugar.'

(3) *Play, Reading, School Subjects.* A variety of objective data (mainly from American sources) is quoted in the chapter[1] to prove that girls are more conservative in their play, participate more in sedentary occupations, or those with a restricted range of actions, girls choose more novels and stories and less adventure and scientific writing than boys. Four times as many girls as boys prefer English as their school subject, twice as many prefer commercial studies, and nearly four times as many prefer languages. In preferences for work, more girls prefer working indoors and dealing with people rather than things.

(4) *Attitudinal associations.* Hallworth and Waite[2] using the 'Semantic differential' technique with boys and girls in the fourth year of Secondary School found that 'boys have more *attitudinal associations* with ambition and study, girls with self and home; boys have a cluster of concepts identified with authority, girls with security'.

(5) *Aggressive and Dominant Behaviour.* Males tend to score higher on measures of dominance and ascendance in tests devised by Allport and by Bernreuter.[1]

(6) *Suggestibility.* Tests tend to show girls as more suggestible than boys.[1]

(7) *Sociability.* Though girls are more interested in personal relationships, and therefore more sociable in this sense, they are often inhibited by introvertive tendencies and inferiority feelings from seeking company. Terman and Miles[1] (1936) found girls more angry

than boys at 'being socially slighted', 'hearing friends unjustly abused'. Girls show more social conformance.

(8) *Emotionality.* The same chapter[1] (p. 977) says: 'The preponderance of evidence from personality inventories indicates somewhat greater emotionality for females.'

(9) *Delinquent and Problem Behaviour.* Except in studies of deceptive behaviour, which have shown girls to cheat more at school, and for the matter of writing obscene notes, boys are deemed delinquent and 'problem children' more often than girls.[1]

(10) *Extraversion and Neuroticism.* In Professor Eysenck's[3] *Crime and Personality* (p. 42) we see that female prisoners, both English and Australian, while considerably more extraverted than normal, are less so than the male prisoners studied in America and Australia; unmarried mothers, as a class, however, scored higher in extraversion than any of these, but lower in neuroticism. As our research group contains budding members of both these female categories, these findings are relevant.

John Gittins in *Approved School Boys*[4] says: 'Variations in physique, in intelligence, in temperament, and in attitude are as wide as in the population at large, but exaggerated traits are more frequent, and abnormalities are more obvious.' This could be endorsed from observation of girls, and 'only more so' could be added, especially with regard to temperament. Furthermore: whereas one can usually visualize an average adolescent girl of a certain age, not meaning a model adolescent, but one with an average degree of gaucheness, an average degree of plumpness, and just average intellect—a rather stodgy I.Q. 100—and average interests in popular entertainment and dancing, it is much more difficult to visualize an average delinquent; the writer found this too with some personality test material. An average adolescent test profile could be found, but not so for the delinquent girl.

As we have seen from the earlier part of this chapter, the most exaggerated feature among the girls in the Approved School population was emotional immaturity, and a marked tendency of dependence and attention-seeking.

To put into statistical terms the attention-seeking conduct of the Approved School girl, the writer used the comments in two sections (mainly) of the Classifying School report to place her on a 5-point scale, together with a further 7-point scale to show the form her attention-seeking conduct (or otherwise) tended to take. As this aspect of the girls' life in the community was, above all, one that inscribed itself deeply on the memory, the writer could substantiate what had been recorded in writing.

The second sample of 100 (1957 admissions) were not known to the writer in the same way, and were assessed entirely from comments in the classifying report. The comparison is most interesting, and suggests these may correspond to definite categories of Approved School girls.

The following tables give the results:

Table 1: Demand for Adult Attention

	Main sample of 500 %	Sample of 100 %
Normal	23·2	22·0
Abnormally detached, or evading attention	23·8	22·0
Rather more than normal attention seeking	31·0	34·0
Definitely more than normal attention seeking	15·0	17·0
Excessive attention seeking	7·0	5·0

Table 2: Kind of Attention-Seeking Conduct

	Main sample of 500 %	Sample of 100 %
Such conduct not outstanding (or withdrawing)	51·6	44·0
Wanting to do useful extra jobs	5·8	6·0
Finding herself nice new roles, just being nice, or 'smarmy'	14·2	14·0
Just hanging around, talking or dumb	11·2	15·0
Being pettily naughty, negative	7·6	9·0
Being rude and anti-social for those she liked	3·4	5·0
Being rude and anti-social generally for attention	6·2	7·0

The degree of demand for adult attention corresponds very closely in the two groups. The slight discrepancies in the kinds of attention-seeking conduct arise mainly from the writer recording some later in the 'such conduct not outstanding' category if she felt it was not quite 'normal', yet not so very abnormal as to fall elsewhere.

The following will give some idea of the comments on classifying reports which link with the above assessments. They do not, of course, give the total picture leading to the assessment.

(1) *Normal.* 'N has been friendly in a warm-hearted way, and generally polite, except when handled too informally, and then she loses regard for the time being. She accepts firm correction and bears no grudge afterwards. She has been trustful and reliant here . . . and has been reliable.' Thus N, while clearly longing for extra attention, could restrain her demands in a nearer to adult way.

(2) *Abnormally detached, or evading attention.* 'D is full of resentment against adults. She wants to get notice, but seems to have no idea how to approach staff in a friendly way, so just stands aside, and then grudges the fact that other girls have more attention. She has improved slightly in this respect.' Or 'B was sullen, reticent and vaguely defiant at first, but she has learned to accept adults to the point where she is only reticent when in direct contact, and shows capacity for childish dependence and warm friendliness. She is at present neither dependent nor independent.'

(3) *Rather more than normal attention-seeking.* 'M has generally been obedient and responsive, and glad of every bit of notice.'

(4) *Definitely more than average attention-seeking.* 'If V is especially enamoured of a member of staff she is unbearably coy; with the remainder she hopes to get her own way merely by charm. She has shown signs latterly of being able to keep a respectful distance, and of being more genuinely cooperative. . . .'

(5) *Excessive attention-seeking.* 'J is perpetually in need of affection, sympathy and notice, and if she gets it once she comes back for more. If refused it in the ordinary way she contrives to steal it by committing petty offences for which she can first be reproved, and then offer an apology.'

The last example would belong to category 4 of the 'kind of attention-seeking conduct', namely 'just hanging around talking or dumb'. With her would be at least a tenth of the population at any given time. In one case this behaviour showed itself in literal *hanging*, suspended by the neck, just for attention—fortunately not for too long:

For her first weeks here R made little positive mark on the community, but she was rejected by the girls, mainly for her unprepossessing ways. Instead of this bringing out minor exhibitionist trends, she went to the length of making what seemed to be a serious attempt at suicide. That the fundamental cause was attention-seeking seemed evident the next day, for she had about her an air of achievement, a quiet satisfaction and a suppressed animation, quite unnoticed in her before. Her contemporaries were anything but sympathetic, but staff endeavoured to give her more attention in an unobtrusive, tactful way.

Finally a picture of the 6 per cent who demanded attention (usually excessive) by rudeness and anti-social conduct:

> Without exception J starts off by being completely bold and regardless, ready to test every response. When she feels accepted, and yet knows she will be kept in her place she is friendly and good-humoured. . . . Once J reaches this point of friendly contact she has, typically, to test out adults, in case they are, after all, too soft for her, but she retains a fair measure of confidence once the initial try-out is over.

(Here category 7 merges, at one point, with 6, where rude demands were made on a favourite member of staff.)

The demanding of attention, rather than just the pleading, wistful waiting for more than the usual notice, seemed particularly typical of the girls who had spent many years in and out of institutions, as had the child of the last excerpt, and who was resentful of rejection by her parents—real or implied. It is interesting that D. H. Stott's[5] figure of 20 boys out of 102 who had been motivated to delinquency because of uncertainty of their parents' affection, corresponds fairly closely to the total for our last three, and most persistent, kinds of attention-seekers (17·2 per cent in the 500 sample, 21 per cent in the other).

Some occasions increased the demand in almost the whole group. Particularly this was so in the absence of the Headmistress (who, in a girls' school, where the group matters less than to boys, is the prop of all props). When, as usually happened, there were too many attention-seekers for comfort, the Headmistress had to depart unobtrusively. As awareness of her absence dawned, all had to be ready to take the back-wash, and the writer, as the Deputy Head during the period concerned, was convinced that the only safe, and eventually workable policy, was to be available for every pressing demand, however challenging, however teasing. After twenty-four hours the pressure abated nearer to what would normally meet the Headmistress herself, and the harassed staff could breathe again. Hints of further rejection at the crucial stage of 'mother' being missing could breed serious revolt. That all Principals of Girls' Approved Schools might not agree with this policy is seen from an excerpt from a follow-up report from a Training School: 'S would have responded to individual attention, but would have been more demanding had she had it.' Reactions to this exaggerated human need did, however, vary in the Training Schools, and—most important to remember—the incidence of attention-seekers varied. The training programme in some cases would have collapsed with pseudo-toddlers in the building. In the Classifying School the bizarre had to be accommodated and tolerated, and was generally enjoyed—within limits.

In a group of more normal adolescents, and much more so among younger children, one would find the braggart, the 'show-off', sometimes weaving tall stories, and there is a good chance that this was an only child thrown much on her own resources, and much aware of her own importance, yet dissatisfied in finding a social mirror to reflect herself. We found this type among our milder attention-seekers, and it was exaggerated where, for instance, a girl had lived as an only child in a home with a physically and mentally deteriorating mother; or where a mother of an only child sought to project false images of the family. But the sub-group of girls who absorbed so much of Staff's time were definitely abnormal personalities, whose attention-seeking was hysterical in quality; one (in the 1957 sample) would lie down in a corridor rather than be ignored. Most of the suicide attempts (or pseudo-attempts, which could have succeeded only by error on their part) were in this section.

Clinical personnel, such as Psychiatrists, who see cases individually, do not always appreciate the group jealousies, and tend to be critical that the clamouring Approved School girl is not settled in a comfortable chair with a cigarette, and given a long session of concentrated attention. Alas, in a group of thirty-five unselected delinquent girls, one could (on the above figures) reckon on having two or three who were excessively demanding (and usually ready to go to ludicrous lengths to attain their needs), five or six who were definitely more than normal in their demands, and seventeen others who, though not so abnormal in seeking, might be just as excessive in their need, and suffering badly from their insistent companions. Anyone who has taught relatively normal adolescent girls knows that they, too, matching the remaining 'normal' ten of our thirty-five, require a goodly supply of notice.

Perhaps this gives some idea of the wear and tear, and the continued need for scrutiny of the staffing situation in Girls' Approved Schools, especially in those receiving the most difficult girls, who have proved resistant to many previous attempts to help them to stabilize. Aichorn's[6] two women workers, when 'entirely worn out' had to be replaced with others! (p. 241).

Through all this description we see in psychoanalytical terminology the dominance of the pleasure principle, instead of the reality principle. The immediate gratification of desires plays a higher part in the more difficult sections of the group than does any need for achievement of status and acceptance in the community. Dr Kate Friedlander,[7] in tracing such phenomena to infantile disappointments in relations with adults, says, 'The wish to be loved and not to be left alone is still present, but is entirely over-shadowed by the constant clamour for gratification, and if satisfaction is not forth-coming, open hatred is expressed.' Most of the workers at the Classifying School, whether verbally or intuitively, subscribed to this cause and effect, but the demands of time and organization (indeed a reality principle!) had so often to rule them. Ideally we should regard all those occasions of *not* meeting demands for notice as failures, even if meeting the demand consists of simulated indifference when the girl is using her needs to deliberately upset the whole community. By steering her calmly away from the group, then in a detached way listening to her demands, and becoming just as personal as the girl's emotional stability at that point makes safe, one can gradually meet some of her needs. The whole process—slow and dangerous in the case of a teenager with a toddler's emotional maturity—can be regarded as a learning process, often a very protracted one, for a girl who has been deprived of learning to adjust socially in a normal family.

That the struggle was still going on, that the vying with each other for staff attention generally took precedence over vying for the attention of other girls, did lessen one grave problem of one-sex institutions. Staff did not hide from the problems of homosexuality. They were aware of the 'crushes' girls had for members of staff, which could drive the girl to excesses of showing off and jealousy, and which were generally handled with sympathy and realism (avoiding, for instance, situations where compromise was possible). They were aware of 'crushes' on other girls, and recognized the exaggerated male or female hair styles or gait or other gestures involved. They were alert to the possibility of bed-sharing, but avoided drawing attention (or those who were wise did) in a shocked way, since this would have made the practice more interesting—just as they had to appear only mildly interested if a mentally defective girl stole the electric light fuses, while endeavouring to stop her through this very 'disinterest'. They believed the problem of homosexuality was kept within safety limits in the school.

This kind of evidence will naturally be suspect to some, but so (to the writer) would evidence from any girls' reports to the contrary: they would certainly have delighted to impress an outsider with 'stories'. The age and emotional immaturity of the majority were in our favour, for most still needed parental figures more than they needed love partners.

In this chapter, and in Chapter IV, the lurid episodes have tended to be overdrawn. While this is not surprising, for the difficult section could monopolize staff attention, an interposed letter from the files may bring some balance to the picture. This was written by the Deputy Headmistress (the present writer) to the Headmistress

of the short-term Training School, who had offered an early vacancy
for a girl.

> Thank you for your letter. . . . As you may, know,' Miss Wannop has
> been away on holiday for the past fortnight, and during this time the
> girls have been organizing and rehearsing a concert as a 'Welcome
> Home'. This is to be on Monday, and as A has played a leading part in
> the arrangements, acting as producer and accompanist, it would be
> very hard to transfer her before the event. Quite apart from A's own
> disappointment, it is quite possible that the bottom may fall out of the
> show without her leadership.

Usually two or three girls could be won over to leadership in the
few weeks of their stay, though the struggle to maintain it was hard.
Once two suggested they might run a Sunday School on their own.
On the second Sunday afternoon word circulated that an unlikely
clique had enrolled, with the intention of smashing the schoolroom
window and escaping; a member of staff dropped in, 'out of interest'.

For the running of the school, quite as much depended on the
mixture of cooperative to non-cooperative, though there were many
blends, between the few positively 'good' and the seriously disruptive.

At each Monday evening Staff meeting, when we discussed until
perhaps 10.30 not only general routine, but also the assessment of a
group due soon to be allocated for Training Schools the main behavioural traits were recorded, according to certain headings and
scales. On these were based the 'Observed Behaviour' section of the
assessment forms which preceded the girl to her Training School.
We did not take easily to this calculation of traits, but their inclusion
in the following tables in this chapter may instil respect in some,
after the discursive account of the Classifying School's population.
Later, in Chapter ¡XXI, we can see how far these observations had
prognostic values for the 500 group. Here the figures for the 100
group are included, for comparison.

Table 3: Behaviour with Group (or Group Participation)

	Sample of 500 %	Sample of 100 %
Participates actively	42·8	34
Participates occasionally or marked swings	50·4	55
Remains isolated	6·8	11

Comment. The 1957 sample of 100 was not a complete group. This
may account for the greater number of isolates.

Both samples may surprise those who see the typical delinquent, girl or boy, always as the extravert. It may well be that many of the second group (half the population) had their natural tendencies to be outgoing confused by early hurts, or by exposure temporarily to a non-congenial group at the Classifying School. Again a girl's isolation might be her most powerful means of gaining attention from girls or staff. The subnormal girl with additional personality problems often resorted to this kind of attention-seeking.

Table 4: Contribution to Group

	Sample of 500 %	Sample of 100 %
Usually positive	26·4	28
Indifferently positive or occasionally disruptive	52·6	59
Usually disruptive	21·0	13

Comment. Table 3 showed 3 out of 10 to be actively sociable; in Table 4 we see that less than 3 out of these 4 were *good* mixers. On the other hand, when we consider the population, this is a surprisingly large proportion; only about 2 out of 10 were habitual disrupters. However, one or two 'disrupters' in each dormitory were enough to cause bedtime fracas. One disrupter at a table for seven girls could irk the others into being unpleasant and quarrelsome. 7 in the whole group of 35, where about half were only indifferently positive, could create unrest and unhappiness.

Table 5: Gravitates towards (i.e. contemporaries)

	Sample of 500 %	Sample of 100 %
To best elements	11·4	7
To no particular types	32·4	38
To worst elements	21·2	22
Varies according to mood	19·4	19
To the very immature	15·6	14

Comment. The problem of who linked up closely with whom was not an academic interest for us, but a pressing practical issue, even if it was a matter of the immature girls ganging up harmlessly with their own kind. But we had to be right on our toes where the severely anti-social or psychopathic gravitated towards others who were in revolt. The inconsistent might be drawn in at intervals, drifting from one extreme group to another, or might ask suddenly to go to bed or help in the kitchen. An experienced staff knew when and how to divert these from trouble. Girls too—and not necessarily the bright girls—could be subtly persuasive with some trouble-makers, through close identification with staff.

Table 6: Expression of feelings in group

	Sample of 500 %	Sample of 100 %
Easily expressed but are under control	23·8	32
Only too easily expressed and rarely under control	40·8	40
Expressed with difficulty if at all	29·4	27
Doubtful if she has much feeling to express	6·0	1

Comment. The effervescent or explosive number as high as 40 per cent in both groups. Here we have the more colourful delinquent type. The 'top' 20 per cent would be nearer to the average adolescent group in this respect. The third group, the inhibited or withdrawn, could also be found anywhere, but would cause discomfort. A case recalled is of a little dull 14-year-old, who held her emotions in check for the six-week classifying period, remained stoically quiet during a day-long journey through her home town to a Training School, and there on the threshold threw herself on the writer's shoulder and sobbed. This is an extreme case, fortunately.

Table 7: Prevailing Mood

	Sample of 500 %	Sample of 100 %
Cheerful	13	16
Serious	13·4	20
Depressed	6·0	6
Sullen or resentful	20·6	15
Careless or regardless	18·2	14
Apathetic	4·0	4
Anxious	23·0	25
Other	1·8	—

Comment. To record these (from the 'observed behaviour' data, and from elsewhere in a girl's file) was not easy, for the range of mood in each could be extreme, but *prevalent* mood is emphasized.

As with the other observations the language is not clinical, nor is it related to clinical types, such as depressive or manic. These headings were used by a mainly lay staff in assessing the girls for the benefit of other lay staff.

The fact that the totals for the two samples correspond so closely, suggests we may have been subdividing in an important way. We shall later find that these groupings had prognostic value, especially when regrouped.

Table 8: General Conduct at the Classifying School

(These headings were not used specially at the meetings for discussion and allocation, but from an analysis of the whole assessment report, and from personal memory of the girls' reactions—hence the greater caution in giving 'top marks' to the 100 sample, whom the writer knew less well.)

	Sample of 500 %	Sample of 100 %
Cooperative	13·8 } 40·6	7 } 41
Just fulfilling obligations, but genuinely so	26·8	34
Superficially cooperative, subversive undercurrent	14·2	17
Openly uncooperative or aggressive	5·8	8
Persistent absconder	8·8	—*
Very childish all the time	15·4	13
Outbursts of very childish behaviour	15·2	21

*Absconders not recorded consistently.

Comment. On about 40 per cent of the girls some reliance could be placed in day-to-day life; of these a proportion might be very weak-willed in emergencies, but could respond to appeals and were ashamed later if others were too outrageous.

Few of the remaining 60 per cent could take such appeals as 'letting the school down', but the 40 per cent could generally take responsibility for about thirty more—and it was the residue, the weak and the warped, that staff had to supervise and manipulate for every waking hour.

The 15 to 17 per cent who were superficially cooperative, over a layer of potential or real subversiveness, was a difficult group to live with, and could undermine the morale of staff who were over-tired. With a stronger subversive personality it was often best to keep her guessing and gradually bring her activities into the open, often to the relief of other girls, who disliked 'two facedness'.

With some of the simpler cases it was possible to be direct and frank without reducing a girl's dignity.

General Comment

That some scientific accuracy can be ascribed to these statistics may be assumed from the surprising matches of the figures for the two samples; where this is not so, the discrepancy may result from the less representative nature of the 100 sample as part of a year's admissions.

If these observations of the 500 sample have some scientific accuracy, and if we are justified in expecting a few weeks' behaviour to provide a pattern of the 'real' girl, our correlations with success up to five years later (see Chapter XXI) should be significant.

We shall, in fact, find highly predictive scores.

Chapter Eight

THE GIRLS 2

A. THEIR PHYSIQUE

In an experiment by Symonds,[1] in America, on 'Sex Differences in the Life Problems and Interests of Adolescents', 784 High School boys and 857 girls ranked fifteen 'major areas of life concern' according to their interest in reading or discussion of them. The largest sex difference was in the place given to personal attractiveness, which was placed, on an average, fifth by the girls and eight by the boys. No figures seem to be available for rating of personal attractiveness in relation to the girls' own personal charm, as judged by the group; the writer's hypothesis would be an inverse ratio—the less a girl's personal attractiveness the greater her preoccupation with it.

To spend much discussion on the statement that adolescent girls are usually deeply interested in personal appearance, in clothes and in hair styles seems a trifle unnecessary; though there is undoubtedly a cultural factor here, seen in latter years in a resuscitation of peacock trends in adolescent males, most parents of teenagers of both sexes in the years 1952 onwards to 1957, with which we are concerned, would agree with Symonds' findings.

Some of our Approved School girls seemed to be pre-adolescent in this, or perhaps our standard schoolgirl tunic, blouse, ankle socks and sandals brought some of those who were emotionally retarded back from their false level of social experience, as we hoped it would, to a more tomboyish phase. In others the lack of physical adornment seemed to exacerbate their need for self-display, and absconding was sometimes an excuse for trying to adapt the school uniform to peculiar twists of feminine fashion. The point here is not that there is necessarily anything wrong in teenage girls wanting to dress more adult than adult, but that girls who had savoured unhappy or precocious experiences needed often to regress before they could progress more naturally. On the assumption that dressing like a lady helps one to act like a lady, we hoped that dressing like a schoolgirl might help them to act like schoolgirls, until their emotional lives had caught up with their physical. That these could be the wrong clothes for the few more mature girls was inevitable.

What a girl feels about her personal appearance, clothing apart, is more important than the reality, and self-consciousness at physical traits, or imagined traits, may have helped to precipitate some of the girls into' their heterosexual experiences—to prove to female contemporaries that they were acceptable to males. When we come to examine measurements of various kinds, we find nothing very extraordinary about their physique.

Lombroso[2] did not find his 'born criminals' attractive. As others have indicated recently, the greater proportion of mental defectives in the prisons of his day may have influenced his observations of degeneracy in the criminal population. One must indeed admit the converse when considering personal appearance of children and young people—that adults are undoubtedly influenced in their judgment by physical appearance, beyond what may be reliable as psychodiagnostic material. Pretty little girls in Children's Homes have sometimes been found in later years to have been less responsive than their admiring housemothers believed; we shall be discussing some of these from our population later. Sadly for unattractive girls without compensatory gifts, the fight against aversion tends to call down pity, which is probably just as destructive of the child's ego.

As Symonds'[1] High School girls ranked personal attractiveness significantly higher than boys, so did the Classifying School staff, while struggling to be fair and undiscriminating, pay far more attention to the personal features of the delinquent girls than did staff of Boys' Classifying Schools of that time, if one can judge by the terser pen-pictures the latter produced. We liked to study the minutiae of a girl's features, of her facial muscles, and her fleeting as well as her habitual expressions. We were interested in these from an aesthetic angle, and also (questionably, accordingly to some schools of thought) as a key to her personality. As we studied her in a life situation (however artificial) we had more checks on our inferences than one has when studying an unknown woman at the next table in a restaurant, or even a case seen once at a psychiatric clinic for a pre-committal report.

Allport, in *Personality*[3] (p. 517), alludes to the slight margin in favour of woman's superior ability to judge people, and explains this partly as coming from the 'signal importance of personal relationships in women's lives'. We discussed our girls intensely over meals, over coffee, in low voices during get-togethers in bed-sitting-rooms when we were off duty. This was not only because we led such inbound lives and lacked variety of interests, but because the girls, their past, and our ever-changing relationships with them and theirs with each other, were on a highly dramatic plane (especially when sweetened by ready-made humorous episodes, or episodes seasoned with humour by the adult later). Indeed it was not easy to find a book of fiction that was vivid enough to compete, and stage drama was viewed critically against our experiences and our awareness of tensions. A portrayal of violence, as in *Othello*, could seem tame after some of the love-hate expression that was often part of our Approved School experience. The social and domestic events overheard discussed by women on the buses en route to town seemed trivial in the extreme. Our predilection for this kind of personal observation sometimes brought us rebuffs, not only from interested visitors or professional assistants who valued only objective data, but from police clerks noting objective data of personal appearance, who did not wish to hear that the absconder was a 'pretty girl', or 'a bit odd-looking'. The attitude of police women to similar data was most favourable!

Often a girl was seen again during an escort duty to her Training School after she had been there for perhaps six months or a year. The transformation could be striking, even if due only to well-cut hair grown back to its natural colour, or to a complexion cleared by rest and good food, or to improved posture. More striking were any changes due to maturer emotions, and to a growth of confidence in adults. Thus hooded eyes (which to some visitors seemed a prevalent feature of the girls) could open more wide to the world. One girl whose expressed interests at the Classifying School had been boyish in the extreme, with ambitions to be a footballer, naturally looked rounder and softer six months later when she wanted to be a hairdresser. One was continually reminded of the part that environment played in shaping the girls physically as well as emotionally, and if the essential constitution was mainly unalterable, one remained optimistic about modifications. Unless staff had some faith in widespread influence on the whole girl through education (in the broad sense) as well as through maturation, they lost their *raison d'etre* except as observers at the one end of a microscope.

How they saw the girls was reflected in the pen-picture on the first page of each assessment report. Though most of those in the 500 sample were in the words of the present writer, she was indebted to comments and discussions of fellow-staff.

Unlike Lombroso, they found traces of beauty and grace in most of their delinquents. Indeed, as you will see from Table 9, page 60, they regarded 60 per cent of our adolescent girls as normal, or fairly normal looking members of the species. Indeed eighty-six of the 500 sample had qualities of physique which would have drawn notice of an agreeable kind to them in a crowd. An example was A who 'strikes one at once as a sensitive, charming girl. She is of about average height and mature build, with a bearing that suggests both modesty and self-assurance. She has thick, dark hair and a round, plump face, with expressive brown eyes . . . Her manner is courteous and deferential and she can converse at a fairly adult level in her soft, well modulated voice . . .' If there was a halo effect from her looks that made her personality the more attractive, this extended through the impact she made on her Training School, which she left in record time, well trained in domestic and social arts, to make a successful marriage.

They saw, nevertheless, in fully 20 per cent of the main sample, less attractive features, which, while being appreciable factors in the girls' social relationships before committal, did not, they hope, depreciate her at the Classifying or Training Schools. Sometimes, indeed, physical imperfections proved endearing:

> She is of about average height, and is fairly broad in build, but rather angular. There is a good deal of boyishness in her bearing and movements, and in the set of her face. She is jerky in most of her muscular control. While she is now much finer in her facial appearance than on admission, S still has straggling fair hair, growing out as if in tufts at the forehead, a large twitching mouth, and a bony, sallow complexioned face. Her eyes can show an agony of nervousness, or can look gentle.

Away from an impatient father, S, though very dull, became a good worker and a good mixer. Two years after licence she was still in the same job, earning more than some of the Approved School staff who had done so much to boost her morale.

A small percentage—six girls—of the 500 sample had the kind of physique which to Lombroso would have seemed typical of the degenerate criminal:

> M is at present a pathetic and almost grotesque figure. She is small, with a short neck and hunched shoulders. Her fair hair is straight and ragged, and her grey eyes, inside their purplish rings, are those of a deprived, anxious person. She has a smallish face, with large, rather bulbous features, and sallow skin. During her early few days here, when she was unhappy and very homesick, these unprepossessing traits were exaggerated by her pitiful appearance. Since she became animated and learned to identify herself with the community to some extent, she looks like an unselfconscious, pre-adolescent girl, though with a strangely old, shrewd expression at the same time.

This girl's physique (and, presumably, her personal appearance) improved greatly at her Training School.

Finally we have Table 9 giving these groupings, according to a subjective estimate of normality of looks. The estimate depends almost entirely on impressions recorded verbally, but were facilitated by the writer's memory of the girl; for this reason the 100 sample, whom the writer did not know well enough to recall, have been omitted.

Table 9: General Appearance

	Sample 500 %
Unusually good	17·2
Fairly normal	60·2
Less good than normal	20·8
Definitely abnormal in looks	1·2

It needs little imagination to see that a girl who looks miserable and deprived, as well as feeling it, will be shunned by most school-mates, except perhaps by one with a similar problem, or by a pretty girl as a special grand gesture, especially under the eye of a sympathetic and vigilant teacher. If a 'pick-up' on the street, the docks or in the dance hall could give an ounce of self-esteem, adults should understand the reasoning of the adolescent emotions behind the rebellion.

So much for the Classifying School staff's aesthetic reactions to a girl's physique. They also viewed her expressive movements as a key (admittedly not always a good key) to her personality. They noted the smaller and larger movements of her face and body, her walk, her posture—her foot-scraping; her hip-swinging; her arms akimbo; her way of laughing, crying, swearing or flattering. One girl might play many parts on our stage in six or eight weeks, for pretence and imitation were among her best achievements. At her most lonely and homesick moments she might simulate an easily broken defiance; in her most anti-authority phase she might be the politest, but most smarmy girl in the school. At a less conscious level she might one day have the exact walk of a member of the staff, and the next have the exact walk of the most aggressively psychopathic contemporary.

The pen-picture attempted to bring a girl's varying moods and poses into focus, but also to give her prevailing bearing within the community, as a mark, however unreliable, of her inner state. When these are brought together in Table 10, we see surprising correspondence between the two samples observed. Since teenagers as an age-group identify with idols (such as pop singers), we possibly see a new fashion in posture, in the poised/casual groupings, where the 1957 girls tended more to take up a casual stance, than the pseudo-poised 1952 to 1954 sample, while the two groupings add up to consistent 26 to 27 per cent totals. Mainly it would appear that the 14 to 17 year-old Approved School population were, if not a 'type', liable to give outward and deducible signs of being a number of special types, during the challenging time while they were under observation.

Table 10: Bearing

	Sample 500 %	Sample 100 %
Alert	7·8	6·0
Apathetic	9·8	10·0
Belligerent	7·8	6·0
Timid, hesitant, or evasive	6·8	8·0
Ungainly	12·6	11·0
Tense	24·0	28·0
Poised	20·6 ⎫ 26·0	13·0 ⎫ 27·0
Casual	5·4 ⎭	14·0 ⎭
Diffident	5·0	3·0
Over-confident	·2	1·0

These, as we have said, denote the prevailing bearing. If only 39 of the 500 girls had appeared belligerent at any time, we should have had little experience in playing down belligerence; a few girls spring to mind as forever spoiling for a fight, and being at a loss when not countered aggressively. Many, many more were in tearing furies at a word from a disliked contemporary, or perhaps if her work was criticized—but was pleased when helped back to her own normal. Those girls recorded as apathetic or tense were predominantly in this or that state.

Such descriptions of a girl's bearing were most often the key which opened the memory, and brought a girl vividly to life, so that not only her prevailing expressive movements were seen, but every twist of her facial muscles, of her eyes, every gesture almost came back. It is difficult not to believe that their bearing was a true indicator of some inner state.

Coming to more objective measures of a girl's personal appearance, we have on record (apart from colour of eyes and hair) only rough groupings for height and weight. This is unfortunate in view of recent renewed interest in bodily measurements of delinquents as compared with normals.

Lombroso,[2] in pursuing his theories of the 'born criminal', did some studies of criminal women and asserted that they were shorter and heavier than the normal. Burt[4] disclaimed that delinquents conform to a physical type, but found that they frequently departed from the normal in height and weight. Healy[5] found 70 per cent of the female delinquents were above the weight norms for their age, and related this over-development to delinquency, particularly to sex delinquency. Whether in the present Approved School samples the physically over-developed were more sexually delinquent than the under-developed proportionately is something the writer would doubt, and something she cannot prove or disprove from available material. Whether the girls' tendency to be over-weight is even related to over-development sexually would, from the present data and past literature, be harder still to substantiate. Apart from a few cases, staff tended to be unimpressed by comments in a girl's papers that she was 'over-sexed', and thought more in terms of her having been over-stimulated, or of her having used sexual promiscuity as an escape from an unhappy home, and/or for gaining notice and reassurance.

In more recent years attention has been drawn again to the significance of physique in the study of delinquents, and, following on from Sheldon's *Varieties in Human Physique*[6] and *Varieties of Delinquent Youth*[7], the Gluecks have paid considerable attention to this aspect, for instance in *Unravelling Delinquency*[8]. In doing so it is stressed that they are not looking for 'delinquent types', in Lombroso's[2] sense, but, as Dr Gibbens[9] says, physique is:

> relatively fixed, and there is growing evidence of its association with susceptibility to disease, choice of career, various skills and other aspects of personality. One of the main objects of research in delinquency should be to throw light upon the 'susceptibility' which helps to determine who will become delinquent in those sections of the population generally exposed to an unfavourable environment.

The Gluecks found that 'absolutely and relatively the delinquents are mesomorphic in constitution (muscular), containing a much higher proportion of all mesomorphic types than the non-delinquents and a far lower proportion of ectomorphs (linear, thin). Ectomorphs, endomorphs (round, plump) and balanced types are decidedly subordinate among the delinquents'.

The only objective measures preserved in the girls' files were the normal height/weight figures. For a large proportion of the 500 sample even this was not available, the only measurement records having been sent to the Training Schools. But there were elaborate records in the pen-pictures on the girls, an impressionistic picture, based on observing her for at least a month, and a comparison with what was known (partly impressionistically, partly in terms of national averages) of average height, build and proportions of her age group.

At the time the data for this research had been collected and punched on to cards, there was no thought of even vague somato-typing, so it will be interesting to see whether there is a rough and ready comparison between our impressionistic material and the exact anthropometric data elsewhere.

We found for our two major samples the following estimates:

Table 11: Height (related roughly to normal population)

	Sample of 500 %	Sample of 100 %
Average	45·2	53·0
Below average	35·4	32·0
Above average	19·4	15·0

Discrepancies are not surprising, as exact measurements, where available, did not always accord with the more subjective description. Even so, we have asymmetric curves for both groups, with more girls estimated to be below than above average in height.

Weight, related roughly to height, is considered in the table:

Table 12: Weight (related to Height)

	Sample of 500 %	Sample of 100 %
Average	67·4	69·0
Below average	13·0	13·0
Above average	19·6	18·0

The two sets of estimates are, considering the lack of statistical refinement in use, very close indeed.

At first sight it might seem that the findings would be in the direction of those of the Gluecks[8] (as above), and with the recent findings in this country by Gibbens[9] with Borstal boys, and by Epps and Parnell[10] with Borstal girls namely that the delinquent groups were predominantly mesomorphs—shorter and heavier in build than the control groups. This would indeed have been in accord with the writer's memory of the Approved School girls en masse—girls with heavy, muscular legs and large thighs, large bosoms and short thick necks. That this conglomerate image is a doubtful one is suggested in analysis.

Of the 177 girls recorded as below average in height, barely a quarter were also recorded as above average in weight, and of those 226 recorded as of average height, only a fifth were recorded as above weight for their height.

This doubt is borne out further by our recording of build in more generalized, but probably more useful terms. These, again, were recorded without thought of somato-typing.

Table 13: Build

	Sample of 500 %	Sample of 100 %
Sturdy, stocky	30·6 ⎱43·2	32·0 ⎱38·0
Stalwart	12·6 ⎰	6·0 ⎰
Plump, 'tubby'	10·2 ⎱12·0	9·0 ⎱12·0
Obese	1·8 ⎰	3·0 ⎰
Tall and slim	12·4 ⎱18·4	15·0 ⎱20·0
Lanky	6·0 ⎰	5·0 ⎰
Slight	18·2 ⎱26·4	21·0 ⎱30·0
Petite	8·2 ⎰	9·0 ⎰

The possible groupings for endomorphs (nos. 3 and 4) are in exact agreement for the two samples, and are close to the Gluecks' findings in *Unravelling*,[8] but a good deal higher then Gibbens'[9] findings.

The possible groupings for ectomorphs (nos. 5 and 6) are again in close agreement for the two samples, but considerably higher than Gibbens[9] (18·4 per cent as against 12 per cent), and higher than the Gluecks',[8] but less than half their percentage for non-delinquents.

The possible mesomorphs seem to be numbers 1 and 2 (where our two samples show some discrepancy, with percentages of 43 and 38 respectively) and give a much lower percentage than the Gluecks[8] (60·1 per cent), and Gibbens[9] (50 per cent), but higher than the Gluecks' non-delinquents (30·7 per cent).

Nos. 7 and 8 are, with caution, considered mixed groups; it is unlikely they could (if more precisely measured) bring the groupings more into line with Gibbens' findings, but rather reduce the mesomorph percentage.

It is perhaps dangerous to have compared bodily constitution on such flimsy evidence as could be presented, but the findings such as they are, may point the way to further work. Certainly the Classifying School population contained girls who, had facilities been available, would have been treated as maladjusted or as neurotic, rather than within a group which had many who were advanced in delinquency. The writer, with her mental picture of predominant mesomorphy, may—typically—be picturing the more extreme problems, some of whom one might predict as later recidivists. A correlation between build and eventual success in treatment and afterwards may throw some light on this.

Gittins,[11] as already quoted, says of his *Approved School Boys* that variations in physique are as wide as in the population at large, but exaggerated traits are more frequent and abnormalities are more obvious. Our objective and subjective findings on our girls' physique accord with this summarizing; there are more odd builds and odd bearings, and the odd tend to be odder than most; there are more who seemed to be just less than normally good to look at and more who were broader and shorter, but the surprise to the average reader may be that generally there was so much that appeared normal. And certainly they would seem on present crude recordings to be more average in physique than some delinquent groups.

Finally there are appended a few further pen-pictures illustrating the type of observations recorded. And since physique seemed correlated with behaviour in the staff memories of the girls, the pen pictures are recorded with this in mind.

Pen-picture I

L is a small girl, with a look of a hungry, neglected street urchin. Her sandy hair is thin, lank, and rarely tidy. Her narrow face has sagging cheeks, a weak cleft chin and a permanently grimy-looking complexion. The least hardened, and the least malevolent of her features are her childish, light blue eyes.

There are two distinct L's—the good little girl in individual situations, who is earnest in her pledges for the future, and the vicious, aggressive girl, with a gift for vituperation of the most brazen, cold-blooded quality. When in this prevailing frame of mind, she taunts others, eggs on the hysterical girls, hates and destroys a serene atmosphere, and sets out to bait staff. When reported for these misdemeanours, she proclaims her innocence in what might well be judged as a righteously indignant manner.

Pen-picture II

E is short, with a thickened, almost matronly figure, and a noticeable double chin, where her meekly bowed head meets her short neck. She has a rolling gait, with a slight limp. Her plump, pale face, with its childish brown eyes and its frame of frizzled, curled brown hair, has a startled expression.

Sometimes she looks most unsure of herself, as if she feels herself perpetually the tool of fate, and can rebel against her lot in just odd spasms of anti-social conduct, along with blatant rudeness and defiance. After individual bolstering up, especially if her good points have been accentuated, and she has been assured that she *is* likeable, E can look serene and happy for a few days at the time. She then livens up in her whole appearance and manner, and is pleasant and attractive.

Pen-picture III

In appearance and in bearing M is a mixture of china doll and farmer's boy. Her round, rosy face, with its perfect contours and features, her bright, rather glassy eyes, and her mass of curled brown hair, contrast strongly with her stalwart figure, her hulking walk, and her strong, harsh voice.

While being fundamentally polite, and displaying a boyish sense of justice and honour, M's manner with adults soon becomes blustering if she is at all unsure of her place in the community—and her verbal intelligence is dull enough for her to be at a loss quite frequently. With a group of girls she fits in very well on the whole, being sociable and helpful, while her masculine traits give her further popularity. Now and then she become the complete 'only' child of the indulged kind, and is impatient and brusquely critical, in a way that can disturb the peace in an irritating, but never serious way.

Pen-picture IV

M is a little thin, round-shouldered girl, whose whole posture and facial expression suggest nervousness, dull intellect and the possibility of antisocial attitudes. Her face is less sallow and pinched than on admission, but the sharp features are still compressed. She has staring blue eyes, which she focuses just beyond the person who is the centre of her attention, giving little darting, seemingly furtive glances back at this person. Though normally solemn, she tends to grin nervously when there is any trouble within the group. Her conversation is staccato, and her manner is withdrawn and secretive.

Pen-picture V

A's appearance is very typical of a crippled girl who is also maladjusted. She is tall and quite well built, but stoops in an ungainly way, and she limps slightly. One leg is underdeveloped, and therefore much thinner than the other. Facially she could be pleasing enough, but her complexion is sallow and blotchy, her eyelids are puffy, and her fair hair is stringy. She has an indefinite jawline, and the semi-anxious lines generally of a child that is both indulged and deprived; her grey eyes reflect this most of all, for they can be ingratiatingly friendly, or can look most venomous. Her voice alters comparably, from a plausible, oily tone to brusque rudeness.

Pen-picture VI

M is like a very drab and disillusioned Alice in Wonderland. She is of about average height and build, but carries herself rigidly, with a poking head, long, narrow face, and straight fair hair that droops stringily to her shoulders. Her mouth is usually pursed, and her voice is grumpy, but has a brusquely humorous overtone. Her small blue eyes, though at times dull and uncommunicative, can add to the whimsicality of her happier expressions.

M's attitudes within the community here are still very much those of the maladjusted child. In fact much of the account given of her, seven years ago, when attending the Hostel for maladjusted children, still holds: she destroys other people's possessions, loves very messy play (or work) and makes loud noises to see what effect they produce.

Unfortunately she has, during the years, built a barrier between herself and adults, so that, though she still craves for affection, she cannot accept it without being demanding and cantankerous in return, while, if handled in a very objective way, she sinks completely into her phantasy world, and is unlikely to progress.

The writer finds it difficult to summarize the mixture of statistical and subjective estimates on physique, though it would seem that an undue proportion of girls were below average in height (relative to their age group) and above average in weight (related to their height). The picture is fairly consistent in the 500 sample, and in the later 100 sample. On the more generalized 'Personal Appearance' data, we find about 40 per cent of each group are either 'sturdy', 'stocky' or 'tubby', and 12 per cent are stalwart or obese.

A consistent percentage of about 8 were petite (a complimentary term); towards 20 per cent were slight (a neutral term) and 5 or 6 per cent were lanky (non-complimentary).

But the difficulty in observing the girls apart from their social adjustment or maladjustment—large paunches or heavy thighs, for instance, apart from compensatory or self-indulgent eating of starchy foods—makes Table 10 more important than the others to the writer. The girls' *bearing* was the haunting, memory-rousing part of her image, linking her name with the written pen-picture. This is true of the 10 per cent who were apathetic, or the 7 to 8 per cent who were timid, as it is of the mid 50 per cent who held their ground firmly (tense, poised, casual) or aggressively (6 to 8 per cent), or the 12 per cent who were hulking, ungainly, yet often endearing.

B. NOISES AND CRISES

We have considered what the Approved School girls were like to live with. In a closed, all-female community, where staff (including the Headmistress) resided amid the bustle, with only a door between them and the main throng, there were always noises, which, even in retrospect, were obtrusive.

The Girls

'*Impression of Pentonville*' by a prisoner, in the Morrises' sociological study of the prison,[1] rouses uncomfortable thoughts:

> This prison is the constant reminder to us all of prison tension, it also signifies how easy it is for one in a crowd such as we have here to loose [sic] ones sense of reason and permit oneself to be easily swayed by the general feeling of a crowd . . . One notices that about the whole population are exhibitionists, given to emotional [sic] gesticulations, and expressions, sudden bursts of song, its noise always catching the ear . . . It isn't because we are on the hairbreath of insanity, rather one can attribute it to the constant inactivity, and closed confindment [sic] hence an emotional relief by exhibitionism.

How far, indeed were similar outbursts and gestures by our girls due not to their basic maladjustments but to the unnaturally confined life? The word 'inactivity' fits to some extent, for in the free quarters of an hour between classes and meals, meals and classes the air was often rent by raucous laughter, by very loud snatches of 'love songs', by studiedly mocking or just attention-winning remarks, made near enough for the staff on duty to hear. But it was nearly always the few very difficult girls, and perhaps their sycophants, who expressed themselves thus. A fine description by a later colleague of one of the 1957 sample, describes the circumstances leading to this kind of noise, emitted by a motherless, institution-reared girl, who had been very difficult to handle for years, and had staged one of these occasionally publicized roof ascents at a Remand Home before she came to us, and enjoyed the attention of the Fire Brigade and the Press:

> She usually has a loud rallying voice, and she uses it in the presence of adults to draw their attention to her achievements or to pour scorn on their attempts to discipline her. She can, however, speak quietly though her voice still has an insistent note and she is ready to be suspicious of all but the calmest of treatment. She has a sense of humour but it is one-sided, and she is only able to take a joke against herself when she is the narrator, otherwise she is soon hotly offended and on the defensive . . . With her contemporaries she uses her voice to make herself the focus of interest. She indulges in cheerfully regardless behaviour, calculated to evoke their admiration or sympathy by its blatant disregard of authority and the emotional confusion into which she lands herself, and her self-assertiveness turns into uncoordinated physical aggression and hoarse screams. After a bout of this kind, she is quiet, although still 'edgy', and physically exhausted and deflated. She is sorry and distressed at the upheaval she has caused and tries hard to conform and make amends.

Such exhibitionism was not a constant feature. The school was rarely without at least one girl who was capable of putting on such a show, but the general mood of the whole community was very important in controlling her. Skilled staff could forestall many scenes by side-tracking, or by giving enough warmth and reassurance for the scene to be unnecessary. A nucleus of more mature girls could humour the very immature, and also give more sense of security within the group. Withdrawal for individual attention was practised as often as possible. Sometimes all circumstances were in favour of outbursts, especially since, as the Pentonville prisoner quoted said, it was easy to allow the mood of the crowd to sway relatively sound members. And not only were the girls having to tolerate staff (with their peculiarly middle-class whims) but each other. 'It's these girls, miss,' was a frequent complaint.

When a nucleus of hysteria-prone adolescent girls is allowed to gain control, the danger is greater than is generally realized, for an anti-authority feeling (dangerous enough in itself) can turn suddenly to hostility between group members. For this reason it was rarely safe to allow such a situation to resolve itself; the integrated strength of the adult had to be gathered up and placed at their disposal, to help calm and restore, for by this time they were usually—like toddlers in a tantrum—afraid of themselves and asking by their very excesses to be stopped. The trouble-makers could then be seen individually, in as therapeutic a way as a situation permitted.

In a simmering mood the whole group would be silent, but bursts of song would be studiedly rebellious: at the earlier part of the research period it was still the song that many had learnt from 'Yankee' boy-friends: *Gee I want to go home.* Songs of an 'average' mood would be *They try to tell us we're too young,* or *High Noon.* The hoarseness or loudness of the singing were the barometer of danger.

Sometimes for days the mood would be wholly serene and friendly, to a degree as unnatural as the other. Such a phase might pass into spontaneously child-like play, when strains of *Ring-a-ring of roses* would come from the recreation room, and Staff would find, on tip-toeing to the door, all thirty-six teenage girls were playing the party game naturally and joyfully, going on shortly to *The Farmer's in his Den.* Happy were the new girls admitted at such times—if they could bear to be happy!

From most of what has been said it might seem that free expression was allowed to individual and group emotions. If Staff gauged these as 'safe' *and* therapeutic, they indeed did so. Mainly they tried to prevent trouble, by conveying as far as they had it within themselves, that they were people of endless resources, endless patience, endless tact, and that it was useless to try to rouse them. If the situation became extreme with a rebel, the shock of being 'shouted down' by a lady who had never before raised her voice in the girl's hearing worked instantly. The preferred way of gaining group attention was by excessive stillness of the waiting adult—not aggressive, but truly peace-making silence. This was not fool-proof, but at least it was worth the occasional failure, to avoid the competitiveness of a sergeant-major régime. 'I thought they were soft here till something happened that made me change my mind', was what a very disturbed pre-psychotic girl wrote to her foster-mother after a few days of testing the Staff out. Her weapon had been, not noise, but mute resistance. The strain of negative silence by individuals could be almost as great as excessive noises.

When the massed chorus in 'free' recreation time had too high a component of hysteria, the member of staff on corridor duty wandered or strode (according to her method or to the challenge) into the large room (the ex-billiard room). There was a reasonable chance that the hysterical note dropped to a bantering one, or with perhaps one defiant singer or banterer still holding forth. If several continued at a clearly dangerous pitch, the wise staff member would find a pretext for lingering, and perhaps charming some of the still cooperative but 'shaky' members into a circle, which could gradually lure the seriously wayward as well. It was rarely wise to be attentive to the trouble-maker at that point, but later to find a tactful reason for giving her the notice she craved. If the mood had reached a point where the staff on duty would only aggravate it by her near presence (or if she were insensitive to the mood), the Headmistress or her Deputy might require to make her presence felt, and a calm, firm entry with a firm waiting stance, without singling out individuals, and usually without speaking a word, generally brought even a temporary lull. If little change followed such tactics, and if devices for side-tracking the rebels and surreptitiously dividing the harder cliques, did not work then trouble could indeed be ahead. Only very rarely did such trouble reach riotous proportions. That the writer, with eight years of experience, was never in the building when this terrifying situation arose, gives some idea of the small incidence. The situation did, however, arise, with a smallish section of the mobile group, three times during those eight years, but was observed by the writer only on the last occasion, when she was a part-time visiting psychologist. There was always the inflammatory material there, and always the danger of someone helping the flames to go up (metaphorically). Above all, the important thing then was not to lose one's nerve, and indeed to keep exceptionally cheerful and affectionate with the frightened, non-involved girls, whilst being as wise and strong as an angel but wily as a devil with the dangerous section. Not surprisingly Staff were afterwards near breaking point.

With Staff as with girls it is not easy to generalize. There were always one or two who did not approve of the philosophy and tactics upheld in this and other sections, but fortunately no one in the research period undermined them. Most were subject to normal swings of moods; this seemed to be not very important as far as the girls were concerned. One was sometimes bestowed a pitying look if one lapsed from good humour—but not always!

C. THE GIRLS' HEALTH

On each girl the School Nurse wrote a few lines for the classifying report, apart from entries on the girl's official Medical Card which went with her to the Training School. From the 'Physique and Health' paragraphs, modified sometimes by notes elsewhere about excessive fatigue or low spirits, we have a record of the general health of the population.

Roughly 30 per cent were in good health; 60 per cent were in fairly good health; 6 per cent were in poor health.

The large proportion of girls described as in fairly good health (and some of those in good health) made as great demands on the Nurse's time as did those who were in poor health. The regular surgery half-hour twice a day saw a steady flow of girls clamouring for notice; some were having tonics, or vitamin treatment, prescribed by the School Medical Officer, who visited once a week and saw each new girl, each girl ready to leave, and any requiring doctor's attention otherwise. Constipation, gingivitis, blepharitis, wax in ears, headaches appeared with particular frequency in the notes. Menstruation periods had to be noted (especially where pregnancy could have occurred) and any irregularities of menstruation. In the 1957 group there was a recurrent mention of systolic heart murmur (about 10 per cent), though this was infrequently noted for the 500 sample. Serious eye-sight difficulties were attended to while at the Classifying School, but more time by far was spent on trying to trace existent spectacles left at home or elsewhere. And keeping track of glasses within the Classifying School was a nightmare; Gittins[1] (*Approved School Boys*) mentions, too, his boys' gift for damaging or losing spectacles.

Most girls had been 'cleaned up' at the Remand Homes, but even so there were records of scabies, impetigo, head and pubic lice—the last mainly after absconding.

It was tempting to head this section 'Smells of the School'. One of the crosses Staff bore less stoically were odours—not only those stemming from female perspiration and menstruation, which responded indifferently to two baths a week plus slap-dash washing twice a day, but also odours from venereal infections. 23 per cent (115 girls) from the 500 sample, and 27 per cent of the later 100 sample had either gonorrhoea, syphilis, or trichomonas vaginalis on admission, or following on absconding from the Classifying School, and many of the forty-three girls with gonorrhoea in the 500 sample also had trichomonas vaginalis. About 1 per cent had syphilis. Staff all developed noses for the different diseases, and sometimes an undetected sufferer was tracked in this way by lay members. The irritant and the anxiety for the inflicted girls (and for their companions) must have added considerably to other causes of tension. Considerable administrative difficulties arose from this problem, even though the Staff were, if anything, too unconcerned about chances of infection; sleeping, laundry and bathing arrangements were seldom altered except for serious cases. There was no visiting venereologist, and so the Nurse (or other available staff when she was on leave) escorted four or five suspects or treatment cases together, with a bus-change, to the nearest General Hospital once a week. As persistent absconders were also the regular sufferers, this duty was no sinecure. After many successful attempts to elude the escort during the journey or from the hospital waiting-room, the privilege of using a taxi for the purpose was obtained. It remained an unpleasant duty, for restlessness, as well as natural fear of pain were aroused in the girls. Some of the most naive were hardly aware of the implications; there were few who were unperturbed, however brazen they appeared to the outsider.

Another odorous problem was enuresis, but this was not a grave difficulty, or rather was not allowed to be an issue, and perhaps for that reason (or just because a girl's nervous system was maturing) some with a persistent history were rarely wet.

For the later 1957 sample some figures were available; about $12\frac{1}{2}$ per cent had a history of enuresis (presumably until they left home, but this is not clear); about 5 per cent wet the bed on two or three occasions at the Classifying School; 1·2 per cent were frequently enuretic, and a further 1·2 per cent were chronic bed-wetters. One girl of the earlier sample—a highly intelligent girl—suffered throughout her Approved School training, an Art School education, and subsequent career, and recovered on marriage. There was an occasional diurnal enuretic, particularly one who came three times for Classification, and whose frequent trips around the building for incontinence were sometimes confused with her trips around to find ways of absconding for excessive sexual indulgence. Far from being the notorious tortured enuretic of institutions, M was totally without shame, whether for her sexual promiscuity, her lack of truth or her wet pants. She could be the sweetest singing Herald Angel on Christmas Day, and at night be off to seek excitement at the lowest level.

Girls were expected to be cleared for pregnancy before admission but every now and then one slipped through the net, or one became pregnant as a result of absconding from the Classifying School. From both eventualities the incidence was only two or three pregnant girls in a year, though it was usual for each to remain at least three or four months before going to a Mother and Baby Home. Their reactions to the condition varied from sublime contentment to acute resentment. One hoped cheerfully that it would 'be a gril, but if not a gril I hope it will be a boy' [sic]—and went on playing outdoor games, and doing handstands in the recreation room. Another made a serene Mary in the annual Nativity Play.

Roughly 1 per cent had a history of epilepsy. The writer never witnessed a *grand mal* epileptic fit. Our studied calm probably helped, though it must be admitted that the girls who had been diagnosed as epileptic were given the prescribed sedative. On the other hand, our very scepticism about genuine epilepsy versus hysteria doubtless caused us to overlook symptoms and to lose interesting data. A very aggressive girl, with a strong incidence of family epilepsy, and an abnormal E.E.G. recording (an 'unstable cortex, potentially epileptic') waited until she reached her Training School to revive her hallucinatory episodes which had been a feature before committal. She had a ghost called Hilda, and was unwittingly sent to St Hilda's School. The Headmistress there succeeded in laying the ghost without hurting its victim.

The fact that Staff so rarely witnessed epileptic fits does not, of course, mean that they escaped the swings of mood and sometimes violent tempers associated with the condition in some.

A further 3 to 4 per cent of each sample were recorded as having had 'fits', 'blackouts', or 'turns', and here Staff tactics seemed to win the day. These girls were some of the best tantrum-throwers, but with care it ended there. 'Fainting', too, could win sympathy when ostentatious misconduct had lost its group appeal. Such simulation, as with lying and prevarication or any other kind of insidious pretence, angered the group, and the uncovering of it was a cruel thing at the time, but ultimately cathartic. A dull exhibitionist who had turned to fainting whenever the group was quietly gathered, was finally told by the supervising staff at meal-time to 'get up'. She did so, in fury, and pulled the cloth and seven plates of soup to the floor. Her contemporaries agreed finally to forgive her—when she had apologized—and the air was much clearer.

Apart from the necessity of professional nursing assistance for minor and major ills, the resort the girls had to the surgery for attention filled a much needed emotional want. Few had had enough consistent sympathy, and some weeks of indulgence often paid dividends. Gittins found the majority of his Approved School boys remarkably hardy, and impervious to physical stresses and irritations. The girls might withstand great duress in midnight absconsions, lightly clad, but expected full sympathy for broken or cut limbs or scratches sustained in the process, and also expected endless sympathy for other bruises and aches. The exception was self-inflicted wounds, such as tattooing of boy-friends' initials with needle and ink, which rarely suppurated and were stoically, indeed proudly, borne. Sympathy was sought rather by her withdrawn attitude as she pricked her hand or arm.

Some insistent demands for nursing care had to be exploded, for the reasons given in discussing simulations, but with care relative to the outcome and the complainant. One outbreak of enteritis sent a stream of girls to bed initially, but treatment all round with rest and drinks of water brought the lead-swingers downstairs within a day for their regular meals. The more seriously neurotic girl's health wants were met with what was felt was a necessary degree of sympathy and treatment.

Nail-biting

The Gluecks,[2] in *Unravelling Delinquency* (p. 129), found a higher percentage of *extreme* nail-biters among their delinquents than among their non-delinquents—21·4 per cent against 15·6 per cent; the difference was barely statistically significant.

Bitten nails, or actual nail-biting was easily observed during the Alexander's Passalong Performance test (see Chapter on Testing), and was recorded consistently during the year 1954, when 140 girls were tested. Only 36·4 per cent of these were *not* observed as having 'badly bitten' or 'very badly bitten' nails. A total of 63·6 per cent were recorded as 'bad' nail-biters, or just as nail-biters. To balance one who said she had bitten her nails only since admission to the Classifying School, another said she bit them *until* she came to the Classifying School.

A more helpful comparison with our girls is a normal sample of 4000 children aged 5 to 16 in schools in South Yorkshire studied by Birch (1955).[3]

By working on Mr Birch's figures for our three age-groups (14, 15 and 16) we find the following comparison:

	C.S.	Mr Birch's Sample	
	Girls 14, 15, 16	Girls 14, 15, 16	Boys 14, 15, 16
	%	%	%
Bitten nails	64	39	53
Not bitten	36	61	47

Though there was found to be a fall-off in nail-biting after the age of 14, at *no* age was the percentage of biters in his sample as high as for the Classifying School. Among boys there was a greater frequency, and at the peak age of 12 the incidence was 62 per cent, still rather less than for our sample.

Professor Valentine,[4] in *The Normal Child*, quotes findings from 15-year-olds in representative High Schools in America, where one third still bit their nails, and a further one third had been 'biters'. We do not have figures for our sample of past 'biters' but, in view of our abnormal sample and our undoubtedly significant differences from the Yorkshire sample, I should question Professor Valentine's playing down of the symptom. At the least it was another example of our C.S. population behaving immaturely or regressively—perhaps because of their anxieties at that time, but even this could be questioned.

A child Psychiatrist, the late Dr Muriel Barton Hall,[5] quoted too by Mr Birch, wrote that the majority of cases of nail-biting 'is an habitual reaction and is otherwise of no particular significance, except perhaps for the fact that children with this habit are often of over-active, energetic, restless nature'. Her observations of many Approved School girls could well have amplified her views about the restless and over-active. She did not have the Shaw nail-biting figures above, or I think she might well have endorsed the comment on immaturity or regressiveness.

Left-Handedness

The manipulations during the Alexander's Passalong Test (see Chapter on Testing) was a convenient, if not scientifically regulated, opportunity for observing right/left-handed movements, the total observation lasting 5 to 10 minutes. The predominantly right-handed girl used the left only for holding the box of blocks, or to help the right hand; at the extreme of right-handedness (or indolence!) she might use the left to prop her head. The converse was true for the left-handed girl. Some used both hands equally for manoeuvring the blocks into place, with greater, less or equal ease when she alternated. These observations were followed up by noticing, or questioning the hand used in writing, and 4 per cent of those recorded were (by these reports) naturally left-handed subjects who had been trained to use their right in the schoolroom.

Referring to the same sample as for nail-biting—the 140 girls tested in 1954 and consistently recorded—we find that 8·3 per cent were recorded as being predominantly left-handed, 76 per cent were recorded as being predominantly right-handed, and the remaining 16·5 per cent seemed to switch hands naturally and with facility. One hesitates to call this last group ambidextrous on such doubtful evidence.

Keeping our estimate of 8·3 per cent in the Shaw group as left-handed, we can make the following comparison with different authors so as to bring possible sex differences into focus:

Table 14: Left-Handedness

Authors	Population Tested	Percentage of left-handed	
		Men	Women
Richardson (Shaw samples)	140 adolescent delinquent girls	—	8·3
Gluecks[2] (*Unravelling Delinquency*)	500 delinquent boys	12	—
	Non-delinquent sample	10	—
Ogle[6] (1871)	8,264 students	8·56	7·17
Clark[7] (1957)	1,273 students	8	5·9

The last two groups (Ogle and Clark) are quoted by Henry Hécaen and Julian de Ajuriaguerra[8] among other very diverse results; they are selected here because of comparable age-groups. Several writers believe that left-handedness is more frequent in males. Again Ballard[9] is quoted by Hécaen (above) as finding, among 10,000 children tested, 4·1 per cent left-handed in a group aged 4 to 14, as against only 2·7 per cent in a group 8 to 14 years of age.

Briefly, this résumé suggests that the Shaw incidence of left-handedness may (a) fit in with the Gluecks' findings that their delinquent sample had slightly more left-handed boys than had the normals, for the Shaw sample tends to have more than the women students; (b) fit in with the findings of Ballard and others that the incidence decreases with age—for the Gluecks' sample was younger than the Shaw sample; (c) fit in with the findings that left-handedness is more frequent in males (cf. with Gluecks' sample of boys).

Any effort at more precise statistical comparison would be unwise at present, for the methods of establishing figures on the subject previously are varied, and none is comparable with the method used for this *small* Shaw sample. Apart from this, there is the doubt whether the 16·5 per cent (above) were indeed ambidextrous, but may rather have concealed a further percentage of predominantly left-handed girls.

As the incidence of left-handedness, linked with reading retardation, has been noted in past studies, to be lower for girls than for boys, and as the incidence in this group is lower than for the Gluecks' delinquent sample and for their non-delinquent sample let us examine the present left-handed group in relation to scholastic retardation. In the small group of eleven left-handed girls in the sub-group of 140, there was no significant relationship with reading retardation; of the total of thirty-six less consistently recorded as left-handed in the 500 sample, six had reading ages below nine—a disproportionately high proportion, but these were also girls of Binet I.Q.'s 82 downwards to 52, so the relation might be to low intellect; the sample is too small for further research.

Four of the twenty-two apparently ambidextrous girls in the sub-group of 140 (again a disproportionately high percentage) had reading ages below nine years, one being totally illiterate, but all of these had I.Q.'s of 75 or less. While there may have been individual difficulties through undefined laterality in the learning processes, especially as they were also very dull, the fact that the remaining eighteen of these twenty-two had reading ages of eleven and upwards would not supply us with more wholesale evidence.

In general, the health picture has been found to be linked with instability and immaturity, and treatment for the treatable conditions was coloured by the perpetual clamour of the healthy as well as the unhealthy for physical attention. The deviance in nail-biting may be largely part of the same under-development of the sample, along with a considerable incidence of social maladjustment.

The deviance in left-handedness, while possibly not accurate, seems to lie in the same direction from the normal as the findings of Kellmer Pringle,[10] who says: 'At present we can only speculate whether, among the environmental stresses to which left-handed maladjusted children are subjected, are disapproval of their left-handedness and pressure to change their dominant hand.' This may have been yet another harsh stroke in this vulnerable population of older girls in the Classifying Approved School.

Chapter Nine

ADMISSIONS TO THE CLASSIFYING SCHOOL

AGE ON ADMISSION

The Shaw Classifying School catered, as we have seen, for girls aged 14, 15 and 16, plus a few who had attained the age of 17 while in a Remand Home awaiting a place, and another small group (not included in the main calculations in this research) who were under 14, and admitted by special permission of the Secretary of State. As we see from the table of age distribution of the 500 sample, almost a quarter were committed between reaching 16 years 6 months and attaining the age of 17.

Table 15: Age on Committal to Approved School

	Sample of 500 %
14 to 14 years 11 months	25·4
15 to 15 years 11 months	32·4
16 to 16 years 5 months	18·2 ⎫ 42·2
16 years 6 months to 16 years 11 months	24 ⎰

Combining 3 and 4 we find a total of 42 per cent committed at 16. This was consistently the peak age for Committals to the Classifying Schools for girls (whilst boys[1] between 1950 and 1953 attained the peak totals between ages 13 to 15, but in 1954 more than equalized at age 15 to 17). But for girls, the second half of the year, when the agencies responsible found there was 'just time', saw the highest proportion committed. The wisdom of this will be discussed.

Certain subjective impressions were formed over the years; some of these can be checked later by comparing findings from this research. First, briefly, the impressions can be stated as follows.

The 16-year-old girls were, by and large, more adult in their interests, with a deal of worldly knowledge and pseudo-sophistication. They seemed, however, especially those over 16½, to be the most

78

deeply resentful towards their parents, or authority, for their Approved School committal, and therefore to be the most evasive, defensive, and the most given to absconding. They (especially the older sixteens) were most often the girls who had been subjected to a variety of interim remedial measures, such as residence in Hostels or Homes, or Committal to Care. They were most likely to have been previously in Junior Approved Schools. Their knowledge of how to evade discipline had been sharpened, as well as their sense of failure.

The 14-year-old girls tended to lightning changes of moods and interests, and a girl who was very difficult one day might be all sweetness the next. They, in their changeableness, welcomed the repeated environmental changes—Remand Home, Classifying School, Training School. They were not, as an age group, the hardened delinquents, or the likely source of persistent troublemaking. The less mature 14-year-olds were the babies, whom the staff saw to need guarding from indulgence by older girls, but not by them.

The 15-year-olds were just a middle group, usually nearer to the 16's in their interests, and less volatile than the 14's. As a group, they were theorized about less.

We may well find our impressions invalid when we check them statistically at the end of this chapter.

THE GIRL'S ARRIVAL

Each week, on average, during the main period of this research, 3·5 delinquent girls were brought from all over the country to the Classifying School individually (or at most two together) by a Probation Officer, a Child Care Officer, or by two Police Officers. Five admissions in a week were quite common. Documentation and domestic preparations for these, as well as for the transfer of about the same number per week to Training Schools, had to be fitted in with organization for giving stability to the institution.

Officers bringing girls usually prepared them well, and it was also important that the greeting at the Classifying School (usually by the Head or her Deputy) should be friendly and tactful, for most arrived apprehensive. There were occasions when the existent group mood was not a reassuring one for the newcomer, but generally a nucleus of reliable girls could be around to help with the ritual bathing, re-clothing, feeding and introduction to the group.

Sometimes for various reasons a girl came in a stormy or sullen mood, and viewed each member of staff with suspicion.

Mrs Anneliese Walker, in an article 'Special Problems of

Delinquent and Maladjusted Girls', in the October 1961 *Approved Schools Gazette*, writes:

> One has to face the fact that once a girl has entered a juvenile court she is introduced to the world of delinquency. From that moment onward what matters to the girl most is to be acceptable to her new group. . . . Once in this group the girl will expect most of her satisfactions to come through this and the adult world has become virtually hostile, though the girl may have to comply with it ostensibly.

This unhappy vision can become reality, but it is an unhappy reality, for it means that the Approved School staff are not working. Approved School girls do not fall easily into group discipline. Loyalty to the gang is tenuous. All but the very few would rather have the attention (even anger) of 'Miss' for five minutes than her 'mates' company for five hours. They do not easily accept another girl's opinion of the staff, but must each harrass her, prod her verbally, with veiled looks, with feelers out for some sign of acceptance. The group must not be allowed to become indifferent to staff. The individual must be drawn out, disarmed, her better self wooed, her more constructive interests brought into the open.

This was not helped by the practice at the Shaw Classifying School of clothing the girls impersonally in navy school uniforms, but the practice began at a time when many were admitted with poor clothing, and unfortunately the practice lingered. Some discipline in clothing was probably necessary at a stage when many of the girls needed to revert in outward practice to match their emotional and social age, but by 1954 the practice, at least as far as older girls was concerned, was questionable.

REASONS FOR ADMISSION

Once the Classifying School had obtained the records presented to the Court (and these generally were handed over by the escort who brought the girl though we tried to have some prior information) one was sure of having a record of previous Court appearances, and in so far as the inquiry had been adequate, a fairly clear record of a girl's earlier delinquencies. As the object was to prove the girl's need for correction or treatment, her Court record could, in this respect, be assumed to be well presented. Failing parental cooperation, there was information from school and from the Police.

What constituted a previous delinquency was another matter, but no more questionable than what constituted a delinquency during the Court procedure itself. Thus, for example, if staying out late in doubtful company, thus clearly being in moral danger, was sufficient for committal to Approved School, then it constituted earlier delinquency, when the possible consequences were similar.

Table 16, giving the circumstances which may lead to a boy or girl being committed to an Approved School (*Report of the Committee on Children and Young Persons*,[2] Oct. 1960) also gives the percentage of our 500 sample who were committed for each of the reasons:

Table 16: Circumstances of Committal

	Sample of 500 % committed
Found guilty of an offence punishable in the case of an adult with imprisonment	24·2
Found in need of care and protection	36·4
Victim of certain offences	0
Beyond control of parents	5·6
Refractory while in care of Local Authority	5·2
Brought before Court by Probation Officer while under supervision	26·6
Approved School Order substituted for Fit Person Order	1·2
Absconder from the care of a fit person	·2
Truancy from School	·6

About 95 per cent of the boys sent to Approved Schools are committed as offenders. Of the girls about 36 per cent are committed as offenders. These are Home Office figures and are quoted in the *Ingleby Report* (1960).[2]

At first sight it is difficult to agree with this from our findings, as only 24 per cent were committed for an offence 'punishable in the case of an adult with imprisonment'.

But section (6) contains one group of offenders, those who have been on probation for an earlier offence, and have been brought back to Court for breach of terms of the probation order; section (6), however, also contains non-offenders who have been placed under supervision and have been brought back 'in his/her own interests', not necessarily through the child's defaulting.

Also we have girls who, though not offenders on this final Court appearance, have been before the Court for previous offences 'punishable in the case of an adult with imprisonment'.

Table 17 gives us the reasons for previous Court appearances; as it was only rare for a girl to appear for more than two reasons, it was not thought necessary to give a table of reasons for yet previous appearances. (A court appearance here does not include interim returns from remand, but the appearance for which she was initially summoned. Numerical appearances in the Court room would often be many, with—sometimes—repeated remands in custody for further inquiries.)

Table 17: Reason for Previous Court Appearances

	Sample of 500 % Committed
Found guilty of an offence punishable in the case of an adult with imprisonment	28
Found in need of care and protection	20·2
Victim of certain offences	·2
Beyond control of parents	10·2
Refractory while in care of Local Authority	·2
Brought before Court by Probation Officer while under supervision	·2
Approved School Order substituted for Fit Person Order	0
Absconder from the care of a fit person	·2
Truancy from school	4·8
No previous Court Appearances	36

The first thing to notice is that a few on this earlier occasion were already under supervision or in care (0·6 per cent).

The second important point about this table is the last entry—that 180, or 36 per cent of these 500 girls committed to Approved School had had *no earlier Court Appearance*. Of these:

23 girls were committed for an offence (mainly larceny or breaking and entering).
130 girls were committed as being in need of care or protection.
20 girls were committed for being beyond parental control.
6 girls were committed for being beyond the control of the Local Authority (who had assumed parental roles).
1 girl was committed for truancy.

The figures for boys' committals would tend to differ in this respect, with fewer committed to Approved School on a first appearance, mainly because the largest proportion of these 180 girls were non-offenders. Why this should be so may be clearer when we have examined conjointly the figures for the later 100 sample, where nine fewer had had no previous Court appearance. In the years 1952–4, if a girl was seriously in moral danger in her home area, no probation officer in the world could keep her from undesirable friends, and suitable vacancies in hostels were hard to obtain. The alternative of taking into the Local Authority's care was used more by 1957, though often with the result of just delaying Approved School committal.

We shall now return to examining the number of offenders, who had committed usually one of the first of two of the following list: (1) Larceny or receiving. (2) Breaking and entering. (3) Violence against the person. (4) Sexual offences. (5) Malicious damage or arson. (6) Other offences.

When the later and earlier reasons for Court appearances were collated, the percentage of offenders was 38·6, i.e. about 5 points *higher* than the figures given in the *Ingleby Report*[2] (see further below), and higher than the figures for the offenders finally committed to Approved School. The following shows how the number of offenders was made up:

(1) *Those Committed to Approved School for Offences*

23 girls were committed on a first Court Appearance.

69 girls were committed who had previously appeared for an offence.

13 girls were committed who had previously appeared as in need of care or protection.

1 girl was committed who had previously appeared as the 'victim of a certain offence'.

9 girls were committed who had previously appeared as being beyond parental control.

6 girls were committed who had previously appeared for truancy from school.

(2) *Those Committed for other Reasons, but with a Previous Appearance (or Appearances) for an Offence*

31 earlier offenders were committed as in need of care or protection.

3 earlier offenders were committed as being beyond parental control.

4 earlier offenders were committed as refractory while in the care of the Local Authority.

34 offenders were placed on probation, and brought back to Court by the Probation Officer.

Total: 193 or 38·6 per cent.

Nor do these represent the total offenders among the girls, except in the legal sense, for quite frequently a girl was known, without doubt, to have stolen while also beyond parental control or in need of care or protection, but—often out of thought for her future record—was committed only on one of the latter charges.

In their 'Evidence for presentation to the Ingleby Committee', the Association of Headmasters, Headmistresses and Matrons of Approved Schools write (par. II) 'A more serious problem is presented by girls, often committed at a very late date as "In need of Care and Protection". In our view this term is wrongly used as they are not usually innocent victims of circumstance, but girls of shallow personality to whom promiscuous living appears attractive. They are often completely anti-social, absconding, refusing training and committing further offences.'

The present writer would wish to clarify the words 'not usually innocent victims of circumstances'. In a sense most of them were innocent victims of their childhood circumstances; she agrees they were not often innocent victims in the moral circumstances which brought them before the Court—a fact which made nonsense of the committal of men and youths for indecent assault against some of our girls technically 'below the age of consent', viz., 16.

Thus we see that not only might an apparent non-offender be a previous offender, but that many of the others, before the Court only on such accounts as 'moral danger' or truancy from school, had been or were petty thieves. We shall see from later figures on misbehaviour and symptoms of emotional disturbance after twelve years, that a total of 43 per cent of the girls were known to have been stealing; 16 per cent were known to have been stealing before twelve years.

The Ingleby Report[2] indeed enlarges on its previous quotation that 64 per cent of the girls received into Approved Schools are committed as non-offenders (Par. 445): 'Almost all adolescent girls sent to approved schools (whether as offenders or not) have a history of sexual immorality, and many of those sent as being in need of care or protection or beyond control are known to have committed offences.' Before the industrial schools for neglected children under 14, and the reformatory schools for convicted children between 12 and 16 were abolished, and the Approved School system was instituted, the distinction between the offender and non-offender was accepted, at least in principle. To those dealing with the two groups the criterion is need for removal from home and fairly prolonged training in new surroundings.

Indeed it was often agreed at the Classifying School that a few offenders, whose stealing resulted from neurotic conflicts, were the easiest people to live with under controlled conditions. As one of the Instructresses said of an unhappy child who was for weeks totally cooperative and very helpful indeed, 'What a good thing for us that

. . . was committed for stealing a halfpenny'. There were always a few girls who had had, and still had, little interest in promiscuity, and some promiscuous girls who were honest with property.

Contamination was one of staff's lesser anxieties; if a younger girl without previous sex experience was drawn into absconding with an older group, it was unlikely to be by their persuasion, but more by reason of her unhappiness. The calamity if she thus had premature sexual experience, especially of a distressing kind, could have occurred if wandering from home, or if absconding from any other Institution. Again and again their histories showed their proneness to such hazards. The pathos lay most in the fact that this child was so basically unhappy, lonely, disturbed, forming such tenuous relationships, that removal from home had become necessary. The same goes for the more usually vocalized dread of contamination by the thieves among us, of the girl who has been committed as in need of care or protection.

In one such case, a girl committed for truancy (more correctly, school phobia), within the time of this research, aroused protests in Parliament and in the Press. Indeed she was a very nice adolescent, but much in need of training and strengthening—and more seriously (and obstinately) in moral danger before committal than was recognized or admitted in the public agitation. Suffice it to say that she appeared from the latest reports available (at 21) to be quite happily adjusted to a far from easy life, and that during her Approved School training she was drawn into no serious misconduct.

Equally the younger children were safer from contamination from the older than might have been believed, except when an older girl was particularly unedifying and unscrupulous. Some younger children of 14 hung on the fringes of unsavoury cliques—and probably understood only what they already knew. Others in the meantime joined one or two of their age in childish interests and romped along corridors or played tag. Often the older girls, helped by a small maturer bodyguard, were actively protective of the morals of the 'babies'.

This large section of moral danger or beyond control cases will cease to be chargeable as such after 17. Thus when Barbara Wootton[3] says there is no proof that the most serious female delinquents have begun their careers in childhood or early youth, one checks this statement on the population studied by looking at the failures (most of whom will have reappeared in Court cases after Approved School) and seeing whether they were early delinquents (see Table 62). The answer is no.

85

AGE AND LENGTH OF DELINQUENCY

We shall now examine the observation mentioned above, that in the Classifying School more 16-year-olds seemed to be more delinquent, and to have become hardened and evasive during previous attempts to treat them. The quotation above from the evidence to the Ingleby Committee[2] also mentions girls 'often committed at a very late date' (Par. 445).

Table 18: Age related to Number of Previous Court Appearances
(% Age Groups)

	Age				
	14	*15*	*16 to 16·5*	*16·6 to 16·11*	*All 16's*
No previous Court appearance	35	37	39	32	35
One previous Court appearance	38	34	34	33	33
Two previous Court appearances	19	18	16	25	21
Three or more previous Court appearances	8	11	11	10	11

We see there has been more tendency to delay committal with these older girls; of the older 16-year-old, 25 per cent had two previous Court appearances, and 35 per cent had two, three or more previous Court appearances, whereas only 27 per cent of the 14's had been allowed more than one 'chance'. But the differences are not significant, and we see that the percentage with no previous Court appearances is almost equal at all ages, with the younger 16's tending to be committed the most peremptorily.

Studying this from a different direction, in terms of the age at her first Court appearance, we find that:

79 per cent of the 14-year-olds appeared first at 14 or 13
77 per cent of the 15-year-olds appeared first at 15 or 14
72 per cent of the 16-year-olds appeared first at 16 or 15

And that of the remainder:

19 per cent of the 16-year-olds first appeared more than two years before committal to Approval School, against 15 per cent of the 14's and 14 per cent of the 15's. Statistically speaking those with early Court appearances were committed at an earlier age ($p > ·001$).

Perhaps the difference lay more in the agencies dealing with the child—in the Probation Officers and Juvenile Court Magistrates for instance, than in the child's persistent, or early criminality, and whether an Approved School Order was made earlier or later in her career.

Let us examine the 'criminality' of a few of the girls with the greatest number of previous Court appearances (4 or 5).

Case A

(1) At 12 A (whose mother was dead and father idle) was taken to Court by the N.S.P.C.C. as in need of care or protection, and removed to a place of safety. She returned home after 6 months.

(2) At 16 she was charged with stealing soap (which she probably needed very badly) from her employer and placed on Probation.

(3) At 16½ she was not reporting regularly and was generally awkward, so was brought to Court on a Breach of Probation Charge. The Order was extended, with a condition of hostel residence.

(4) Soon after, as she was generally uncooperative, the Probation Order was extended and the place of residence changed to another hostel.

(5) A further breach of the same kind led to a further extension and another change of hostel residence.

(6) Further awkwardness, brought to Court, and at 16 years 11 months she was committed to Approved School, and admitted to a Remand Home to await a vacancy. A created such a scene there that she spent a night in a police cell before admission to the Classifying School. She was so cooperative and happy, and so afraid of further changes that she was retained (by special permission) for over a year, for Training, and subsequently did quite well.

Case B

(1 and 2) The early Court appearances were mentioned but no details given.

(3) At 15 B, whose violent father had left the family, stole tulips from the Park. She was placed on probation. During this period the mother was evicted and B went to a friend's to sleep. The mother provided her blankets, but reclaimed them later, so B had to go voluntarily to a hostel.

(4) She was in Court for stealing a powder compact. Probation to continue, with residence at a hostel. B soon absconded and

(5) after larceny was again before Court, but was conditionally discharged and returned to the hostel.

(6) She absconded again and, still barely 16, was committed to

Approved School. At first she was cooperative, but absconded later from her Training School, broke and entered and stole, and was committed to Borstal.

Case C

C's delinquencies are nearer to the expectations of an early criminal career.

(1 and 2) At 13 she had two separate appearances, for housebreaking, and for breaking and entering and stealing. The first time she was conditionally discharged, the second time placed on probation.

(3) She was brought for breach of probation; Court decision not given.

(4) She was brought to Court for truanting from school and running from home and pawning goods.

(5) Still only 15 she ran away with a boy-friend, stayed at a hotel, and in an argument with the proprietor hit her on the head with a vase. Committed to an Approved School. Did well. Employed first as a clerk, then as a nurse.

Case D's delinquent career is best described by herself, though the several previous Court Appearances are not detailed:

My life story is not very interesting but up to now I have remembered bits about my life. When I was at school I used to be bad at doing lessons, and I used to stay away from school when we were having games. I used to get bad reports and my father use to ask my mother why I had not been to school, she used to say she know nothing about it, and I used to get hit at times, this was when I was twelve years old. My brother X and my brother Y, also my sister Z, had been away for getting into serious trouble but my mother said that if I did as I was told she would give me money and she used to leave me in on a nightime while she went drinking with my father and friends with my two brothers and my sister who are a lot younger than me, I got into the habit of staying in so much that I used to go out and leave home and I used to go down to my Aunty—I used to tell her what my parents were doing and she used to go and fetch my smallest brother down to their house and look after him my mother did not bother about this because she did not look after us as it was, and so we were all chucked onto my Aunty—.

But once we had to get out of the house because my mother used to tell my father that I had given the rent man it and I used to have to tell lies to save her from getting into a row.

I thought my mother was the only thing that mattered and I used to tell myself that I would do any thing on the earth for her. But I soon changed my mind for when I was sent away she promised me she would write and send me things also that she would come to see me, this was

before I went away to the Remand home at —— She went to see my
sister because she had come out of that school at —— ——, and now
she was getting married she sent our —— to the Remand home to me
to ask if she could have my costume But when my sister sat down at
the table opposite me and said that she wanted my costume I just flared
up in a temper she told me my mother had sent her so I told her she
could have the costume but before she went she said my mother did not
want me home that I would be better away. I went up to her and I
smacked her across the face and I said these words, 'You can tell my
mam that when she has told me the thinks I know if she does not write
or come to see me I will show her up in front on the Court on Monday.'
However she did come to court and she knew I would tell the court what
she had been doing to the family if I made up my mind, I was sent away
for three years to —— my mother did not come to see me at all while
I was away but I was not bothered I worked myself up in those three
years to be the oldest and the head girl of the house, I had some good
reports I used to write to my Sunday School teacher —— and she used
to help me a great deal, I left —— last 29th March and I went to a
Hostel in —— I was not very happy so I was allowed to go home again,
I was at home nine months and doing well and then the last month I was
sent away again to a remand Home, I was sent to court after a month
and got three years again and I was sent to —— (another Remand Home)
and I got to be the head girl there 5 weeks after I came to the Shaw
School,

Indeed study of the eighteen cases who had had more than three
previous Court appearances, reveals only three girls who at the
Classifying School were regarded as very difficult to live with; they
were *not* among the five of the eighteen who eventually were committed to Borstal. Perhaps the number of previous appearances
influenced the Court which eventually sentenced these five to Borstal,
like the girl who, remanded for lifting a ball-point pen from a hospital
supervisor's desk was, on coming before the Court again, sent for
Borstal training.

Until Approved School and Borstal become (and deserve in fact
to become) more fully accepted as supplying a kind of training
suitable for certain kinds of delinquents, rather than as steps on the
downward path, or as grades of punishment earned, then some cases,
often the ones who need the right treatment quickly, will come too
late, or come when they should not come at all.

Forceful attention is drawn to this in paragraph 2 of the 'Evidence
from the Association of Managers, and of Headmasters, Headmistresses and Matrons of Approved Schools for presentation to
the Royal Commission on The Penal System' (1965):

The key question for our present purpose is whether children who have
offended against the law need to incur a stigma in obtaining the treatment they need; and secondly, whether the Committal to Approved

89

Schools should arouse in magistrates and all persons concerned, such feelings of severity and punishment that committal to Approved School is deferred until all other forms of treatment have been tried and have failed—even though the treatment available in an approved school was obviously desirable from the beginning. The sad comment on this procedure is that deferred treatment makes the rehabilitation of a child more difficult and sometimes impossible.

One could sense the charity behind many of the delayed Court judgments; two of these eighteen girls had witnessed tragedies that would impress a Bench readily; one at 5 saw her mother burned to death, the other at about the same age saw her favourite brother drown. Most of the eighteen had particularly disjointed family lives and it was easy for the Court to discern that they needed kindness, not punishment. That they received kindness eventually in Approved Schools is suggested from the fact that one of the girls, running away from home *after* Approved School training, was apprehended near the former Training School on one occasion, and near the Classifying School on the other.

But if one is looking for toughness in the Approved School girl, it may be necessary to look as often among those with no previous Court appearances, as among persistent appearers in Court.

A case which springs to mind is a girl without an earlier Court record, who had become a successful prostitute. She was committed at 16 years 9 months—a fine looking blonde of normal intellect and pleasing personality, who liked us despite her contempt for our lack of economic 'know how'. She had no wish to change and no scruples about winning others to her point of view; her subsequent addresses in corrupt quarters were in the keeping of some Approved School absconders for years afterwards. She herself was as successful at absconding as at prostitution, and was little within A.S. walls.

The condition of a girl and her needs had to be studied in preference to her offences or her misdemeanours or lapses. On paper it is ridiculous to read on an Approved School Order 'that the said —— stole a chocolate bun valued at 3d', but as the last of a series of petty thefts over fifteen months, it may be one of several potent indicators of niggling unhappiness, and a need for a new environment. When one reflects that just over a hundred years ago she might have gone to the gallows, or been transported, one can feel grateful for our insight and charity. Whether we are much nearer to knowing the 'right' environment is another matter.

LENGTH OF DELINQUENT HISTORY

As well as examining the frequency of Court appearances, let us examine a less standardized measurement, and one where our information may be far from complete—namely the age of the girl's first delinquency. This *may* coincide with the evidence of Court appearances, but may refer to reports of earlier misdemeanours, or of offences in the legal sense which were not the subject of Court inquiry.

In statistical terms we find the following from the Shaw figures:

64 per cent of the 14-year-olds committed their first delinquency at about 14 or 13.

65 per cent of the 15-year-olds committed their first delinquency at 15 or 14.

56 per cent of the 16-year-olds committed their first delinquency at 16 or 15.

We see then that considerably more of the 16-year-olds were known by some one to be delinquent two or more years before their committal to Approved School (p $> \cdot$001) (see Chapter XXI). Furthermore, when we look at our two categories of 16-year-olds (those committed before 16½, and those committed after), we find that 13 per cent of the latter had been delinquent before 12-years-old, as against 8 per cent of the younger 16-year-olds. This shows clearly that our belief that they were being 'rounded up' at the last minute could be supported from statistics.

Let us examine the 16-year-olds again in the light of other headings, and see whether our description as more sophisticated holds.

We find, on relating the degree of attention-seeking (recorded in Chapter VII) to age, that the older 16's comported themselves, on the whole, with more normality. Most excessive attention-seekers were 14, and most 15's were evasive and detached. The whole represents a tendency only, for the probability score was not at statistically significant level (about ·2). According to the Gesell Institute this corresponds to the age differences in response to their procedures of child study.[4] They are *not* according to our subjective impressions earlier in this chapter.

Giving the benefit of the doubt, what happened to the different age groups? When we look ahead at our 'success' figures (Appendix, Table IV) there seems to be some indication that those committed later (16½+) or earlier (at 14) were rather more successful than the 'evasive' and 'detached' 15-year-olds.

Chapter Ten

WHERE THEY CAME FROM

HOME AREA

During the three years 1952-4 covered by this research, 562 girls came from thirty-one Counties and fifty-four County Boroughs. As we have seen in Chapter 2, since the Reformatory Acts of 1854, the central government has partially supported the Approved Schools. By the Childrens' Act of 1921 the proportion of contributions was settled as half from the local authorities and half from the State. The responsible Local Authority (usually that where the child is normally resident, but sometimes where the offence is committed or the circumstances leading to his committal arise) may ask the parents of a child in Approved School to contribute to the cost of maintenance, up to age 16. During 1954 the flat-rate contribution (fixed by the Secretary of State) paid by each Local Authority for a girl at The Shaw School was 10s. 3d. per day. Her total maintenance cost was therefore £1 0s. 6d. per day, the remainder being paid by the Exchequer to the School Managers.

Of the thirty-one Counties sending girls during those years, twenty were within the catchment area for the Shaw Classifying School, and eleven were in the southern half of the Country. Of the fifty-four responsible County Boroughs, forty-eight were within the normal catchment area, and six without it. Four girls came from Scotland or Northern Ireland, because they had been committed while resident away.

Girls might be sent from the other Classifying School's area (i.e. from the southern half of England and Wales) to avoid association with an earlier bad associate; or she might have been committed while resident at a Probation Hostel in the northern area, and by design or otherwise been allocated accordingly. A few of those recorded as from the south had become such serious problems at a Training School that a classification elsewhere seemed desirable. Twenty-nine girls were admitted from these southern authorities during the three years, including five from (then) London County Council.

Of the County Councils responsible for girls admitted in the three years, the most populated was Lancashire, and not surprisingly the

County sent forty-three girls, or 8 per cent of the School's intake. West Riding sent thirty-three (6 per cent of intake), Derbyshire twenty-eight (5 per cent of intake) Co. Durham twenty (3·5 per cent), Northumberland sixteen (3 per cent), Staffordshire fourteen, Cheshire eleven, Nottinghamshire ten, East Riding and Salop each seven girls, North Riding sent six, Cumberland five, and London C.C. sent five (though outside the catchment area). The remainder sent diminishing numbers, the only Northern County area not being represented being Westmorland; even Rutland sent one. Ten Southern and South Midland County Councils (apart from London) were responsible for seventeen girls in the school's care in those three years, mainly odd ones, but Worcestershire and Middlesex each had three.

The County Councils were responsible for 238 girls or 42 per cent of the admissions in the three years.

It is well established that delinquency is a greater problem in dense urban areas, so, not surprisingly, 58 per cent of the population came from County Boroughs.

7·3 per cent of the intake, or forty-one girls (almost as many as from the whole of Lancashire County area) were from Kingston-upon-Hull, while Manchester (almost two and a half times as large) contributed 6·5 per cent of the Classifying School's population. Indeed Hull sent many more than Nottingham (twenty-three girls), Liverpool, Leeds and Sheffield (seventeen girls each) which were larger cities. Other County Boroughs sent proportionately to their population more or less, except for Stoke-on-Trent and Bradford (under 300,000 population, like Hull) which sent only eight and seven girls respectively in the three years.

Hull, the top producer of adolescent Approved School girls in those years, had the temptations of a seaport, and a fishing-port, and was one of the most bombed cities during the childhood of many of the 500 girls. The first two possible causes remained, but admissions from there dropped considerably in subsequent years. It is understood that this coincided with the appointment of Women Police. Less certain is a reported fact of change in educational policy, namely that during the earlier time, when a blitz was being made on female delinquency, a change of school occurred for one year at age 14, causing upheaval in the girls who could least take the change.

Delinquency per head of population is held by the experts to occur less frequently in rural areas; adult influences are more powerful where the child is known personally by a wide circle; prestige and affection come from more than the family. To a lesser extent (but

93

variably) a tightly knit working-class urban area spreads a net-work of concern; in each environment there is the odd one not contained by the net, and this person can flounder badly.

The following table shows the contrast in figures for the Shaw School intake between densely urban and more scattered areas:

Table 19: Area Distributions

Area	Total sent in 3 years	No. per annum out of 100,000 population
East & West Ridings	40	·3
West Yorkshire conurbation	36	·7
North West England	59	·3
Merseyside	22	·5
S.E. Lancashire conurbation	54	·7
Northern England	42	·4
Tyneside conurbation	35	1·4

Thus the East and West Ridings had ·3 Protestant girls aged 14 to 17, out of 100,000 population, committed to the Classifying Approved School per year, while the West Yorkshire conurbation's proportion was ·7. The North West region had a proportion of ·3, but the S.E. Lancs conurbation a proportion of ·7 again, and Merseyside ·5.

The Northern region had a proportion of ·4, but Tyneside conurbation's proportion was 1·4—four times as high.

The seaside features, it is believed, appear in the relatively high proportion for Newcastle-on-Tyne, and again for the Tyneside conurbation, which is double the proportion for the other conurbations. 'Going on ships' was very much a recurrence in the histories of older girls from this area.

Girls might have slept on the ships, linking up with other girls who were insecure at home and then resuming the friendships and all the unsettledness this could arouse, at the Classifying School.

Yet Merseyside, also with seaport temptations, has, like Liverpool itself, a lower proportion of committals to the Shaw in these years. Caution must be exercised here—Merseyside has a high Catholic population, and these are Protestant Approved School girls only.

Relations between C.S. and L.A.

Along with the maintenance account when the girl was transferred to her Training School, the Children's Department of the Local

94

Authority received a brief summary of the girl's condition and response during her stay. Intermediate contact with the Authority was made when necessary: to elicit further information about home background; to check on any dubious information given by the girl (for example, if she'd 'heard' that her brother had been killed, or that her mother was ill); to ask for a home visit if parents were not writing to the girl. The more personal contacts were made with the Probation Officer, if the girl had been on probation or under supervision; sometimes Probation Officers wrote regularly to their girls.

The Local Authority's interest in the girl was, of course, going to be elicited for some years after classification—during training and after care—so that it was the usually pleasant duty of the Classifying School to communicate the girl's present and future needs in relation to her predicament.

At the period of the research, the Children's Officers had had less personal contact with individual Approved Schools, and suspicion had to be broken down more than was the case with the Probation Departments. This was an inevitable part of the evolution of relationships and a minor contribution towards the ultimate welfare of the girls.

The Managers of the Training Approved Schools had power to assign any after-care agent for Approved School children on licence. This was, of course, arranged after the girl left the Classifying School. At the later period concerned in the research, the Children's Department of the Local Authorities concerned supplied after-care services for about 39 per cent of the girls released (i.e. released in 1956) as against 30·8 per cent by probation officers. For the after-care of girls released in 1966, the probation and after-care service were asked to help in 59·6 per cent of cases, and the L.A. Child Care Service in 31 per cent (White Paper on Statistics relating to Approved Schools, Remand Homes and Attendance Centres in England and Wales for the year 1966).

SITUATION OF HOME

34 per cent of the Gluecks'[1] 500 delinquent women lived in rural areas or in small towns. The classification in the present study is different, in that rural is rural, and urban is urban, whether large or small. In the last section on Home Area we see that 57 per cent of the girls came from cities or County Boroughs. Also the heavily populated areas (the conurbations) sent more girls than did the more scattered, mixed rural and urban authorities.

Only 7 per cent or 32 of the 500 girls had lived in truly rural areas, three of these having lived in very isolated places. Table 20 gives the distribution of location.

Table 20: Home Area

| | Sample of 500 | | Sample of 100 | |
	No.	%	No.	%
Poor working class, congested area	146	31·5	41	45·5
Good working class, congested area	115	24·8	16	17·8
Council Estate	147	31·7	24	26·7
Suburban, or good residential	23	4·9	6	6·7
Rural	32	6·9	2	2·2
Other (e.g. various institutions)	1	·2	1	1·1
Not known	36		10	
Total	500	100·0	100	100

Of the Gluecks[1] 500 delinquent women (p. 455) 3·8 per cent lived in childhood, and 5·1 in adolescence, in a suburban neighbourhood. In our main sample the percentage is 4·6; in the 100 sample (1957) it was 6·7 per cent. This seems, then, to represent a fairly constant figure of such committals from 'good neighbourhoods'. For the Courts this had been very much a last resort; one girl of this group was a very serious problem indeed before she was finally brought before the Court, and she had been seen by many doctors, psychiatrists and had been twice in a Mental Hospital as a Voluntary patient, yet the parents may have had no more insight than working-class parents whose daughter might be given 'one chance'.

QUALITY OF HOME

In the Records of Information for the Court, and in additional information, some Council estates were described as 'good', and some as, perhaps, having many problem families. This was not noted with sufficient consistency for grouping to be attempted. Thus as far as home situation is concerned, only the 'poor working class, congested area', and 'good working class' tell us much about the neighbourhoods' cultural status. No figures are presented for typically delinquent areas; this would have been a hazardous undertaking, from so many witnesses bringing information to local Courts which, after all, would usually know from the streets or estates how respectable the particular zone was held to be.

Figures for recent studies in Britain show a tendency to accumulations of social problems, including delinquency, in certain areas, but not by any means concentrated in the poor, congested and dilapidated parts—Morris (1957),[2] Mannheim[3] (1948), Mays in 1954, in his Liverpool Study; Jephcott and Carter[4] (1955). Another recent writer, who concentrates on the inadequate homes themselves, is Harriet Wilson.[5] In *Delinquency and Child Neglect* (1962), she formulated standards of adequacy in present-day Society (standards which would indeed be rather higher at the time she wrote than in the period covered by the present research) and made a careful study of fifty-two families scoring, in forty-nine cases, 'five or more points of performance inadequacy' in terms of solvency, health and education.

Within these neglected families, where the only shared characteristic of the parents was 'being unable to cope with the demands made upon them by the community', the rate of delinquency among the girls averaged 10 per cent per year from age 8 to 16, whereas with the boys it was 28 per cent per year—this ratio of 1:3 being considerably higher than the delinquency ratio of girls to boys over the whole country.

It would be an impossible task, on retrospective data, collated for a different purpose, from very scattered observers, to do a comparative study with any of the above writers on this topic. But some figures are available, and bearing their limitations in mind, a picture may emerge of the proportion of girls arriving in the Northern Classifying School for Girls from various economic and social backgrounds.

Table 21 gives us some data, based either directly on information in the girls' Records of Information for the Court, or culled from a variety of information. Neither method is of course, as reliable as a standardized form of collation on the smaller number of homes in other research mentioned.

Table 21: Material Condition of Home Normally Lived In

| | Sample of 500 | | Sample of 100 | |
	No.	%	No.	%
Comfortable	174	36	39	44
Fairly comfortable	207	43	36	41
Extremely uncomfortable	104	21	13	15
Not enough known	15	—	12	—
Total	500	100	100	100

We should expect the second sample (1957), with an average of four years more of welfare state and relative affluence to have more comfortable surroundings; at the same time, expectations of comfort may have been higher in at least some of the later home visitors.

In both sets a very sizable percentage of girls came from extremely uncomfortable homes. That an uncomfortable home is not of necessity an impoverished one is seen from two examples:

> Mr and Mrs —— and the remaining three children live in a desolate, unkempt, dirty but roomy house on a main city road in a working class residential district of Manchester . . . Mr —— is a labourer, earning £8 per week (Note: this was in 1954) and Mrs —— is a cleaner, earning £2 10s. per week. The elder daughter pays £2 per week board . . .

> Mrs —— is a part-time cashier in a cafe . . . The six-roomed house is in a good neighbourhood, but has been allowed to fall into a bad state of repair, and is comfortless and chaotic.

On the other hand, it might be a home with the inadequacies typical of the homes said to breed delinquents:

> The home, consisting of a kitchen and two bedrooms, is in a shocking condition. The Probation Officer reports that there are rat holes in the ceiling, insufficient drains, and that the food is kept on an open shelf in the living room . . . Mr —— suffers from asthma. He is not employed . . . Latterly he has been in hospital for treatment . . . Mrs —— has bronchitis . . . There were marital difficulties, in which she (the girl) took her mother's side, and the father accused her (the girl) of being cruel to him, though (she said) she had never touched him . . .

> When Mrs R—— began her association with Mr H—— the family (4) lived in a four-roomed house. H has spent most of his time in prison and soon after this association began, the family were evicted from their home for non-payment of ¬ent. Since that time they have lived in furnished rooms.
>
> When H is in prison Mrs R usually obtains employment, and at such times the position in the home is always better. . . .
>
> They occupy two rooms . . .; the property is in a dilapidated condition, and situated in a working class district.

As social workers rarely feel the need to describe in detail a reasonably comfortable home, there are no examples to quote.

Of the Gluecks'[1] *500 Delinquent Women*, 43 per cent were said to have lived in a physically 'poor' home in childhood, and in adolescence. Their criteria differ, and 'cases of extreme overcrowding' belong in this class (the 'poor' class) even if the home is good or fair in other respects. Such terms as 'desolate', or 'comfortless', and 'chaotic' may have weighed with the investigators of the Shaw cases as much as sheer physical neglect.

It is probably true that few of the readers would be 'fairly comfortable' in the homes so described, while they would be not wretched, but perhaps somewhat critical in most of what are recorded as 'comfortable' homes.

Possibly most girls, even the ill-supervised in comfortless homes are much more within the home than are most boys. They are also much affected by the aura of comfort or discomfort, and extreme dinginess and disorder may affect them more than having to wash in a chipped enamel bowl or sleep under coats on an old sofa. Lack of privacy may affect both sexes equally. The girls were often compensated for a long time by their maternal interest in the babies of the household, but big brothers were frequently 'hated' for their teasing, or their criticisms of the food prepared by Cinderella sister.

But, as will be confirmed by figures later, 40 per cent of the girls had more than one home environment, and while the physical state of the home might be comparable at each change, it was sometimes not so.

The girl who lived in the 'desolate, unkempt, dirty but roomy house' described above, was evacuated at 4 to the Lake District. She writes:

My sister—came with me but lived at my other Aunty across the way from me . . . It was a nice village with nice people who were nice to my sister and I. My Aunty kept me well dressed and looked after. I was never short of anything. I never knew my parents or my home in Chorlton, Manchester . . . I was very happy there, but one thing spoilt my happiness, and that is, whenever Christmas came around my father sent me paper hats but my Aunty burnt them, she would have nothing to do with Manchester, she said it was dirty. . . . Well the time came when my mother wanted me home with the rest of the family. . . . My father had flitted from Chorlton to Moss Side. . . .

Another who had the shock of wildly conflicting standards had been evacuated at 2 or 3 from London to a 'convalescent home' in the North. At the 'leaving age' she went to a 'strange place and a strange woman'. . . .

At first I called her Auntie but then gradually I began to call her Mum. . . . I don't think I had more than anyone else but I couldn't help but take care of the things she gave me. We lived on a farm too. . . . Two years had gone before I knew it. Then I was given a choice between staying with Mum and going to live with my parents. . . . When the joy was over I lived in a small neglected house, quite unlike the one I was used to and wore patched clothes and shoes which badly needed cobbling. My father drank every night practically and my real mother couldn't help herself because she was suffering from a disease in the mind. . . . I was soon picking up the habit of eating off the ground and running around the place in a filthy state. . . .

Here there is a flavour of melodramatic fiction in the writing, but the facts agreed with the major ones in the official record.

Another child dwelt on the happy breaks she had with a well-doing Aunt and Uncle, who had wished to adopt her. But at home she and the parents latterly shared a four-roomed cottage (three rooms habitable) with an elderly eccentric, 'living in filthy, comfortless conditions'. She shared a bed, covered with a sheet and old coats, with her mother, who was 'of loose moral character'.

Data on material comfort in the home must, before they are meaningful, be supplemented by other data. We have seen that all comfortless homes were not impoverished, but many were, or were on the brink of penury.

The economic status of the parents is given in Table 22.

Table 22: Economic Status of Parents

	Sample of 500 No.	Sample of 500 %	Sample of 100 No. and %
Professional	4	·8	1
Clerical	17	3·4	4
Farmer	1	·2	—
Trades	71	14·2	16
Semi-skilled	97	19·4	22
Unskilled	172	34·4	31
Dependent on Welfare Services	68	13·6	9
Other	15	3	4
Not known	46	9·2	10
Old Age or Widow's Pension	9	1·8	3
Total	500	100	100

Comparing the percentages for the two Approved School samples, we again find a fairly even balance, but, as with home comfort, there is a statistical improvement in the dependent families; instead of the 14 per cent of parents dependent in 1952–4, we have 9 per cent dependent. This is, however, based on a section of the 1957 intake, and must not be over-stressed. It does not seem to match the family health situation, which we shall see later.

Again, with data collated much later from records not planned for a social study, it is not well to overdo comparison with other writers, who have tabulated social class more precisely (e.g. Dr Gibbens,[6] 1963) but just to state, with some reserve, that the proportions seem not too different from the usual findings for large groups of delinquents of either sex in this country; even within this country standards of living and of judgment vary, and comparisons with groups in the South East might be question-begging.

Groups of unsocialized girl delinquents did occur, as well as some whose social standards at one time in life had been in conflict with those at another. There were girls who had lived in decrepit surroundings, been the worst dressed in the class, possibly infested with lice and sent home occasionally for cleansing; thus social downgrading was part of life, and might be succumbed to or struggled against. Unemployed fathers, sometimes drunken fathers, and frequently unsympathetic fathers and overburdened or inadequate mothers did not stimulate verbal communication in the home, and school education often passed over their heads. Some of these absorbed wider social norms in sex, cleanliness and decorum, perhaps from a favourite teacher, but some did not.

This explanation, however (in line with Harriet Wilson's[5]) covers only a section of the total population of the Classifying School, and experience there, as well as follow-ups in the Training Schools where such cases predominated, suggested they were not a difficult group in the short term, and in the longer term much depended on the seriousness with which the Training School concerned regarded 'character training' as its main role, rather than putting on a veneer which would soon chip on return to the old setting; on the other hand, Training Schools receiving the more neurotic girl would clearly have to concentrate less on creating patterns of behaviour, while those receiving the materially indulged girl might well use a more pressurized life with some hardship as a corrective.

The following brief summaries give a sketchy picture of some categories of delinquent girls from socially inadequate or unfortunate families. To see this at its extreme, only those families dependent on Welfare services or dependent on Old Age or Widows' Pensions are being traced.

There were 77 girls of our 500 group coming from such families. Thirty-three of these (43 per cent of this sub-group) lived with both parents; twenty-seven of the sub-group lived with the mother alone, and of these four were on widow's pension, not on National Assistance; seven girls of the group lived with the mother and a new partner, legal or otherwise. Of the four living with the grandparents alone, three of the latter were, not unnaturally, on Old Age Pension, and therefore not 'dependent' quite in our sense, but perhaps too materially needful for an adolescent girl's ambitions.

As the twenty-seven living with the mother alone (i.e. with mother as head of the household, in which a variety of siblings, and husbands or wives and children of the latter could be installed) the poverty or inadequacy has largely come upon them by way of death or a marriage break-up.

To the extent that 'inadequacy' (physical or social) has its true connotation where father is unable (for any reason) to keep employment and mother is unable (for any reason) to manage on the welfare resources, we shall return to the 43 per cent (thirty-three girls) the 'dependent' group living with both parents.

12 of the 33 lived in homes in poor working-class areas.

11 of the 33 lived on Council estates.

8 of the 33 lived in homes in good working-class areas.

Of the twelve in poor working-class areas, nine belonged to families larger than four, and three to families larger than six; of the eleven on Council estates, eight belonged to families larger than four, and three to families larger than six.

Of the thirty-three girls who had lived with both parents in 'dependent' state, eleven had seriously detrimental health backgrounds in the families, and, of these, all were of a sibling group numbering four or more. Five of these families had a tuberculous history, and here the sizes of families were five, six, seven (twice) and nine. Two families with an epileptic parent were of six and seven, and three with a mentally defective parent numbered four, five and eight.

Though concentrating here on the extremely unfortunate subgroups, we can find plenty that was sordid or ineffectual or both in other economic groups. For example:

P's father and mother and the youngest three children live in a dilapidated, poorly furnished, dirty three-roomed slum house in ——. Mr —— is a labourer, earning £7 or £8 a week (Note: this was in 1954) and giving Mrs —— about £6. He often suffers from cystitis and nerve trouble and is frequently unemployed. He is described as equally weak mentally. Mrs —— is also of low intelligence and is illiterate. (A neighbour writes to P for her.) She had a cleft palate, and is of poor physique. She earns a little as a part-time cleaner. P says the youngest sister is bronchial, as she (P) was earlier in childhood. . . .

That this sub-section of home-centred, rather than area-centred delinquency exists, with the pattern of emotional insecurity almost inevitably accompanying the particular brands of economic deprivation, is clear from the present research records. Further figures on the families will highlight this even more. With fewer sordid conditions in the home such a girl, with a history of staying out late, might not have been brought before the Court at all; but then she would also most probably, have been a more socialized being.

But the real point of issue is that 36 to 44 per cent of girls came from comfortable homes; 21 per cent of parents with a profession or skill.

This section has dealt with the civic authority sending the girl; the economic area from which she came; the physical comfort of her home; the economic status of her parents or guardians. While we have emphasized the considerable percentages from poor urban areas, of unskilled working-class parentage, who have sometimes been dependent mainly on Welfare Services, we are also faced with the fact that over a third were from comfortable homes, and over a fifth had guardians with a training or skill—though the percentage from professional and administrative or farming classes was small or non-existent. It may be that we have hereby a rough division into types of delinquents, with the cultural tail of society needing basic conditioning and straight-forward education, the staff involved requiring less training than for the more complicated emotional problems; indeed we shall find that the socialization job was generally well done in the Girls' Approved Schools.

The importance of the material factors in the girls' lives need the emphasis given above. Cosy middle-class parents complaining of inevitable emotional tensions in their circle, need reminders that the rain isn't coming through their roof, and that their children don't often suffer from malnutrition or tuberculosis. We shall see, for instance in Tables VI and VII of the Appendix that, even in this unrepresentative sample of the country's population, intellectual dullness (verbal and non-verbal) as well as scholastic attainment were significantly related to poverty and discomfort. Home relationships were also linked—large, poor, slackly disciplined families—for whom troubles 'piled up'. These girls tended ($p > \cdot05$) to be the truants rather than the thieves, and they also tended to respond to our pseudo-mothering at the Classifying School; if awkward they at least were more openly awkward.

Raising the competence of Approved School girls to the point where, from sheer good habits of management, they can be better mothers (and perhaps mothers of manœuvrable families) has been a recognized part of the curriculum for years; it has not always received enough credit.

Chapter Eleven

THE PARENTS AND OTHERS.
PRESENT AND ABSENT

A factor which leaves no doubt of its importance in the backgrounds of these Approved School girls is the broken home. Calculated merely from those broken by death, separation, divorce and desertion, without including splits due to illegitimacy, and causes such as parental imprisonment or illness, the figures are 52·2 per cent for the 500 sample, and 51 per cent for the 100 sample. From what the writer can trace this seems to exceed the figure found in any major research into male juvenile delinquency. Dr Epps' Borstal Group[1] containing 45·7 per cent Approved School failures, had only 30·6 per cent with homes broken by death, divorce and separation; her subsequent study of 100 recidivist Borstal girls[2] had 35 per cent with homes broken by divorce and separation alone[1]. (Figures for broken homes for these reasons given by Charlotte Banks[3] for samples of boy delinquents in Table IX of Stephanos: *Studies in Psychology*, pp. 173–203 show totals of 33 per cent (Burt):[4] 44 per cent Borstal and Detention Centre Groups and 9 per cent (Douglas) for the normal population.)

When those Shaw girls whose parents were apart because of illegitimacy are included, the two percentages for prolonged parental absences are 60 and 65; 40 per cent of the 500 group and 35 per cent of the 100 group lived with both parents through the years leading up to their Court appearances, or lived with them apart from many considerable absences of a parent for illness and other reasons, or many absences of a child for an even greater variety of causes.

These figures must be examined in detail.

ILLEGITIMACY

A relationship between illegitimacy and delinquency tends to be assumed. In most studies with experimental and control groups a significant difference has been found between the proportion of illegitimate children in each.

In *Young Offenders*[5] 1942 3·7 per cent of the London delinquents were illegitimate at birth, against 0·8 per cent among the controls.

The Gluecks'[6] delinquents in *Unravelling Juvenile Delinquency* 1950 had 18·6 per cent illegitimate juveniles, against 13 per cent among the controls. Litauer[7] (I.S.T.D., 1957) in a London area sample found 11·1 per cent of 'illegitimate (or doubtful) cases'. Dr Epps[2] (1954) found 10 per cent illegitimate among her Borstal girls. Of Gittins'[8] (1952) 100 cases, eleven were illegitimate. The Gluecks'[9] *500 Delinquent Women* (1934) had 8 per cent whose illegitimacy at birth was established or questioned. The formalities at the time of a Court appearance and inquiry are possibly more likely to ascertain a child's legitimacy than the earliest interviews at a Child Guidance Clinic. On the other hand the Approved School population is more likely to contain children whose legitimacy is in doubt, or whose illegitimacy has been concealed within an apparently normal family.

How far illegitimacy was a blot on the mind of the adolescent girl in the Approved Schools could be judged mainly by her frequent avoidance of the subject when writing about herself, compared with the readiness with which a girl could write about parental divorce or death. One illegitimate girl (born in 1938) said her father was killed in the Great War. More than one glamourized the situation by giving her father high rank in Army, Navy or Air Forces. Most difficult seemed to be the need for adopted girls who had absorbed 'respectable standards', to accept the maternal lapse. One such girl, obsessed by her ignorance of her mother's personality and status, became obsessed with the whole topic of birth, so that it intruded into unlikely intelligence test responses, and had intruded into her social pre-occupations so much that she lost jobs because of her 'dirty talk'.

Two consecutive entries in one girl's Personal History at age 15 read:

April: A had discovered that she was illegitimate by going through her mother's papers in the latter's absence and she was once more pilfering from home. She also began to eat enormous quantities of food, so much so that her mother had to lock the food cupboard. *August:* By now A had begun an immoral association with a man named ——

This is not to say that all illegitimate children are, or were so inhibited or evasive about their origins—nor indeed that all of our Approved School girls were; it may have been more insidiously linked with the maladjustments of these particular girls who were. But neither did 'areas of illegitimacy', or ethics or economics of certain areas seem to have much to do with a girl's feelings, except for the adopted girls who have been discussed. Derogatory remarks, having little relation to the speaker's own ethical standards, are cheap ammunition in childish quarrels, and an overheard dispute between mothers over the back fence might bring knowledge and shame. One adopted girl was told by a play-mate, 'You were a dirty baby and your own Mummy didn't want you'. More than a dozen girls learned with some shock of their illegitimacy or their consequent adoption. One met the shock tangibly, when her second parent died and relatives, learning for the first time that they had not been married, righteously refused to look after the child.

A girl might be soaked in illegitimacy, and yet not be impervious to gloating school-mates or over-heard slights. A few girls in particular, came from families where it was the rule; in one case the girl concerned was the legitimate exception, there being three older and three younger who were illegitimate, and the mother's one legitimate liaison had brought little joy, only violence and hatred. Another was one of two older illegitimate children, prior to two unsatisfactory but more permanent cohabitations. The girl was finally recorded as 'illegitimate and eldest of between five and seven illegitimate children'. Another girl was one of five even less discriminate illegitimate births. Quite a few girls, themselves legitimate by a father who later deserted, had to face the confusion of younger illegitimate brothers or sisters by longer or shorter associations. So often poverty became a combined cause of resentment where liaisons had been brief and irresponsible. There were, of course, also satisfactory unions at least as far as mother and the new family were concerned.

Table 23 gives the figures for known legitimate and illegitimate girls in the group, and the consequence of lack of normal parentage in terms of care for the child.

There were 10·6 per cent or fifty-three illegitimate girls in the 500 sample. The figure compares fairly closely to others of the delinquent samples named. The national percentage of illegitimate births in 1938 (the average year of birth for these 500 girls) was 4·2 per cent.

There were 15 per cent illegitimate girls in the 100 sample. The national percentage of illegitimate births in 1942 (the average year of birth for the 100) was 5·6 per cent. Thus the increase in our sample is rather greater proportionately than the national increase. (Our later sample, however, was not a whole year group).

We are most concerned with those who, by reason of illegitimacy have been deprived of a parent or parents. These totals are forty girls, or 8 per cent of the 500 sample, and 12 per cent of the 100 sample. Rather more than half of each deprived group was without mother and father.

Of the forty girls of the 500 sample who were deprived of their own father in this way, ten were adopted—five before 6 months, four between 6 months and 3 years, and one after 3 years. (Twice this percentage of the 1957 sample were adopted.) Two of the 500 sample

Table 23: Legitimacy/Illegitimacy

	Shaw Sample 1 500		Shaw Sample 2 100
	No.	%	No. and %
Legitimate, not adopted etc.	435	87	81
Legitimate, institutionalized	1	0·2	2
Legitimate, adopted by relatives	2	0·4	1
Legitimized by marriage of parents	4	0·8	1
All legitimates	447	89·4	85
Parents together, cohabiting	13	2·6	3
Parents not together, and child illegitimate			
Illegitimate, but adopted	10	2	4
Illegitimate, reared by mother alone or with grandmother or relative	6	1·2	4
Illegitimate, reared by mother and step-father or cohabitant	9	1·8	1
Illegitimate, reared by grandmother or other relatives or family friend	11	2·2	1
Illegitimate, fostered out to strangers	2	0·4	2
Illegitimate, in institutions (whole of childhood)	2	0·4	—
	0	100	100
Total with Mother absent	25	5	7
Total with Father absent	40	8	12

were fostered out, and two spent their childhood in institutions. (Five times the percentage of the 1957 girls were fostered out and none of the illegitimate children spent all of childhood in an Institution, due no doubt to the drive to give deprived children a substitute home.) But a sad feature of the girls' lives, as we shall see more fully, was the repeated changes, and the repeated shocks of change. A girl classed as spending her childhood in foster-homes may have spent longish interim periods in a variety of Childrens' Homes or other institutions.

Much has been written, fictional and otherwise, of the adopted or fostered child discovering her origins. We had our full share of cases who were or were not recovering from such traumas. One girl learned during an angry quarrel with her foster-mother at 12 that she was not their own daughter. Not only did she lose face, but, following further misconduct, lost her christian and surnames and had to resume the inelegant names to which she was born. The far-seeing Head of her Training School arranged for her name to be legally changed back, and gradually, with restored morale, she was reconciled with the foster-parents who had originally lent her that name.

Of the remainder who lost their natural mother as well as their natural father by an illegitimate birth, eleven girls were reared by a grandmother or other relatives or friends of the family. In these cases mother would usually be seen occasionally but the relationship (especially in the nine granny-reared cases) would often be disguised and the girl correspondingly confused. Sometimes she would spend brief spells with the mother (perhaps married, with children) but most of these girls tended to have a mawkish, self-indulgent attitude to life, and there was 'nothing to get hold of', in the way of character —though the personality might be very delightful as far as it went. Where there was a tussle between mother and grandmother for influence, the effect, though less pleasant, seemed to be more solid.

Six (1·2 per cent) of the 500 sample, and 4 per cent of the later sample were reared by the mother alone, but usually in residence with the maternal grandmother, or another relative. Then, usually, the mother went out to work, and dual standards of upbringing could creep in, with grandmother often indulgent, and showing before neighbours and relatives a mixture of devotion and pity for this by-blow. Again one tended to find mawkish sentiment and little realism in the girl, and a pleasant personality but an intangible problem.

An interesting point is the larger percentage of the mothers in the 1957 sample who had brought their child up alone or in the grand-maternal home. This will be seen also in another connection; whether money was easier, or step-fathers scarcer by 1957, it is hard to say.

Nine (1·8 per cent) of the earlier illegitimate group and one of the later group were brought up in a home with a step-father or an unofficial cohabitant of the mother. Six of these nine children when at school had to cope with two surnames, while their class-mates had one. Perhaps this was one of the things that brought them bang against their irregular birth—this and (sometimes) having siblings with a constant name and a more clear status in the home. Others of these nine girls alluded to their illegitimacy, thus:

When I was three my mother got married to my stepfather. I hate him as he made her life a misery. He's good-looking even though he was a cripple and had been going out with other women. I accidently gave a letter to my mother when it was for him. It was from a lady with lovely blonde hair. When she read it she cried for a long time, I have realized now why he never liked me and what that letter meant. He did to that blonde girl what someone did to my mother. She was having a baby and my father did the same thing as the man who was my real father; he left her and we moved to . . .

Another:

When I was born my mother was not married. My mother's name was —— and so I took her name until later on she married my father who was a Scot that had taken to the roads like my mother . . . I was about 2 years old when my mother and father parted and mother was going to have another baby, which was born in a house-boat in ——. While living in the house-boat mother met Mr —— I think that he was the child's real father, but I do not know if that was the reason for my mother and father parting. When Mr —— had married my mother and my name was changed from —— to ——, we again took to the road sometimes sleeping under trees and on hay stacks.

It must not be assumed that this latter girl (with her acceptance of her status) was in a fine state of adjustment; she had identified with her mother's lack of adherence to conventions, and while she could love and admire 'normal' adults, could not accept their way of life without conflict; which she in turn abhorred, for she was a girl who needed to be loyal. Her later adjustment was at a more luxurious level than roads and haystacks—as the mistress of a foreign restaurateur—a role which, if unsuccessful, she could sever, as her mother had done before her.

A girl could, with a weak step-father, and an indulgent, thoughtless, pleasure-loving mother, be more or less indifferent to her illegitimacy. This was so with a girl whose mother took her on weekend coach trips, dancing and drinking, sometimes remaining away overnight. But such a state, contrary perhaps to popular ideas of slap-happy delinquents seemed to be rare among the subjects of this research.

A brief word on those living throughout childhood with unmarried parents. Some parents were living together with little tension in themselves about the irregularity, and thus left the children unmoved. Should the situation be less happy, and if neighbours were 'talking', or many social agencies visiting, then the child might be ill-at-ease. Of one case our visiting Psychiatrist wrote: 'She talks freely about her problems, and it is evident that she has suffered a great deal as a result of the uncertainty about her parentage and the irregularity of her mother's union. The whole family have been at cross purposes, and this girl has developed an air of independence in self-defence.'

90 per cent of the girls admitted to the Classifying School in 1952, 1953 and 1954 were, as far as had been established, legitimate, or had been legitimized. We shall see that of those with a birth-right to live with both parents, a further 50 per cent were deprived by

ill-luck or ill-guidance of this opportunity, before finally being removed by the Court to new parent substitutes—the Managers of a Girls' Approved School.

DEATH OF A PARENT OR PARENTS

Prevention of delinquency has recently hung a good deal on the prevention of a break in the home, by early concerted effort of social workers. Marriage guidance and other agencies may prevent a parent's departure on emotional grounds, but even the best health services in the world cannot prevent some girls losing their mother or father by death. And the best insurance and pension schemes can lessen the economic hardship, but help little in the sphere that matters most:

> On my eleventh birthday we were going to have a party. I was excited.
> Father and I always got on the same bus in the morning . . . As I got off
> the bus I kissed my father good-bye as usual . . . I came home from
> school only to find my family weeping. I was told my father had been
> killed . . . I felt as though my world was falling to pieces, although I had
> a sister and three brothers to play with, I was very lonely.

Though the writer of this was later called by a Headmistress 'a monument of bluff and insincerity', the story was factually true.

Or, from a solemn 14-year-old:

> I lived with my parents until I was 3 years old. My mother and father
> died with T.B. when I was 3 years old. When they died I had to go in
> a Childrens' Orphanage until I was 6 years old. My aunt who was my
> mother's sister adopted me and took me away from my two sisters and
> my brother. . . . When I went to live with my aunt I did not like her as
> she was always hitting me. I have got a scar on my leg where she threw
> a poker at me and I have a scar on my arm were she cut me with a
> knife . . . I hated my aunt and I wanted to get away from her so I went
> and did what I wanted and that's why I am here.

A child's memories:

> When I was about five year old my mam was very ill she had to go in
> hospital, and the next mooning my dad got a lettle sain that she had got
> a little baby boy. and my dad was very pleased so he whent to the
> hopspital to see her and the baby was a beautful baby it was like my
> farther, and he ponhoed every day to the hospital to see if my mam and
> the baby was all wrighth. In a few days latter my dad got a litter sain
> thant the baby had died and my dad was very upset he whant strigth up
> to the Hospital to see if my mam was all wrigth and he seen the baby
> the doctor tolled my farther that my mam will be coming home sone
> When I was going out to play I see my mam and I run up to her and I
> kiss her she did not look very well at all, she asked me were I was going

110

and I said that I was going to play with my friend, my mam whent in the houes And as soon as my dad seen my Mam he ran and kiss her and minit I came in crien and mam said what or you crieing for love and I sered that I had fell down and heart my leg and she put some bandage on and I stop criein My mam sat down and and had somthing to eat, My dad was keep look at my mam and he said to her you dont look feery well, mam said to him I am all wrigth my dad did not like the look of mam alt all. so he whent to the doctor And he told him, and he said that she was all wrigth, and my dad said to him if you dont come and see her I will get a police doctor and as soon as my dad said that he came strigth away, the doctor give her som tablets and meddison it was about twelev o clock when my mam tooh bad again My dad said to her, I will pohoe for the doctor and my mam said no she said if you do I will cut my thrut my mam ask for a racer my dad said dont be silly youll be all wrigth, the last words she said is goodbye borney. We were all criein in the bedroom, my dad whent for the dortor he tolled him my dad said to the doctor it was you you should of sended her straigth to hospital, the docto did not no what to say. When I was about sixes year old my dad got married again we did not like her at all put we had to call her mam. . . .

Perhaps most tragic of all was the granny-reared girl who, already at sixes and sevens with her father, and the confidante of her more frivolous mother, absconded for the third time from a Remand Home (this time because it was her mother's birthday) began to climb into the dark house, and was stopped by a neighbour who asked, 'Don't you know your mother's dead?' The latter had gassed herself. The girl stopped writing her 'Life Story' before this point.

Burt, *The Young Delinquent*, p. 94 wrote, 'With delinquent boys it is the removal of the father and his disciplinary influence that figures most frequently.... With the girls it is separation from the mother that accounts for the highest percentages.'

We shall see from Table 24 that numerically this was not so for losses by death, nor, as we shall see, from other causes, and in depth of feeling one would not judge it to be so either. In this we are in agreement with David Wills[10] *Throw away thy Rod* (p. 104): 'Girls need fathers. I incline to the belief that once infancy is well behind they need fathers more than they need mothers; certainly they need it as much.... They need not only a living father ...; they need a strong father who can on occasion be stern and hold them firmly in check....' An aggressive 14-year-old girl at The Shaw, whose father had died a year or two before, sewed on to a tray-cloth for her mother's wedding anniversary the words: 'A mother is lovely, she clothes and feeds you, but all a father can do is die and leave you.' Rejection could not be more eloquent.

Of the Gluecks' *500 Delinquent Women* (1934) 26·1 per cent had breaks in the home in childhood or adolescence through the mother's death, and 28 per cent through the father's death. The Juvenile Court statistics of the U.S. Children's Bureau (U.S. Pub. No. 245) give, for annual samples averaging about 30,000, around the 8·5 per cent mark for fathers dead and about 3·6 per cent for mothers dead in the years 1934–6. (The age range for the Gluecks' study was older than our Approved School group, and the U.S. Children's Bureau statistics covered a younger range.)

Table 24: Death of Parent(s)

	Shaw Sample 1		Shaw Sample 2
	500		100
	No	%	No. and %
Both parents alive	318	63·6	64
Mother alive	427	85·4	64 + 23 = 87
Father alive	378	75·6	64 + 8 = 72
⎰Mother dead before 6 months	7	1·4	0⎱
⎱Father dead before 6 months	4	·8	1⎰
Mother dead before 3 years	20	4	1
Father dead before 3 years	17	3·4	3
Mother dead 3 to 11 years	21	4·2	4
Father dead 3 to 11 years	36	7·2	6
Mother dead after 11 years	19	3·8	5
Father dead after 11 years	18	3·6	4
Total: Mother dead	60	12	10
Total: Father dead	71	14·2	13
Not relevant: Mothers (e.g. deserted, unknown)	13	2·6	3
Not relevant: Fathers (illegit. or deserted or unknown)	51	10·2	15

Dr Gibbens'[11] figures for 200 Borstal Lads are 9·5 per cent for fathers dead and 9·0 per cent for mothers dead. Dr Epps[1] with Borstal girls, found 5·3 per cent with parental deprivation by death.

For the 500 sample and the 100 sample we have a higher percentage of fathers than of mothers dead. Until the age of 3, the loss of one parent balances the other—though in the 100 sample we may be seeing a result of better health services in the reduced total of maternal fatalities. The fact that the maternal losses in this early period are about equal to those in the 3 to 11 period, which is three times as long, seems to support Bowlby[12] and others who have claimed the seriousness of maternal deprivation in early childhood as a cause of emotional maladjustment. Greatest proportionately of all are the maternal deaths before 6 months (included subsequently in the 'before 3 years' total); in these seven cases institutions had often been the only solution, or the solution until a substitute mother was found.

But the proportionate importance of mother and father deaths stands out in the 3 to 11 years period, where we have twenty-one mothers and thirty-six fathers dying in the 500 sample, and four against six in the 100 sample. This, mainly in the latency period, may be important for the girl's greater need both of the strong father, and for the building up of a satisfactory image for later tender male figures in her life. Her precipitate search for affection, quite often from older men, could be a result of her deprivation. After 11 years losses tend to be greater among mothers, but the difference is small. Finally we have a total of sixty girls without mothers by the time of Approved School Committal, and seventy-one without fathers because of death, and a further forty because of illegitimacy—over one-fifth fatherless before we come to study absences for other reasons.

Gibbens[11] gives the stages of the Borstal lads' lives when the parental loss by death was incurred. The boys in that sample likewise sustained most parental losses in the early years, with 14 of the 18 maternal deaths before the age of 5, and nine of the nineteen fathers. We can roughly compare the two samples by grouping those under 11 and over 11.

Table 25: Comparison with Borstal Lads /Parental Deaths

Borstal Lads Sample of 200			Approved School Girls Sample of 500		
	No	%	Age	No	%
a) Father dead	19	9·5		71	14·2
Age at Father's Death					
0 to 11 yrs.	14	7	0 to 11 (incl.)	53	10·6
11 to 16 yrs.	5	2·5	12 to 16+	18	3·6
b) Mother dead	18	9		60	12
Age at Mother's Death					
0 to 11 yrs.	17	8·5	0 to 11 (incl.)	41	8·2
11 to 15 yrs.	1	·5	12 to 16+	19	3·8

Allowing for the slight overlap in timing, it would appear from these figures that the increased incidence of paternal loss for the girls was mainly in the pre-adolescent years, the loss there being 50 per cent greater than for the Borstal lads.

The very marked increase in the maternal losses for the girls is, however, after the girl was 11. This, again, is very understandable as a link with delinquency. A girl at this stage tends to be particularly sentimental. She is more advanced in adolescence than a boy at the parallel ages, therefore tending to be preoccupied with death, as well as with birth. She is not taken up so much with gangs, or with physical activity. She is lonely, and longs to confide, and her mother (she thinks, at least) would be the ideal confidante. Often too the mother-less girl at this stage was expected to keep house for her father—and society, as well as her father, expected her to keep a job as well, whereas her mother, with many years more of experience, would have been slightly frowned upon for doing the same. One delicate girl, much attached to her widowed music-hall father, was under criticism for having 'four short-lived jobs' while caring for him before and after his serious illness. When, in his weakness, he became less cheerful and companionable, she turned to an older man, who had come to lodge with them. When he, in turn, lost interest she attempted suicide and was committed to Approved School.

Causes of Death of Parents

For one year group of the 500 sample, fairly reliable figures were attainable for causes of parental deaths. The official form (M.H.) sent to all parents on a girl's admission asked for this information, and surviving mothers supplied it with efficiency; surviving fathers supplied it with fair efficiency.

In 1954, 155 girls were admitted. 12 mothers had died, of the following causes:

Tuberculosis	4
Heart disease	2
'Chest'	1
Cancer	1
Not known	4
	—
Total	12, or 8% approx. of year's intake (i.e. lower than in 1952 and 1953)

17 Fathers had died, of the following causes:

Tuberculosis	4
'Chest' (Pneumonia or bronchitis)	5

114

Heart disease	3
War casualties	2
Cancer	1
Stomach trouble	1
Not known	1
	—
Total	17, or 11% of year's intake.

The high incidence of death from tuberculosis (5·2 per cent of the parents of the 1954 intake) and the 3·9 per cent from chest trouble (mainly pneumonia and bronchitis) may be found to correlate with the quota of overcrowded, ill-managed homes we mentioned earlier. Comparisons are difficult, because between 1939 and 1949, when most of these parental deaths had occurred, there was a national drop of 23 per cent in tuberculosis deaths. Even so, the rate for the parents of the Shaw girls was clearly disproportionate as was the total number of parent deaths.

The important thing for these bereft girls, if they genuinely revered the lost parent, was to help them to be grateful for an experience that many of their fellows had not enjoyed. Then they had to be encouraged by knowing that many normal adults had lived through such losses. If bereavement had left them more or less alone in the world, this fact had to be squarely faced, and the future, with all its difficulties, pictured in realistic terms. Here we are talking about the more straightforward 'off-the-rails' cases; the problem for a girl with a load of guilt about a parent's death was one that should be discussed in connection with other neurotic trends in adolescent Approved School girls.

DIVORCE, SEPARATION OR DESERTION

Table 26 gives the stark facts of parental absences through divorce, separation or desertion.

The most serious feature is the considerable increase in the later 1957 sample (admittedly not a complete yearly sample) with a final 42 per cent of parental absences for this reason. The major increase is in the intermittent separations (10 per cent) and will not alter our main discussion of the longer term partings of the 500 sample.

One thing that needs to be emphasized with most of this group is that the child was deprived of one parent, but also sometimes the remaining parent might be already, or might become inadequate socially or emotionally. For this reason the almost equal absences of both parents before 3 years does not cut across the theories of early maternal deprivation, as the mother in her misery could be withdrawn from her small child—and might also have to go to work to fend for her.

Before three years the loss is about 1·2 per cent per year for each parent (with the father's absence rate greater in the first six months), and from three to eleven it is half this rate for the mother, but almost the same yearly rate for the father. We do seem to have support here again for the loss of a father incurred in the latency period being a

Table 26: Divorce, Separation, Desertion

	Shaw Sample 1 No	%	Shaw Sample 2 No and %
Both parents (or adoptive parents) living together (i.e. not separated or divorced)	293	58·6	49
Above not relevant (e.g. illegitimacy)	45	9·0	9·0
{ Mother absent before 6 months	2	0·4	2 }
{ Father absent before 6 months	7	1·4	1 }
Mother absent before 3 years	18	3·6	7
Father absent before 3 years	19	3·8	5
Mother absent 3 to 11 years	26	5·2	4
Father absent 3 to 11 years	45	9	8
Mother absent after 11 years	8	1·6	2
Father absent after 11 years	14	2·8	3
Parents separated intermittently	19	3·8	10
Adoptive parents separated before 3 years	2	·4	1
Adoptive parents separated after 3 years	11	2·2	2
Experiencing Separation Total	162	32·4	42
Total with mother absent	52	10·4 }26	13 }29
Total with father absent	78	15·6	16

more serious deprivation for the girl in her adolescent years; this is seen also *in* the adolescent years, where 14 of the 500 fathers absented themselves, as against eight mothers.

Troubles indeed knocked at these doors by hordes. 13 of the 500 who had had to make a second (perhaps third) adjustment in early childhood to adoptive parents, later found this new house falling round their ears as the adoptive family in turn broke up. Naturally the figures for these breaks are highest after three years.

For the subsequent comparisons we shall leave the Shaw figures at the point of finalized separation, divorce or desertion (26 and 29 per cent respectively) rather than include the intermittent separations (which are probably not all recorded anyway) and the separations of adoptive parents, where the child has already been included among the victims of illegitimacy or parental death.

Herewith are a few comparisons:

Table 27: Home Broken by Divorce, Separation, Desertion

		%
Shaw Sample of 500 (born 1936–40)		26
Shaw Sample of 100 (born 1941–43)		29
Gibbens' *Borstal Lads*[11] (born about 1937)		26·5
Epps' *Borstal Girls*[1] (born about 1931)	1) Main group	25·3
	2) Borstal recall group	35
* Charlotte Banks[3]—*Detention Centre Boys* (born about 1942)		25
N.B. These last 3 groups were older, with average ages, about 18–19, hence longer time for parental separation.		
The Gluecks' *1000 Juvenile Delinquents*[6]		13·3
Burt[4]: *The Young Delinquent* (born about 1908)		12 (Controls 3%)
Gittins[5]: *A.S. Boys* (100 Sample)		21
N.B. These last 3 groups are rather younger than the Shaw Sample, hence less time for separation.		

* *National Survey* (Douglas)—children born 1946 (quoted by Charlotte Banks)

Dr Gibbens[11] (p. 69) says of his figures for Borstal lads' broken homes: 'Separation when he is 16 usually has been preceded by years of quarrelling and temporary separations. The unbroken home may on occasions be as bad as any other.'

Tappan[13] (1949, p. 134–5) says:

A major part of scholarship devoted to the family has been concerned with the broken home and a lesser, but quite extensive, amount to parental discipline. It now appears that neither of these factors is so important in itself as is the child's reaction to them. Tension, discord, and conflict in the home are often found in the delinquent *Gestalt*; it is these rather than a formal breaking of the home, that possess significance in the child's maladaptations. In fact, it is undoubtedly true that a child's adjustment has often been improved when the desertion, divorce, or death of a parent has put a decisive period to a family atmosphere made morbid by hostility.

The staff's feeling about the total of about 30 per cent (150 girls) of the 500 sample, and 40 per cent of the 100 sample was that the break itself was often catastrophic, the terrible finality of the departure of a parent, sometimes without so many memories of quarrels. And it so often happened that both parents were still seen, separately, so that the separateness was thus whetted, as was the child's feeling of rejection. One case particularly is recalled where the child was sent each Saturday to collect the maintenance money from the father in his separate household. In such cases where regular contact was kept by the child with both households, tale-bearing often became a feature, and undermined the child's security further. Also one felt that girls, in any case, were much disturbed by the individual difference of not having real parents, like their confederates.

But in Chapter 22 we shall see that girls with parents *together*, on the whole, did worst; this may be related to many things other than quarrelling, but may, too, confound our theory.

That there were cases where a parent was 'a good riddance' is illustrated here:

> I have not mentioned my father because I can't really remember him he is a Chief Petty Officer in the Navy he was hardly ever at home, I remember coming home from school one day it was raining I had on my mackintosh and wellingtons the water in gutter was rushing in the drains I was walking in the water and puddles wondering what I was going to have for my tea, I arrived home about a quarter past four, I opened the middle door that leads into the living room, Then I saw my father I felt proud of him at first he somehow looked very bussness like in his uniform. He told me to go and sit on his knee, and with him not being at home for a long time I felt shy, eventually he persuaded me to go and sit down, he than gave me a gold bangle which he said was from Africa I felt very proud of having something from there, he also gave me a big tin of chocolates. I felt on top of the world. About seven oclock he asked my mother what time the public house opened. It was from then I found what a rotter he was he thought of nothing but drink. I once caught him going to throw a saucepan at my mother it miss't and hit the pantry door the saucepan to this day has a dint in it.

The forsaken mother suffered ill-health and self-pity. At an early stage she enclosed a note with a letter to her daughter:

> To the person who opens these letters: When you have read ——'s letters you cannot know what a worry —— was, and she seems to have forgotten all that happened she used to say I ought to drop dead and call me a Bl—— dog and if I asked her where she'd been she'd tell me to mind my own business. She said she would never write to me and never wished to come home. . . . If I did as my mother and sisters tell me I should not write to —— because they know what a worry she's been.

But few of the girls could be so objective about their past. One, who said very tenderly what some others must have experienced, wrote:

We had lived at my Grans for nearly thirteen years, then my Mam and Dad had a argument and my [mother] left my Grans, so my Dad went to look for her and could not find her so he came back, the next day he went out again looking for her but still could not find her so he rang up my aunty —— in —— to see if she was their but she was not so for a few days my dad carried on with is work, and I could tell he was worrieing over her but he kept saying to me though your Mam doesn't love me anymore you do don't you so I kept on saying yes because he thought a lot more about me while my Mam was away but this did not last very long has four weeks after on a thursday night my dad went for a dring with my Grandad and they were not in long when some body came to my dad and said there is somebody to see you outside so my dad want out and there was my Mam she asked my dad for he cloths and my dad came back home, and I could tell there was some thing wrong because he told me to get all my mams things out of her drawer, so I did so and I packed them all in her case when I had packed the case my dad said to me (as I was the only one in) do you want to go and see your Mam she is at the corner of the street as I can't stop you from seeing her, so I started crying and my dad said allright I will upset you any more I won't be long, so he went out and about half a hour later he came back, by now the other kiddies were back from pictures, so he didn't say anything till the children went to bed, then he said to me your mam is missing you very much but she will not be coming back to your Grans. ever and that started me of crying again so my sat me on is knee and said you love your mam more than anybody don't you so I said yes (as I do). Well my Gran and the family came in then so he saked if I wanted to play cards with and I did and won him. . . .

Another, indulged and petted by her mother during the father's years in the war, wrote: 'When my daddy came out of the army my mummy ran away with another man who used to come and stay at our house very often. Daddy and I went to the Football Match one Saturday and when we came back we found my mother had gone it was quite a shock to me and I went into hospital with a nervous breakdown, I was very poorly.'

Sometimes the girl must clearly have wished more to be with the other partner than for a repair of the broken marriage. One intelligent girl, sick of her mother's nagging, and of her irrational tempers, cried in distress at receiving a letter from her mother on her birthday evening, and said it would have been a lovely birthday (at the Classifying School) otherwise. In her bitter hatred, and despite the father's plea from his separate address, she refused to write to her mother.

MAJOR DEPRIVATIONS

Finally we have a table with the summing up of reasons for parental absence. The totals are in respect of girls, not parents.

We shall later find (Table 29) that the percentages of girls not living with both parents were respectively 60·4 and 63·0; this is because 4·8 per cent of the 500 sample (twenty-four girls) and 8 per cent of the 100 sample had lost both parents in these ways. There were of course, other reasons for losing both parents, so that 18 per cent of the 500 sample and 20 per cent of the 100 sample were living with grandmother, relatives, foster parents, adoptive parents, or in institutions before further moves were made because of the Court procedures (Table 30).

Table 28: Reasons for Absence

Parents absent (all reasons)	Illegitimacy (reared by non-parent)		Death		Divorce, Separation		Total	
	Sample of 500 %	100	Sample of 500 %	100	Sample of 500 %	100	Sample of 500 %	100
Mother absent	5·0	7·0	12·0	10·0	10·4	13·0	27·4	30·0
Father absent	8·0	12·0	14·2	13·0	15·6	16·0	37·8	41·0
Total girls with parent absent							65·2	71·0

What bedevils any statistical procedure with such groups is that tragedies were sometimes heaped up, and moves were not simply a matter of a change of job and removal expenses, but of the dispersal of the child's universe. In fact no attempt was made to record household removals of the kind most of us know—such upheavals seemed so minor in comparison, and besides they did not seem to be so large numerically. But the following table, with the number of different home environments is concerned with the child's *roots*; this usually was based on changes of mother-figure, including foster-mothers, unless the fostering was a short-term arrangement, as for illness. An institution where a girl was expected to be 'at home' was counted.

The increase in parental absences in the later 1957 sample is reflected in the even smaller percentage of girls living consistently in one home environment—48 per cent as against 59·6 per cent in

Table 29: Number of Different Home Environments

Number of Environments	Sample of 500		Sample of 100
	No.	%	No.
1	298	59·6	48
2	93	18·6	18
3	56	11·2	15
4	24	4·8	5
5	13	2·6	8
6	9	1·8	3
More than 6	7	1·4	3
Total	500	100	100

the 500 sample. More serious is the fact that the percentage of those with more than four environments has gone up from 5·8 per cent to 14 per cent. This often reflects moves between foster-homes (intentionally long-term) and institutions, and does not speak well for a growth of society's understanding of the female child and—especially—of the female adolescent in the mid-twentieth century.

Linked up with the plurality of homes is the plurality of catastrophes in the child's life. Both can best be illustrated by a few examples.

This girl is recorded as having only two home environments (though she may have had a period in an institution). She retained her adoptive father but her mother died, her father deserted, and her adoptive mother deserted;

My mother died of tuberculosis six weeks after my birth, leaving my brother who was three years old and myself. My father Mr —— I don't know and would not like to know as I loathe him, for he was always hitting my mother and causing trouble. That is all I know about my own parents.

I was adopted . . . when I was just turned two years of age. They both loved me very much, dressed me beautifully and gave me everything possible a child of my age could have. My father went into the army the day I started school. . . . Nothing very interesting happened very much in the next three years except that I saw daddy less and another gentleman was coming to our house and I thought he liked mummy a little too much, and was taking her out quite a little more than I thought he should, my mummy told me to call him Uncle ——, so I never thought there was anything wrong in his visits and taking mummy out, till mummy started leaving me by myself sometimes all night, and smacking me if I said I was frightened and making me get myself ready for school

121

not bothering if I was neat and clean or not. Then daddy came home and we were very happy for about a year, all though mum and daddy were often quarrelling, and suddenly my mum went away while daddy had taken me to Rhyl for a day. Daddy said I wouldn't see mummy any more as they were going to be divorced, at the time I didn't under stand him, but I remember crying and I have not seen my mum for seven years this month, and I don't think I would recognize her now . . .

When I was twelve daddy was taken to hospital with yellow jaundice and kidney trouble, he was very ill, but he got over this illness and came out of hospital . . .

. . . In my last year at school I had started going with boys and coming in late at night, my school work was suffering . . . and I hated school, my reports said 'unreliable, has ability but doesn't use it', so I wouldn't go to school and I went worse I absconded from home four times in eighteen months . . . There is not much more to say except that my dad died six weeks ago of heart failure and a broken heart too. . . .

He died alone in a four-roomed wooden hut, poorly furnished and dirty, while the adopted daughter was on remand after stealing £1 17s. from a girl's wage packet.

The next girl had only three home environments as such, but the confusion and distortion of relationships might have accounted for a dozen. She was born illegitimately, for her mother, who had married a bigamist, left him to marry a man by whom she had two children, but returned to the first man and bore a third child. It was after this that she cohabited with a third man and bore our subject, plus two siblings. This man was killed when the girl was four. From this point her story (dictated) best recounts her vicissitudes, though she possibly did not know that there had been a fourth 'husband' in the home, before the fifth whom she disliked so much on her return from evacuation; this last proved eventually to be a happy marriage for the mother.

The first thing I remember is sitting under the table counting my mother's money. I remember when I was three years old I watched them carry my father past the window on a stretcher. They took him to the Infirmary and he died about a week later. I was only three when it happened, but I can remember it as plainly as daylight. He had collapsed and bumped his head against a lamp-post.

Afterwards I lived with my mother and brothers and sisters and then there was the War and we were bombed out of four houses. My brother was taken to Hospital, and they said they were taking all children to Hospital, so they took me as well. I had measles in hospital. I had my fifth birthday in hospital. I was in about a month and then I went to an evacuation place. I lived in a house with a woman—oh she was wicked and left us by myself in the house for nights on end. I was there about four months. She used to hit us, but not much, and she used to ask neighbours to look after us, and I used to sit for hours by myself.

122

The second place was a teacher's house—the teacher's house at the school at ——. When I was there she asked me if I could say my prayers properly, and I lived with her for about two months, and I was upstairs and she was getting ready to go and the bell rang and I forget what happened after, but she said there was a lady—Miss —— wanted to see me, and I went to live with her after that; it was in ——, and I stayed there for ages—until I was about nine or ten or something like that. I was very happy there, but I still cried for my mother. After that I came home. You got all your own way with Miss ——, and that was the cause of my bad temper. In the summer we went to the seaside to a hut owned by Miss —— and was there for weeks on end by the seaside. It was lovely. I came home for a holiday when I was eight, or something like that. We lived in —— Street. It was a terrible street. I stayed at home for a week. Miss —— thought I had gone home for good and got another evacuee and when I went back she kept me for a while, but she didn't want two, so I had to go home. . . . I had forgotten what my mother looked like and did not know I had any brothers and sisters. My mam used to mention them in letters and I did not know who they were. I can remember that we were all marching and all the parents were waiting for their children; we were all marching in fours and my mam shouted my name and I just walked straight on and did not know her. The teacher said 'there's your mother' but I said no.

I knew my mother went out with a man and I knew she was getting married. It was round about Easter time that I first saw him. He was quiet and cunning. It was on a Good Friday. We did not want to go out and he said 'go on out', and that was when I first didn't like him, and I never spoke to him hardly ever after that. And he seemed to have a spite for me after that. We could be having just an ordinary argument in the house, but he used to point to me and say 'will you shut-up', and I used to argue with him and he threatened me, and I was terrified to go to bed. He used to hit me and he knocked me right against the fireside. My mother used to stick up for us and did not like him to hit us. She used to say 'check them by all means, but don't hit them—I wouldn't hit them myself'. My brothers and sisters used to get on all right with him. One day I was arguing with my mam and he said 'Are you going to shut-up. Oh I'm going to see about this—your'e making everybody in the house ill', and there wasn't nobody ill, and he went down to see the Probation Officer, and she said I think this had better he passed on to Court and have a court case about this. He told her how I was cheeky and he wouldn't let my mam speak. He said no he couldn't do anything with her. He used to threaten he would get me away for three years. He used to say I'll see you away. Anyway he got his wish—there was a Court case on the Tuesday, and then I went to —— Remand Home for three weeks, and then I went back to Court and they said you will have to go away to an Approved School. I went back to —— until they could find an Approved School for me.

When we lived in —— Street, my mother used to take us with her when she went out and would not leave us in the house. It was a terrible house—that was when I was young—before I was evacuated. I was in the air-raid shelter all the four times when the houses were bombed, but I can only remember about once. I ran out of the shelter and started to scream and somebody said 'get that bairn in'. I remember screaming in the shelter and my mam saying 'Sh'. My mother was very good to me and never hit me in her life—she has been a mother and father to us.

She married again last year, in 1951. I hate him; it's him that got me here. When we left —— Street we lived at —— New Estate, and then we moved to —— Street.

I used to cheek the teachers at school, but I never played truant, except once, when I went with —— to the pictures.

My stepfather is still living with my mother. He said before I went away that if he found out I had a good report when he enquired—he has the nerve to say he will enquire—there will always be a welcome for me at home at any time. It's more my home than his anyway. There wouldn't have been all this trouble only for him.

My mother wants to try to get me home as she didn't think they would send me away for two years—she thinks a year will be enough for me to learn to behave myself.

That the second Training School was able to give this girl security and self-respect, and even make her into a graceful toe-dancer, says much for their technique. At the Classifying School she was vicious, jealous, and vituperative, as described in Pen-picture I on p. 65, flying off the handle at the least hint of criticism. She was transferred from the former Training School after serious violence.

Our girls were failures of some institution, be it the home or otherwise, but children who were early in Orphanages or Local Authority Nurseries and later failed, were abysmal failures. Usually the initial rejection could be pin-pointed as 'the cause'. Two outstanding problems were rejected illegitimate children. In one case the mother kept the child's existence secret from all but her parents. The child was in four Children's Homes, four foster-homes, one hostel, two residential posts, one 'refuge', one Mental Hospital, and spent two weeks in Prison as too unruly for normal remand before she reached the Classifying School. She was there two memorable weeks, survived a few days at a Training School and went to Borstal.

The following is the snakes and ladders exercise of another institution child:

Born youngest of five children.

At 2 her mother died.

At 3 admitted to a Children's Home, as the father could find no one to care for the children while he was at work (2nd environment).

At 5 moved from the Local Authority Nursery to a Cottage at the main Children's Homes (3rd environment—but in fact there would be at least two mother figures at the Cottage, counting the 'relief').

Soon after she was boarded out, but was naughty, so returned to the Homes (4th environment—but not known if returned to same Cottage).

At 9 she was boarded out with foster-parents (5th environment).

At 10 she was returned to the Homes, after petty pilfering in the foster-home. (Not known if same cottage and back to 4th environment.)

Six months later she was returned to the foster-home as the other child there had been found to be the pilferer, not our girl (back to 5th environment).

At 14, the foster-father was found to be an epileptic whose fits were now followed by violence. The Children's Committee instructed that our girl should be removed. She returned to the Children's Home. (Same cottage? Doubtful if same Housemother anyway after four years. Probably 6th environment.)

The girl now contacted her father, who had remarried and had four more children.

At 15 her father applied for the girl to be returned to his care. This was granted by the Children's Department. (7th environment— new mother-figure.)

One month later the step-mother disappeared. The girl stayed away from work and cared for the younger children and cooked their meals. They were later joined by an older sister when her husband turned her out. This sister subsequently vanished. When 16, after two of the younger children were in court for breaking and entering, and were admitted to care, our girl was incestually assaulted by her father, who was later sent to prison. She was remanded, then committed to Approved School as being in need of care or protection.

She was allocated after Classification to a Training School for the E.S.N. type of girl. From there contact was renewed with successful ex-foster-mother and (epileptic) ex-foster-father. They wrote and visited regularly.

At 17 the girl was all set for a home leave with them. Three days before it was due, the ex-foster-father telephoned to say that ex-foster-mother had gone off with another man. After permission was refused for her to spend her leave with the husband, no more was heard of foster-father or foster-mother for a year, by which time the foster-mother was remarried.

The other cases belonged to the 500 sample; this one belonged to the later sample; one would wish it belonged to the Dark Ages.

We shall later be searching for the statistical significance on personality and behaviour of these multiple changes.

We shall find that the girls with more than three 'lives' were, not surprisingly, more in evidence among the extreme attention-seekers (searching for their identity?), but the result was not significant, p being between ·2 and ·1.

After the break

A further Table (No. 30) gives the percentages living *mainly* with various adults after the parental breaks due to an illegitimate birth, to death or to divorce or separation. It is a simplified version, since, in more than 20 per cent of the 500 sample, and 34 per cent of the 100 sample, we had more than one change of environment to record, and in more than 5 per cent of the cases the changes were multiplied beyond normal statistical treatment. However we may see some of the outstanding features.

Table 30: Residence Following Break in Home

Persons with whom girl is mainly resident, after:	Illegitimacy %		Losing Parent(s) by Death %		Losing Parent(s) by Sep. or Divorce %		Total not living with both Parents %	
	500 Sample	100 Sample	500 Sample	100 Sample	500 Sample	100 Sample	500 Sample	100 Sample
Mother alone	·2	3·0	9·2	8·0	8·2	14·0	17·6	25·0
Mother and Grandmother	·8	1·0	1·2	2·0	1·6	2·0	3·6	5·0
Mother and other rel.	·2	—	—	—	—	—	·2	—
Father alone (mainly after 11 years)	—	—	3·8	5·0	2·6	2·0	6·4	7·0
Father with Grandmother or other rel.	—	—	—	—	·6	—	·6	—
Mother and Step-Father or Cohabitant	1·8	1·0	1·4	1·0	3·8	—	7·0	2·0
Father and Step-Mother or Co-habitant	—	—	3·6	1·0	3·4	5·0	7·0	6·0
Grandmother alone	1·8	1·0	2·8	2·0	2·6	3·0	9·4	7·0
Other rel. alone	·4	—	—	1·0	1·8			
Foster Parents	·4	2·0	—	—	—	—	·4	2·0
Adoptive Parents	2·0	4·0	·4	—	—	—	2·4	4·0
Institution(s)	·4	—	3·8	3·0	1·6	2·0	5·8	5·0
% not with both Parents	8·0	12·0	26·2	23·0	26·2	28·0	60·4	63·0
% with Parents							39·6	37·0

The Parents and Others. Present and Absent

The anomalous percentages of those with parents absent (see Table 28, Reasons for Absence) is accounted for mainly by the cases with both parents dead; these numbered 9, or 1·8 per cent of the 500 sample. Other reasons for apparent discrepancies are certain dual deprivations, such as we shall read of later in this section, as in a number of cases where the parents separated and the remaining one then died.

We see that, for whichever of the reasons, the greatest number of girls—88 and 25 respectively—lived with the mother alone after a major deprivation.

Statistical calculations showed there was a tendency for girls whose mother was absent for much of childhood to be particularly attention-seeking; this is not surprising with so many substitute mothers available in the Classifying School. Those with both parents absent also had proportionately more attention-seekers—but the chi-square result was not at significant level, p being between ·2 and ·1. Still, it is interesting that in all-female community those whose fathers were absent made relatively fewer demands on us.

However there was no relationship between the age of first being delinquent, and the role of the adults supplying early influence.

Finally Table 31 shows multiple deprivations, or what we have called 'Major detrimental situations' for fate was in fifty-eight cases not satisfied with dealing one large blow. To sift whether the kind of losses we have covered were 'major' to the girl would require a life-long study of her, or perhaps psycho-analysis. It may be that some of the later so-called 'Minor detrimental situations' were the more serious in some cases, but a firm line must be drawn in such probings. We have included the categories above—parental death, divorce, or separation, or illegitimate birth.

Table 31: Major Detrimental Situations

(Loss of one parent, or both, through illegitimacy, death, or separation or divorce).

Sample of 500

	Number of Major Detrimental Situations				
	None	1	2	3	Total
Total girls suffering	199	243	50	8	500
Percentage of girls suffering	39·8	48·6	10·0	1·6	100

Examples of experiencing three major detrimental situations:

(1) Child born illegitimately of co-habiting parents of whom one dies, and the other remarries, but subsequently separates from the step-parent; or the child is born illegitimately to the mother who dies, and the adoptive parents later separate.

(2) One parent dies. The other deserts his children. The second dies.

(3) Both parents die. The adoptive parents separate.

W. Litauer[7] found 63·3 per cent of his 'Court and Previous Disposal' guardians who were husband and wife (compared with our 39·6 per cent in the 500 sample). He found 23·2 per cent living with two heads of household, not both parents or husband and wife; we found 16·8. He found 13·5 per cent in families with one head of household; we find *37·8* per cent. (The remaining 5·8 per cent were in Institutions.) Yet he found that his sample contained more broken homes than did Carr-Saunders, Mannheim and Rhodes in *Young Offenders* (1948). The Gluecks[6] in *Unravelling Juvenile Delinquency* (1950) found 50·2 per cent of delinquents with their own parents, and 71·2 per cent of the controls.

A further comparison, which emphasizes the instability of the lives of our delinquent girl samples: Ivy Bennett[15] *Delinquent and Neurotic Children* (p. 218) found that 44 per cent of her delinquent group of fifty had broken homes (much fewer than our groups, even though more causes, of the kind we shall call minor, were included in her count), while only 11 per cent of fifty neurotic children, also attending Child Guidance Clinics, were thus hampered. Dr Kellmer Pringle,[17] in an investigation covering 2,593 children in schools and hostels for maladjusted children, found one parent absent in about 28 per cent of her sample, compared with 14 per cent among the general population. Their children were younger on average, which may be important, yet our adolescent girls seemed to go on collecting catastrophe points until they faded from our ken. A pretty child whose mother deserted her at 5 was in a Home until 8, when her father remarried. At 11 or 12 she began to truant and be difficult. At 16 she ran away instead of going to work. Beaten by her father, and remanded. Approved School committal. Relationship with father poor. At 17 her mother (remarried) advertised for information about her daughter. Contact was made, and became warm and 'sloppy'. At 18 she went on licence to her mother and step-father. She wrote newsy, interesting letters back to school. At 19 the mother's second marriage broke up, and the girl had to go into lodgings. Her ex-Headmistress wrote: 'J writes quite often, and her letters are always very interesting and nicely composed. I write as often as I can, as one way of minimizing the loneliness and disappointment upon the break-up of another home'.

Some writers have included less prolonged absences of mother or father in their assessments of broken homes; illness necessitating parental absence, or the withdrawal of parental care, or the imprisonment of a parent will cause a longer or shorter break in the family, and in the child's relationship with, and supervision by that parent. For the group we are dealing with yet another frequent cause of parental absence and home disruption was a father's departure to the Armed Forces between 1939 and 1945. During these intervals it would be rare for the remaining parent to be the same sort of person as before. In the case of an ill partner the other would be worried, and probably spending much time on hospital visits. One partner's imprisonment might well lead to bitterness in the other, and to evasions or strained relationships with neighbours and relatives. A husband in the Forces in war-time could make the wife troubled and absent-minded, or might lead her to pursue the offer of alternative affections, and so bring a very confusing relationship into the child's life. In all cases there would tend to be a withdrawal of affection from the child, mainly in so far as the remaining partner had lost the fount from which he or she drew, or should have drawn, affection.

The shorter parental absences for lesser illnesses, for 'going home to mother' after a marital quarrel, for the child being sent to auntie (or to an institution) while mother had another baby—these all constituted breaks in the mother–child relationship. A father working away could also constitute this.

Ivy Bennett,[15] in her study of fifty delinquent and fifty neurotic children, found highly significant differences between the two groups for interrupted mother–child and father–child relationships; of the former her fifty delinquents had a total of thirty-six such interruptions, and of the latter they had forty.

Yet another cause of such breaks is the child having a lengthy illness and hospitalization. And, in the case of our delinquent samples, there was the possibility of the child having been evacuated without mother during war-time.

We shall examine figures for what we call 'Minor detrimental situations'; to the child each of these could be a major situation, but compared with the seriousness of our major detrimental situations, involving total absence of a parent, we have assumed them to be minor.

Parental Illness

The accuracy of the figures in Table 32 cannot be vouchsafed. Some illnesses, such as recent ones affecting the supervision of a girl on probation, or recurrent illness of a neurotic nature, or of a kind likely to undermine the home's economic security, were due for mention in reports from Probation Officers for the Court. The official Approved School Form MH queried certain illnesses, such as TB in the family, and there was a space for further remarks, often extended by an accompanying letter. Causes of any parental death could supply a clue to long illness. This aspect of the home life was also a recurrent theme in the girls' 'Life Stories', as having affected them deeply.

The figures may be exaggerated at some points, for instance from a girl's inaccuracy about facts, and the time involved, but on the other hand there are likely to be many omissions. The figures refer not only to a parent being bodily absent from home but, to being unable to give the child reasonable attention and care during the illness.

Table 32: Parental Illness

Illness	Sample of 500 %	Sample of 100 %
Mother ill before 6 months	2·0	1·0
Father ill before 6 months	1·0	1·0
Mother ill before 3 years	2·8	1·0
Father ill before 3 years	1·0	1·0
Mother ill after 3 years	8·2	12·0
Father ill after 3 years	4·8	11·0
Mother ailing frequently	3·8	3·0
Father ailing frequently	11·2	4·0
Mother with recurrent nervous illness	2·4	1·0
Father with recurrent nervous illness	2·2	0
Guardian ill, or some doubt	1·6	3·0
Both parents reasonably healthy as far as known	62·0	64·0
Mothers ill or ailing	17·2	17·0
Fathers ill or ailing	19·2	16·0

The two samples show minor discrepancies especially in the large number of fathers ill after three years, and the smaller number ailing frequently; one explanation may be that there were fewer fathers, because of more permanent absences, in the 1957 group. Improved health services may be another reason.

Mothers in the 500 sample were recorded more often as being ill, and fathers more often as ailing. All told, eighty-six (17·2 per cent) of the 500 girls had mothers either ill or ailing, nervously or physically. As these refer (as far as we can know) to rather long periods of insecurity in the home, with mother away, or laid low, or the child being cared for elsewhere, it is not difficult to imagine the disruptions in the family, especially in one already disorganized for other reasons. We shall see that such a minor detrimental situation often went with major ones, such as the later death of the sick parent. The forty-six ailing or ill fathers (19·2 per cent) of the 500 cases would have a serious effect on the family finances over a period, or intermittently. Bronchitis was often given as the cause of paternal sickness and recurrent inability to earn.

Nervous illness was definitely mentioned for only twelve fathers and eleven mothers. All cases where a parent was described as 'neurotic' were not included, as the usage was sometimes suspect. Those included had usually had some hospital attention.

W. Litauer, at the Portman Clinic (1957) who found a larger percentage of illness recorded in his 'Court and Previous Disposal' cases, likewise discarded some of his reported 'nervy' families. His explanation of his low percentage of parents with 'normal' health (only 52·7 per cent in the homes with both parents, as against 73·8 per cent of Carr-Saunders, Mannheim and Rhodes *Young Offenders*) is a likely one in relation to the whole Classifying School samples as well—that 'the investigations in a psychiatric clinic usually reveal extensive information about the health of parents both physical and mental'; since our samples contained so many families with a missing parent, the sum total of parental illness was less verifiable.

As an example of the impact illness could make on a family, no history could compete with that of a 15-year-old child who came to us after failing to respond in her aunt's home when her father had been imprisoned for numerous offences of incest against her and her younger sister.

The mother was a diabetic:

My mother just started to not take her injections and my father was then demobbed from the army . . . I attended —— High School . . . but almost every week I had to stay of school because my mother was so ill, each time I went back I used to have to say I was ill. Mother would not

131

have a home help, so I had to do all the work, washing, ironing, baking, cooking and looking after my mother. My two sisters used to help me too, my mother kept going into diabetic combas, and was continually in and out of hospital. Then she atarted to have terrific pain and was told ... she had colitis ... and of course I used to have to keep cleaning her and vaselineing her because she was red-rore she used to scream in agony of pain, her legs started to swell and she was painfully thin so we suggested getting her a wheel chair ... and we all used to take her out round the town.

(In moments of confidence the daughter told of sudden mad impulses by the mother to be taken out in the chair during the night, and her demands that the daughters invade allotments to steal cabbages, which had to be explained away to the father! On other occasions the mother would order them out of bed to fry chips in the early hours.) 'Then she cried all night long, in pain and my Grandad, dad, and sisters and myself sat with her all night long, having sleep every so long.'

During these night watches, while one girl sat with the mother, the other shared a bed with the father, who, over a period of two years, demanded intercourse with each, unknown to the other. After the mother's death our girl began to run away from home, and was found by the police in a churchyard. She then told the story, and Court action ensued, leading to a prison sentence for the father, who, unable to take the further strain, was admitted to Mental Hospital. The girl could not settle with her aunt in a good home, and she arrived at the Classifying School, looking 'anxious, fidgety and emotionally starved'. She swung between extreme cooperativeness and irresponsibility, so that she lost face with girls and staff, and her fears of insanity grew. This pattern of conduct persisted for most of her period in a Training School, during which, despite all other possible care and devotion, queries by the Headmistress about her state of mind brought forth no offers of psychotherapy for her in isolation, or in conjunction with her father, as a means of dissolving some of the mountain of guilt standing between them. Meantime she alienated all her other relatives by misbehaving during home leaves. When last heard of she was leading a wandering, promiscuous life in London, and telling one fantastic tale on top of another during her brief returns to her home area.

The more serious known hereditary and infectious illnesses in families are classified in Table 33 opposite, for the two samples.

Caution has been exercised, and only if a parent was diagnosed as mentally defective was this recorded. Siblings, aunts, etc. are not included, hence perhaps the low figures compared with what Dr Epps found with her Borstal girls (1951).

Table 33: Detrimental Health History in Family

Defect	Sample of 500		Sample of 100
	No.	%	%
Epilepsy	12	2·4	3
Mental Illness	12	2·4	2
Tuberculosis	53	10·6	13
Other	2	0·4	1
Mentally defective	9	1·8	1
Not seriously detrimental	412	82·4	77
Not Known			3

We have already mentioned the frequency of tuberculosis in the samples (even higher in the 1957 group) and have instanced cases of very large families with father economically dependent for this reason. The following case has a slight variation: the mother, after many years of ill-health, died (a year before the girl's committal) of pulmonary tuberculosis, at the age of 45. Chest X-rays of the whole family after the mother's death showed that two younger brothers were infected. They were admitted to a Sanitorium. A younger sister, epileptic and mentally defective, was already in hospital. The father, though of good character, was in poor health, and was a cripple who, in our girl's memory, had never worked. Not a bracing environment for a 15-year-old.... She was a child of his second marriage, and there were three older half-siblings, to one of whom she returned on licence twenty months later. Within two months she was returned to the Training School, on the recommendation of the Children's Department—though reports say that no officer of the Department had seen the girl in the meantime. She joined the Forces, and, still virtually homeless, did well. Not only was such a home physically insecure, but it was enervating, removing stimulus to work and to life itself.

The main problem with a child of a mentally disturbed parent was her terror of inherited sickness, and if she possessed as violent and murderous a temper as two of the twelve girls in this category, each loss of control was followed by severe anxiety which had to be allayed; both were intelligent girls of good strong character potential, and stalwart physique—and it was fortunate that each serious out-burst occurred when a stronger adult personality was available to prevent serious injury, and to calm and reassure afterwards; there was no pretence about such outbreaks, and no one who witnessed them wondered how murders came to be committed. Fear was a strong element, in children who had not learned the measure of an adult environment, both girls having been reared in unnatural institutional worlds. They learned a measure of control, being ambitious to do well, and were known to be reasonably adjusted by twenty-one.

Separation from Parent Through Child's Illness

After the disasters piled up behind us, one might query the significance of a little spell in hospital. Dr Bowlby, and many writers quoted by him, found that any considerable period of maternal separation in early childhood especially before about 2½ years, could leave marks of emotional deprivation on the personality. Dr Trasler (*In Place of Parents*, 1960), after investigating a group of children who had been taken into the Local Authority's care, writes:

> Our investigation suggests that the degree of psychological disturbance which the child suffers is not greatly influenced by the objective circumstances of separation. A much more important factor appears to be the quality of his environment both before and after the event. The soundness of the child's resistance to anxiety and panic depends to a considerable extent upon the character of the relationship which has been established between him and his natural parents. If he can meet the disaster equipped with a secure knowledge of his own value, and a well-founded trust in the genuineness of his parents' affection, it will be easier for him to understand the reasons for their separation from him.

We have seen that a proportion of our Approved School girls must have been in grave doubts of their place in their family and thus of their own worth. On Dr Trasler's assumption we should expect more of our subsequently delinquent girls to have a record of early hospitalization (or other briefer separations) occurring alongside homes marked by severe detrimental situations, such as parental separations.

Our records of the child being in hospital are doubtless very incomplete. We had to rely mainly on careful completion of a form sent to each available home on a child's admission. For some children the parent who had their physical care in the early years was not available. Sometimes a distraught father would write: 'I have done my best with the form, but I was away in the army when she was small, and when I came back my wife had gone away'. Ivy Bennett[15] notes the difficulty of obtaining data on the early history of delinquent children, even where the child's own parents were available. Memories seemed to be vague and confused for the details of illnesses among the members—often of large families. This was so mainly with our dull, inadequate, but thus far cooperative mothers. Rarely could a Children's Department supply information about the early physical state of a child once in their care, since her moves had usually been many, her stays often brief, and staff in the Homes rather fluid.

We generally asked a girl if she had been in hospital, but details depended on her verbal facility, her sense of time, on her memory, or, perhaps sometimes, on her wish to forget yet another paragraph of a disrupted existence. Against our deficient information is the fact that we may have recorded briefer hospitalizations than could be considered damaging—though we omitted tonsillectomies, unless linked with other reasons for admission to hospital. But, as Dr Gibbens[11] (p. 78) says, 'Sometimes of course, the parent's incompetence or poverty makes it necessary to admit the child to hospital for almost every ailment'.

The following figures were obtained for the two samples, with a total of 26·2 per cent (or 131) girls and twenty-two girls respectively admitted to hospital. It may be that their similarity is a confirmation of a pattern of early childhood hospital detention of our delinquent girls:

Table 34: Separation from Home through Girl's Illness

	Sample of 500			Sample of 100	
	No	%	% per Year	%	% per Year
In hospital before 6 months	8	1·6	3·2	3·0	6
In hospital 6 months up to 3 years	10	2·0	0·8	3·0	1·2
In hospital 3 up to 5 years	18	3·6	1·8	3·0	1·5
In hospital 5 up to 12 years	62	12·4	1·8	11·0	1·6
In hospital after 12 years	34	6·8	2·0	10·0	3 (approx)
Not known to have been in hospital	368	73·6	—	70·0	—
Totals	500	100·0	—	100·0	

Admission after twelve years was often for treatment for venereal infections, usually after Court investigations had been held. However blasé the girl may have appeared, the physical and emotional experiences of the treatment must have been unhappy, and lowering to her morale. Inevitably, especially as a Court case, she would sometimes be treated as of less dignity than had she—say—had a fractured limb or appendicitis. She was also if in hospital in contact with a less desirable cross-section of society in Wards treating the disease.

Bowlby, *Maternal Care and Mental Health* (p. 28), says:

While there is reason to believe that all children under three and a very large proportion between three and five suffer from deprivation (i.e.

135

from maternal separation) in the case of those between five and eight it is probably a minority and the question arises—why some and not others? Contrary to what obtains in the younger age-groups, for children of this age the better their relation to their mothers the better can they tolerate separation.

This would mean, generally, that our Approved School girls between 5 and 8, and perhaps later, would be likely to show the classic effects of deprivation from a fair period in hospital. However, in assessing 'minor' detrimental situations (Table 31), a whole point has been scored for hospitalization before 5, and a half point after 5.

It is interesting that in both samples the highest incidence per year of hospitalization is before the age of 6 months. The formation of the mother–child bond would be weakened, with a possibly damaging effect on the child's early learning, and hence his mental and physical growth, while an unhappy or inadequate background thereafter would weaken this still further. On examining this (admittedly) small group of eight girls among the 500 sample, four prove to be illegitimate girls, three of whom would have in any case been able to achieve little relationship with immoral and rejecting mothers.

Case 1. Illegitimate Child. Was kept in hospital about a month because 'they were afraid she would not live'. She was cared for by her grandmother until a year old. Then her mother took her to live with her and her new husband. The child was totally blind in one eye about this time. At three the step-father was called up, so she was with her mother and grandmother. At 5 her mother commenced co-habitation with another man and took the child there. She failed to settle then and continued to find human relationships difficult, but was at least attractively sad.

Case 2. Weighed 2¾ lbs at birth and was kept in hospital for some months. Illegitimate, second of mother's eventual five surviving daughters, but eight more children all died. Most were legitimate, within a respectable marriage, before and after which the mother lived immorally, to the extent finally of imprisonment for brothel-keeping. The girl was a moaner, whose favourite bible-reading was from Jeremiah, but she was quite winsome, and was harmless.

Case 3. One of five illegitimate daughters of a trouble-making mother. Born in hospital and moved from there as an infant to another hospital, a hundred or more miles away, for investigation of elephantine legs, which remained hugely swollen. At five months she was fostered out. Removed later to a foster home where she was cruelly treated. Returned to the other, which, despite the mother's allegations, seemed helpful and good. Returned to her mother at 12 and says 'the trouble began'. Miscarriage at 14. Madly preoccupied with men and sexual matters, and converted the interest to 'sloppi-

136

ness' with her friends at the Classifying School when she was not moaning most insistently to staff.

Case 4. Child of gipsy parents, detained for unknown reason in hospital until adopted by intellectual cranks, who mismanaged her existent emotional problems to an indescribable degree, and created many more. Wandered from home persistently. Soiled herself. Developed a good vocabulary but reasoned almost at defective level. Remained a rejected child, though usually parental duty was seen to be done, and if the adoptive father failed to visit at the Classifying School it was because of 'work of national importance' nearer home. If a label must be used, this was the most psychopathic child of the four, who after her training still feebly rejected her noble home and had to be ascertained and institutionalized for her own safety.

Only for two of the remaining four girls who were hospitalized before 6 months, was there a home background not marred by physical loss of one parent at least; one, dropped by her sister at 2, and sustaining a fractured skull, was indulged by her mother throughout childhood, and lived to be jealous of the looks of her careless sister; the other was pampered for eight years after cataracts had been removed in infancy, until three younger children arrived to make the little home grossly over-crowded and mismanaged. The other two of this group of eight were ravaged by sickness, death, separation, and the one by years in an Institution, after which she had to adjust to a step-mother and five step-siblings.

Thus early hospital stays occurred, as Dr Trasler suggested, in these cases along with such other difficulties as to cloud the effect of the hospitalization. Indeed in only one case of the eighteen girls recorded as in hospital before the age of 3, was there seen to be a truly stable home background; if we count the two indulged girls described we have three. Even where the emotional stability of the home could be argued to be reasonable, the cause of the illness could be questioned as much as the separation. Certainly of those hospitalized before 6 months, 7 out of 8 seemed to be a particularly peevish, gloomy bunch. Those known to have been in hospital from 6 months to 3 years contained a few with classic rejection symptoms; the only one (where the home background seemed unimpeachable) that was probably traceable solely to the rejection, had been so aggressive with her mother for a year or two before committal that the latter could not be happily alone in the house with her. Even here there was again the complication of a head injury, the cause of being in hospital. With us she just looked boyishly pugilistic and behaved fairly normally.

One of the toddler group had grown into a teenager whose appearance varied between that of cherub, demon, and mere imp.

137

She was almost as overbearing in her brief deferential phases as in her regular destructive phases, when she was the most expert tantalizer we ever knew. We diagnosed her as 'to a large degree a child. . . . At some early phase she has obviously missed the firm discipline her temperament required, so that she is now unconsciously seeking punishment from those to whom she becomes most attached'. She was in hospital at 9 months; she had meningitis; a couple of years later her father was in the R.A.F., and was killed. When she was 10 her mother remarried, and the daughter claimed her stepfather treated her harshly; this was sad, but very understandable. She broke, entered and stole, was jealous of her sister, was unstable at school, and had Child Guidance treatment for six months. She stole again. When boarded out with her aunt she was 'dirty'. At the Remand Home she managed to swallow twenty half-grain tablets of phenobarbitone, and was admitted to Mental Hospital. At her Approved Training School 'her dreadful outbursts of temper frightened the girls and upset everybody. She found an outlet in ballet but unless she was always given the leading parts she upset the whole class'. Nine months after licence she was before the Court for larceny . . .

To sum up:

132 girls were recorded as having had a fair period (some a long period—one a period of nine years) in hospital, but ninety-six of these (about 80 per cent of them) had been over 5 at the time.

Of the eighteen in hospital before 3 years, eleven returned to homes where they were illegitimate, or where there was parental separation or death, then or later.

Of the eighteen in hospital between 3 and 5 years, thirteen returned to such homes.

Of the ninety-six in hospital from 5 to the time of committal, fifty-two returned to such homes, but in the remaining forty-four the hospital separation was linked with parental illness or a parent's imprisonment at some stage in twenty-three cases.

Separation Through Evacuation

Although the 500 girls were infants or young children in the early war years, and though a goodly portion lived in bombed cities, only 10 per cent were recorded as having been evacuated.

Of these fifty girls, twenty-eight were evacuated without their mother, usually for well over a year, some for much more. Thirteen were evacuated with their mother, and nine were evacuated to relatives.

We have heard in Chapter Ten of two who were evacuated from problem homes for a long period, until they identified themselves with the comfort and the love there, and found it impossible to settle at home on their return. We also have the other side of the coin:

> I remember arriving at the Farm . . . and then I remember my elder sister and my brother being wrapped up in big heavy coats that didn't belong to us, and being taken across to a neighbouring Farm (3 miles away) . . . You see there are five girls and one boy in our family . . . Then I remember my Mother coming to each one of us and telling us to be good and she'll be seeing us soon. She was going home. Oh how utterly dependent we were on her, who would plait my hair, who would make sure that Brian didn't frighten Rita (who was rather nervous). For the first time we really felt we couldn't do without her.

Few of our number were so articulate, and a good many received less mothering before and knew less what they missed, if they missed anything.

Again this experience, which has been advanced, especially by workers of psychoanalytical views, as being emotionally crippling to a child, stood alone in only three of the fifty girls evacuated in childhood. Of the twenty-eight girls evacuated without their mother, sixteen had a major detrimental experience besides—illegitimacy, parental separation or death. Ten more had at least one other minor detrimental experience. A girl who had a period in hospital at 2 with tuberculosis, was shortly afterwards evacuated to strangers for two years 'on health grounds'. During this time the mother separated from her co-habitant (the girl's father) and married. At 9 the girl was again in hospital (? TB). She was frequently in trouble for poor school attendance . . . When, later, she was out of hand and missing from her step-father's home, her own father died . . .

Father's Absence in H.M. Forces

Only 137 of the girls' fathers were recorded (in her official papers, in parents' reports or in the girl's story) as having served in H.M. Forces during the Second World War. This from 500 girls born between 1936 and 1940 suggests gaps in our records (even adding fathers lost from the start). The kind of industrial workers and the number of miners may have accounted for a proportion of excepted cases, indifferent physique for others, and a few fathers, where the girl was at the end of a large family, were too old.

But if the total number seems small, the proportion of those whose absence in the Forces was linked with parental separation, during the war or later, is considerable—42 per cent of the fathers who served. These were, of course, divided mostly between unfaithful wives and unfaithful husbands during absence, and failure to adapt to happy marital relationships later. This is no new story, but perhaps a grotesquely and tragically enlarged version.

The Parents and Others. Present and Absent

In thirty-two of the families where the father was away, a death of one parent is recorded. Not many fathers died on active service, but a good many were recorded as being in ill-health later. Illness of one or other parent is recorded in the case of about 40 of those 137 families. Only in 19 of the 137 was the father's separation from the family in the Forces recorded as the only detrimental situation. If it is questioned as being detrimental (in view of the thousands of young people who had undergone this deprivation without becoming delinquent or neurotic) we can justify it on the grounds that, in 86 per cent of instances, it was one more link missing from a rather frail chain.

Many of these girls recalled their father's return from the army with gifts from abroad. The impact was not always recorded. Sometimes the family had struggled (often with granny's help) to close the ranks, and father's impact was only gradually noticed—mainly if the quarrelling started. A few girls welcomed discipline of a kind they had missed. 'My father saw I was cheeky and took me in hand'. Sometimes—or often—a father's return meant that an only child, or one of two, became, after a gap of five or six years, the eldest of a string of little siblings, who crowded out the now inadequate home, swallowed up mother's time and any surplus money, and harrassed father. While the father adjusted to these new children as such, he sometimes found it very difficult to adjust to daughters whom he had not known during their formative years, and who were reaching dangerous adolescence. An unhappy return and unhappier sequel are seen in this story. The girl concerned was the younger of two daughters for six years, but became the second of eight:

I will start ny life story by going back to the time I was six years old I can rember the time my father came home from the war my sister and I were siting in a big shair near the window When my mother came in and said you father is coming home to day and I would like you to be good

Well we sat there fore one hour then all of a suden there came a loud bang at the door and my mother went to open it and there stood my father

He came in and we got up and said holo and then we sat down again because we were very frightened then two weeks later when we were at are tea my father got very made fore no reason at all and at that time my mother was having a baby. Well we all said nothing till my father got up and tryd to strangl my mother Then they started to have an argument then all at once my father struck out at my mother then he tryd to strangl her again but my Uncle Tommy got hold of him and made him let go and my mother ran into the kichen and I told my sister to run and get (Auntie Bell) the lady next door but she started to cry and by this time the house was up side down and my father keep on swering at my mother. Then going towards Bed tim he went quiet for a bite then he went to bed well this is all I can think of.

Well I will tell a story starting about two years ago when I was 12 year old about two years a go my mother was having her last baby Then one night my father went to a party and when he cam back he was drunck and that was the very first time I had ever seen my father drunk and it was the last.

He had not been in very long when he started to shout at me and he keep on saying that I was not his daughter and he said that if I did not die he would swing for me and when he said that he made me cry But the next day after that he would not leave me alone. Then one day my sister said that she had pains in her stomach so my mother took her to the doctors to see wat was the matter with her and he said that she was having a baby.

Then one day my mother ask who the baby was and she said it was my father's so he was sentencs 4 year inprion ment and when he come hom I will not liv with my mother because I hate my father and never will forgiv him of the shame he as brough upon my mother and sister
The end

It should be said, however, that of the eight fathers in the 500 sample who had incestual relations with their daughters, only three were recorded as having been absent from the home in the Forces, and one of the three (dealt with in an earlier chapter) had other precipitating causes. In another case there were allegations against a father whom the daughter resented from the first time she saw him —at the age of three. When he returned from the Forces and showed preference for the ensuing new baby, she resented him more than ever. Though at Secondary School 'nothing but good was known of her', she spent Saturday afternoons illicitly with a man in his late fifties, who paid her. When eventually she was taken to the Police Station by her father she accused him there of having interfered with her sexually three times. The overt problem in this case was doubtless present in a less obvious form in the minds of some other girls to whom father was a stranger on return.

We also met the problem of the father so imbued with the idea of unquestioning army discipline that he expected the same response 'at the double' from his children when he returned. Some fathers were bitterly hated for this reason.

Parent in Prison

Absence of a parent, a break in a child's care and supervision, and, most important, a break in what should be a cohesive relationship, are the points in mind at this stage in giving figures for a parent in prison. 'Delinquency in the family' is a favourite factor in causal works on delinquency; the Gluecks[6] found the families of delinquents fully twice as delinquent as those of the controls: 44·8 per cent of the delinquents and 15 per cent of the controls had criminal mothers; 66·2 per cent of the delinquents and 32 per cent of the controls had criminal fathers. Of Dr Epp's 300 Borstal Girls,[1] both parents had served a prison sentence in four cases, the mother in five cases, and the father in eight. Since at present we are concerned with breaks in the daughter/parent relationship, we are not quoting for delinquent siblings, and we are quoting periods spent by a parent in prison, not criminality, which seems a strong deduction to make from some of the incarcerations. Our totals of parental imprisonment—11·4 per cent—are higher than Dr Epps' which would, with the dual imprisonments, reach 7 per cent.

Table 35 gives the totals:

Table 35: Parent (or adoptive parent) absent through Imprisonment

Imprisonment	Sample of 500 %	Sample of 100 %
Mother in prison before 6 months	—	—
Father in prison before 6 months	1·2	—
Mother in prison before 3 years	—	1·0
Father in prison before 3 years	1·8	1·0
Mother in prison 3 to 11+ years	1·4	3·0
Father in prison 3 to 11+ years	2·4	2·0
Mother in prison after 11+ years	1·2	1·0
Father in prison after 11+ years	4·6	8·0
Neither parent known to have been imprisoned	88·6	84·0
Total mothers in prison	2·6	5·0
Total fathers in prison	8·8	11·0

Again these figures cannot be guaranteed; however the Record of Information for the Court contained a section for parental Court records, and this information should have been generally available from Police records.

In the 500 sample alone, we have yet another group of forty-four fathers who, at least for part of the girl's life, sometimes for longish terms, left the family circle incomplete. In twenty cases this was the only reason for incompleteness, the parents not having separated at

142

other times, except where the father had served in the Forces, or where (in one case) he had alternating periods in Mental Hospital, in Prison and at home, where—it would seem—a new child was invariably conceived.

In thirty of the fifty-seven cases with a criminal, neglectful, or sexually perverted history, leading to imprisonment of one partner, this was linked to a ruptured marriage. In a few cases the father elected to be imprisoned rather than maintain a wife whom he loathed. In most of these cases the marriage break was part of a pattern of psychopathy—aggressive or inadequate.

In seven instances one parent had died before the other went to prison. In two cases the shock of illness and loss of the partner seemed to pave the way to prison; one was our case of incest against the two daughters, the other the quoted case of death from childbirth. In the others it seemed as likely that the criminal or inadequate partner hastened the other's departure from life.

Of the fifty-seven cases where imprisonment was established, the following rough assessment has been made:

Table 36: Reasons for Imprisonment

	Cases	Father	Mother
1. Criminal group (Larceny, house-breaking, etc., forgery)			
(a) Habitual Criminals	21	17	4
(b) Isolated criminal offences	4	4	—
Total	25	21	4
2. Sexual offences			
(a) Incest, with girl committed to A.S.	8	8	—
Incest, with another daughter	2	2	—
(b) Brothel-keeping, procuring	4	—	4
(c) Bigamy	2	1	1
(d) Carnal knowledge of minor	1	1	—
(e) Practised illegal abortion	1	—	1
Total	18	12	6
3. Neglect (one with cruelty)	9	5	4
4. Non-payment of maintenance, or failure to send children to school	5	5	—
Total Imprisoned	57	43	14

Some of the twenty habitually criminal fathers (who form only about 35 per cent of the prisoners, and 4 per cent of our main sample) seemed to live a surprisingly normal family life while they were present and to take fatherly responsibilities quite seriously. Others, who were misfits there as outside, were often rejected and scorned by the daughter. In some cases, because of separation, or death of the other parent and consequent fostering, the girl did not know him well. One girl, who lost her mother at 3 months, lost the father when he was sentenced to prison two years later for neglect, and the children were boarded out—our girl in two separate homes, the sister in a succession of them. Her father seemed to drift. When the girl was asked if he had married again, she said no, and added, without malice, 'I don't think anyone would have him'. An inadequate, anti-social father could at this stage be shrugged off, if mother had been able to give some solidity, and if mother had not openly expressed fear that the daughter was 'bad like her father'. The problem that remained always was to build up some confidence in men, for the sake of a successful marriage in the future.

The ten girls with incestual fathers, eight of whom had come to Approved School as a result of being the junior partner in the incest, had a very difficult readjustment to make. In nearly every case the home relationships were in an upheaval; the mother either refused (sometimes justifiably) to believe the girl's story, or she was bitterly jealous, especially if she herself had aged prematurely. In one instance the mother had refused to the last to believe the story, and even then parental relations seemed to continue normally, while conflict raged round the girl's absence of guilt, or possession by guilt. Psychiatric and social witnesses found her severely troubled, while teachers dealing with her day by day were concerned that the affair had left no mark!

The girl who had been the victim of incest and had come to Approved School for care or protection, at least left the scandal behind. The two children who had lived through an experience where an older sister was the victim, who had seen the mother's distress, and heard the talk at school, and seen the neighbours whispering, were psychologically less disturbed but had much hatred to quell.

The proportion of mothers to fathers imprisoned in both groups is far higher than is usual between the sexes, being 1 : 3·4 in the more representative group of 500, against a proportion of about 1 : 12 in the Prison and Borstal Statistical Tables for 1954 (Publ. 1963).

To accept a reduction in a mother's dignity was often a very serious step. This could be so when a girl learned she was illegitimate, and if she learned from statement or innuendo that mother was 'no good'.

It lessened her own status, and the more so if the mother had been in prison.

I was 14 and had only 12 months to do at school. My mother got me and my two other sisters together and told us she would be going away for about 12 months and would we help her by going to live with my Father till she came back my two elder sisters flatly refused they were by this time old enough to go their own way in life, but my younger sister and brother and myself had no option, so we went to live with my father and his housekeeper. . . . My school work began to go wrong, and above all I found something out that I never knew, nor to this day would I have wanted to know. My headmistress asked me where my mother was. It then dawned on me that I didn't know. How could I tell her, I didn't know, she knew I was always with my mother. So I told her a lie. I said she's living in —— with my Grandmother, but all the time I didn't know. I then set about finding out. I found out rather crudely from my father, she was in Prison. What on earth had she done, it was a few weeks later that I found out she had helped some one with an ellegal operation and in return had received eighteen months imprisonment. Then I started, I done something foolish, and in return received 2 years Probation. I done eighteen months. Meanwhile my mother had come home and had gone to live with my two elder sisters, I only saw her once, and then she asked how was I, and never mentioned us coming back to live with her. She seemed to have gone older and lost all the love she had had for us. I could see she was ashamed of me. She didn't actually say so, but by her conversation, one could sometimes understand. Then I just about got fed up, and on impulse ran away from my father. . . . I was only away for a few hours, when I found myself in a remand home. When I appeared at court I was found to be in need of care and protection, and the court thought it wise that I should go to a Hostel in Birmingham. I didn't, within a month, I was of once again, this time not alone, there was a girl who seemed to be in the same position as me. . . . I thought girls in them places were all there for the same thing. When we were picked up I later found that I'd been dealing with a girl who was responsable for £100 or more worth of stolen goods. I was charged with receiving 4/9 worth of sandwiches, not know to me to be of stolen money. I was then committed to an approved school, but on waiting for a vacancy (there seems to be Hundreds waiting) I was remanded in ——. I got fed up with my selve there, and became mischeifous. The Matron took me back to court, I was then remanded to Birmingham Prison. *I now know why my Mother became bitter.*

The other two groups of parents with prison records belong mainly to the irresponsible, the feckless, the poor managers, who fail to care for their children at home, or fail to send them to school, and fail to pay maintenance when they have been 'sent away', or to maintain the wife from whom they are separated. But these comprised only 3 per cent of the 500 sample—though, of course, many others had been neglectful without being subject to imprisonment.

Leaving the concept of absence temporarily, and returning to the concept of criminality of home background, which we dismissed early in the chapter, we are now reminded that not all delinquent parents go to prison.

This research also showed that, in the 500 sample, 9·2 per cent had fathers, and 4 per cent mothers, who were known to have been in trouble with the police, and 1 per cent had both parents, while six girls were reared by relatives who had been in trouble, making a total of 16 per cent. This is only 3·8 per cent more, or nineteen girls more, than those who went to prison.

Nor would one say, on recall, that the daughters of the delinquent parents were necessarily our most delinquent girls; especially was this not so of our neglected girls, except where the neglect occurred in infancy and led to the child being institution-reared. This brings one to a conclusion by Harriet Wilson, *Delinquency and Child Neglect*[16] (1962) (pp. 146-7) 'The delinquencies he commits are not behaviour patterns instilled into him by his elders; they are the only method by which he can get what he wants, a method learnt in infancy.... The type of delinquency which is born out of neglect is different in nature from delinquency arising in a home that is well aware of the moral standards of society.' She found the neglectful parents were alike in a negative way only, and that the children's delinquencies were not closely linked with the personalities of the parents. On the basis of our brief examination at this point of a small section of our sample, this would seem to be a fair picture.

We shall find later that, in accord with the 'delinquent family' thesis, multiple delinquent siblings tended to be in families with a delinquent parent or parents.

We have now come to the end of a fairly detailed account of the nature of the parental and other homes our Approved School girls had experienced. We rated the following as major detrimental situations:

1. Illegitimacy.
2. Death of Parent(s).
3. Separation, divorce of parents.

We have seen that 8 of the 500 sample managed to suffer all three, and 50 suffered two; 199 suffered none.

The following, rated as minor detrimental situations were:

1. Serious illness of parent.
2. Imprisonment of parent.

3. Father absent in Forces.
4. Child evacuated without Mother.
5. Child been in hospital for a period (half-point if after 5 years).

We have noted that our girls seldom had their troubles singly. It is, indeed, surprising to find on coordinating the major and minor detrimental situations that 57 of the 500 suffered none of those listed, and 19 more suffered hospitalization after five years only. Top place was taken with three major disturbances and two minor ones—both parents died; the adoptive parents separated when the mother deserted; the adoptive father was away in the Forces, and later he had two severe illnesses and could not supervise the girl. Yet she was one of the most successful girls who passed through the Classifying School at this time. We have already read her own account.

When we come to statistical relationships between broken homes and other factors especially success in and after Approved School training, we shall find the accumulated major and minor detrimental situations have been used for the purpose. This was because sorrows had come in twos and threes to some, while others seemed to have escaped relatively slightly. Did this affect the girl's nature, her cooperation, her responsiveness to others, her eventual success?

The grouping of the situations for the contingency tables was this:

Table 37

	Cases
No major and no minor detrimental situations	57
1, 2 or 3 major, but no minor detrimental situations	72
No major, but from $\frac{1}{2}$* to $2\frac{1}{2}$ or more minor situations	144
1, 2 or 3 major and from $\frac{1}{2}$ to $2\frac{1}{2}$ or more detrimental situations	227

* $\frac{1}{2}$ = hospitalization after five years.

This grouping was necessary for statistical reasons. Inevitably the insolated cases, and indeed whole groups lose themselves. So that this does not happen prematurely, there is a more precise picture in Table 38, page 148.

To continue in cold statistical terms, we shall see in a later chapter that the four groupings above (Table 37) were inter-related with a number of factors.

It was found, that the piling up of difficulties in some cases did not link significantly with early committal to Approved School nor with the age of the first known delinquency. There was a significant link with the cause of her committal to Approved School, mainly for

Table 38

Detrimental situations	Cases
No major, no minor	57
1 major no minor	60
2 or 3 major, no minor	12
No major, $\frac{1}{2}$ or 1	82
1 major, $\frac{1}{2}$ or 1	110
2 or 3 major, $\frac{1}{2}$ or 1	28
No major, $1\frac{1}{2}$ or 2	45
1 major, $1\frac{1}{2}$ or 2	52
2 or 3 major, $1\frac{1}{2}$ or 2	16
No major, $2\frac{1}{2}$ or more	17
1 or 2 major, $2\frac{1}{2}$ or more	21
Total	**500**

those committed as being beyond control of parents, guardians or other 'fit persons' in whose control they had been placed. Not surprisingly, disproportionately more of these were girls who had one, two or three major detrimental situations in their lives. In the same way, for the small category of those committed for absconding from the care of a fit person, or having an 'Approved School order substituted for the fit person order', more were in fact girls living mainly in institutions, having suffered the gamut of early major *and* minor disasters, and to some extent healthily rebelling at being in Homes or other people's houses.

Other statistical connections are more surprising, especially that the girls with *no* early separations tended to do *worse* in later years (see Chapter XXI).

Chapter Twelve

EARLIEST ABNORMAL
ENVIRONMENTAL EXPERIENCES

We have talked hitherto of what the difficulties were and the measures resorted to by Society, but as so many things happened to these girls, we shall go back to the earliest break with the home environment of any proportions and see what this tells us.

The heading, borrowed from the Gluecks'[1] *500 Delinquent Women* is defined by them (pp. 387–8) as follows: 'This refers to the nature of the first departure of the offender from the home or environment in which she was reared, a departure caused by a situation sufficiently serious, unusual, or marked in character to denote a breach in the family and/or community ties.'

Apart from those on whom a break was imposed, a sizable percentage took the step of their own accord; perhaps 'driven to it by circumstances' is a truer account.

The age at which the break happened is more important, and a comparison with the Gluecks'[1] *500 Delinquent Women* will be interesting.

In Table 39 we compare the ages for this first marked breach in family and/or community ties. Unfortunately the age groups are different, but rough comparison is possible. We find a sadly regressive feature in the later Shaw sample, where 29 per cent of the children had been removed from the natural home setting for a considerable period before 8 years of age; we shall see in the next Table (No. 40) that the increase was more due to instances of neglect than to complete break-ups of the home. The figure would seem close to that found by the Gluecks thirty years earlier, allowing for different age-groupings. 22 per cent of the 500 sample removed before eight years is still sizable. At the other end of the scale, we find 13·4 per cent of the American prison women who experienced this first major disruption after reaching nineteen.

This table will be found to correlate significantly with behaviour at the Classifying School and Training School.

The reasons for the disruption from the family are seen in Table 40 to be again remarkably close, especially for girls running away, or leaving home of their own accord (which in the case of a girl who is older, but not old enough, can be done with economic but not legal impunity—if the parents or police decide to charge the girl!).

Abnormal experiences of broken homes likewise run parallel. Descriptions on the right are in the Gluecks' terminology.[1] Discrepancies for delinquency are even greater than they seem, since the first Shaw group, who left home only as a result of the recent Court procedure, was also delinquent (nominally, at least).

Table 39: Age first left home (or Age at time of First Abnormal Environmental Experience)

Shaw Girls	Sample of 500	Sample of 100	Gluecks' 500 Women	
	%	%	%	Age
Never till present committal or prior remand:				
(i.e. age 14 to 16 inclusive)	25·6	13·0		
4 years or under	12·2	20·0		
			25·3	Under 7
5 to 8 years (inclusive)	9·6	9·0		
			13·4	7 to 10
9 to 12 years (inclusive)	12·8	12·0		
			17·1	11 to 14
13 to 14 years (inclusive)	13·4	15·0		
15 to 17 years (inclusive)	26·4	31·0		
			30·8	15 to 18
	100·0	100·0	86·6	
			13·4	19 and over

What we have here seem to be roughly parallel situations in the lives of two young female populations which, when the concomitant behaviour impinges on the adult outside world, lead to somewhat parallel decisions being made—except that both the English sections seem to have been dubbed delinquent at an earlier stage in the proceedings, and to have been treated more punitively (since a penal institution cannot pretend about its punitiveness, in the child's and parents' and society's eyes). As Dr Bovet[2] says in *Psychiatric Aspects of Juvenile Delinquency* (p. 10), 'It must be rare for decisions with serious coercive consequences to be taken with so little supporting evidence as in the case of juvenile delinquency.' And if, as he says, the emotional state in which workers and society approach the

Earliest Abnormal Environmental Experiences

Table 40: *Reason for First Leaving Home (or Reason for Earliest Abnormal Environmental Experience)*

Shaw Girls	Sample of 500 %	Sample of 100 %	Gluecks' 500 Women	
Did not leave home until recent Court procedure	25·6	13·0		
Evacuation	3·8	—		
Previous delinquencies	23·2	26·0	15·7	Delinquency of offender
Break-up of household through death, separation, illness, poverty	16·4	15·0	17·8	⎧Death of Parent(s) ⎨Separation etc., ⎩Illness of parents—
Parents, guardians unable to continue care	3·4	16·0	12·5	Neglect of offender or home for other reasons unsuitable
Child left of own accord to live with other adults, boy friend, or live promiscuously or wander	17·8	19·0	17·1	Ran away from home
To seek employment	2·4	—	6·0	To seek employment
Other reasons (usually child's illness)	7·4	11·0	7·9	Other reasons
			23·0	Migration

problem is even more responsible for the paucity of objective information, then certainly it is even more true of girls, that there is much heat of emotion in those workers discussing them, and far more serious paucity of information.

Chapter Thirteen

RELATIONS WITH SIBLINGS

SIBLINGS

We have hitherto spoken of the child versus parent, parents or no parent, as if no siblings, half-siblings and step-siblings existed. They certainly did: our Classifying School girls had amassed an unseemly number of siblings of one kind or another.

To the writer's surprise, there were 37 per cent children with first place in the family, and this was so for the 500 sample and the 100 sample. Of these 11 per cent of the 500, and 18 per cent of the 100, were first and only children—or were so until a parent remarried, or co-habited elsewhere, and then 66 per cent of the only children became the eldest or youngest, or even the mid-child of quite a sequence of half-and/or step-siblings. Finally, then, only 4 per cent (twenty girls) of the 500 group remained only children, but 10 per cent of the 100 group were in this category.

Sometimes the erstwhile only children were illegitimate babies. The way such complications could arise is illustrated in an essentially kindly 16-year-old girl who was committed to Approved School after falling foul of a woman with a criminal record and convictions for prostitution. The girl was born illegitimately of her parents' co-habitation, but two months later her mother abandoned her and she was cared for by her father, until, a year later, he moved to another county where he lived with a divorcee, whose own children (number unknown) were in their father's custody. The girl was well behaved at school, but often late 'due to home conditions'. She had to dress an increasing number of her seven little half-siblings for school. She had no pocket money and no free evenings, and eventually rebelled and stayed out late with undesirable youths. After 12 months' residence at a Probation Home she returned home to find her place as eldest sister taken by a 17-year-old step-sister—one of her step-mother's prior to the second marriage. These two girls eventually ran away together and lived in diverse questionable company. Mean-time—though not directly impinging on her life—her own mother had three children by another association. Thus she had, not seven half-siblings, but seven plus three, and some step-siblings. Her family position in a comfortable house with stable parents and a daily woman could have been delightful, but her father, step-mother, seven younger children, the elder step-sister and our girl lived in a five-roomed house—poorly furnished and untidy—in derelict property. They lived mainly on National Assistance, for the father was rarely employed.

The 26 per cent first children who became eldest of a family of full siblings (with or without half-siblings) were distributed fairly normally among the varying sizes of families, except for a bulge, where twenty girls (4 per cent) were the eldest in families of five. One was the eldest of ten, and one of eleven; but the initial surmise that these eldest girls were the drudge of the large families was not proved —except that an analysis of brothers and sisters (if completed) might have revealed 'eldest girl' positions.

In both samples, 22 to 23 per cent were second in a family of anything up to eleven children with a rather disproportionate tendency to be second of three (6·6 per cent).

If a genuinely significant position occurred in our sample, it was for girls to be fourth in a family of four (5 per cent); third and fourth in a family of five (each 5 per cent); third or last in a family of six (about 2 per cent each), or in the middle of families of seven, eight and nine, of which there were naturally not so many. 42·8 per cent of the 500 sample, and 35 per cent of the 100 sample, were from families of five or more (without counting half- or step-siblings), compared with 45 per cent of Dr Epps'[1] Borstal sample in 1951; the dates of the three samples may account for the steady drop from 1951 to 1957.

Thirteen of the 500 sample were from families with more than ten full siblings—six families with eleven and the remaining seven ranging up to seventeen. Of the Gluecks'[2] 500 Delinquent Women (30 years earlier) 20·6 per cent were from families of ten or more.

During 1952–4 the average size of family in England and Wales was about 1·9*. Our girls' families of full siblings average 4·3 in the years 1952–4 and 3·9 in 1957.

The Gluecks,[2] in *Unravelling Delinquency* (p. 120) found that lower proportions of the 500 delinquent boys were only children, first children or youngest children, and a significantly high number (compared with the control group) were middle children. This was 'contrary to general expectation' because 'only children, first children and youngest children are thought to be especially vulnerable to the development of behaviour difficulties, because they receive preferential treatment'. Another more recent view would be that only children and first children are handled by a less confident, less experienced mother. Much has already been written in this study to

* For women married once only, aged under 45, and married up to 10 years.

show the multiple shocks and changes in the lives of so many of these delinquent girls. By the time we reduce our only girls by the number who attained half-siblings, we find our numbers nearer to the Gluecks', where step-siblings were included. Generally the figure for all the groups have much in common, and the tendency to certain over-represented mid-positions in the 500 sample at the Classifying School has been emphasized. In these large families—over-crowded often, sometimes with a mother who could give adequate mothering to two or three but whose emotional resources dwindled under stress of sheer hard work and demands on her patience—we can see that the conditions of partial maternal separation could occur even where illness, imprisonment, gaps in the family, divorce and death and all the other factors mentioned did not intrude.

One peculiarity in the Shaw group was for the very large families to belong to fathers unemployed either for real reasons like tuberculosis (as instanced in Chapter XI) or for less clear reasons. One girl was the second youngest of her father's twenty-two children, ten being by his second marriage, and of these all but two had been in trouble. The father, who lost one finger in the First World War, never lifted another outside their three-bedroomed Council house, but presumably increased his pension for dependents as he went along.

Half- and Step-Siblings

The following figures give the distribution of half- and step-siblings:

37 (7·4 per cent of the 500) *only* children later had half- or step-siblings.

32 (6·4 per cent of the 500) in families of *two* had half- or step-siblings.

51 (10·2 per cent of the 500) in families of *three or more* had half- or step-siblings.

All told, 23·8 per cent had half- or step-siblings.

The average number of half- or step-siblings possessed by a girl was about 2·2; over the 500 it was 0·2 per girl. In addition thirty-four girls lived in homes where there were children of other adults (e.g. of an older sister, or of a lodger).

Sibling Deaths

Some of the sibling groups were not intact. Only for the intake of 1954 were careful records kept of the entries on Form MH, which the parents (where available) had filled in conscientiously. Fifty-four deaths of siblings or half-siblings (apart from a few recorded still-births) were recorded for 156 families; but fifty families were affected, because of multiple losses to a few mothers, Table 42 shows the causes, as recorded.

Table 41: Comparison of Family Place, Size, etc. with other Research

	Shaw sample of 500 %	Shaw sample of 100 %	Epps[1] Borstal Girls %	I.S.T.D.[3] %	Lees and Newsom[4] sample	Gluecks[5] Unravelling Delinquency	Gluecks[2] 500 Women
Only	11·2	18·0	13·3	11·8	5·2	4·8	3·2
Eldest	26·0	19·0	21·6	26·2	21·3	15·6	22·7
Intermediate	42·6	36·0	36·5	38·5	51·1	60·0	Not known
Youngest	20·2	27·0	28·6*	23·5†	22·3	19·6	,, ,,*
	100	100	100	100	100	100	100
No. of Cases	500	100	300	187	502	500	500
Average size of family	4·3 (full-sibs)	3·9 (full-sibs)	—	3·9 (with step-sibs)	—	6·85 (With step and half sibs)	About 6·3 (? full sibs)
% of Only Children with step or half-sibs	7·4	8·0	6·7	—	—	—	—

* *An older group.* † *A younger group.*

Table 42: Causes of Sibling Deaths

Cause, as given	Under 1 year	1 to 5 years	5 to 16 years	Age uncertain	Total
Pneumonia, bronchial pneumonia, bronchitis	11*	4	—	—	15
Fits, convulsions	3	1	—	—	4
Gastro-enteritis	4†	—	—	—	4
Meningitis	1	1	1	1	4
Congenital defect	3	—	—	—	3
Infectious diseases (e.g. measles)	1	1	1	—	3
Scalds or burns	—	2	—	—	2
Accident	—	4†	1	—	5
Other, or no cause given	5	2	1	6	14
Total sibling deaths	28	15	4	7	54

Total girls in 1954		156
Total cases with dead Sibling(s)		50

* Three in one family.   † Two in one family.

The losses in these fifty families could have occurred, on an average perhaps, at any time within the years 1938–53; this makes comparison with national figures impossible, as it was a decade within which deaths for gastro-enteritis and meningitis were strikingly reduced; this does not seem to have been so for the bronchial group, which is the highest, as it was for paternal deaths, and may partially have been linked with smog, bad housing, overcrowding, and—sometimes—incapacity to give normal home care.

Gaps in Families

Another feature with our sample was large gaps in families, due often in our main sample to a father's long absence in the Forces, and the enlargement of the original family, or a new family by a second wife on his return. Jealousy and resentment could thus arise, because of the gradual reduction in standard of living, when a modest income and living space were subdivided again and again. Of the 156 families of the girls who came to us in 1954, forty-two had gaps of six years or more. One family, with four children before the father's absence, and three subsequently, was riddled with jealousy and resentment which wore them and the parents down; the eldest three girls (all pre-gap) came to us.

One might expect a girl placed in an unfavourable position in a large family to have made greater demands for our attention;

statistically this was not so. There were, however, other interesting relationships. The large families related significantly (p > ·001) with poor economic status and poor material condition, even in this unrepresentative economic sample. Scholastic attainment in reading was, as expected, significantly worse in the largest families (p > ·01).

SIBLING DELINQUENCY

Out of sheer quantity, in these teeming families we could expect more girls to have one delinquent or troublesome sibling. That the numbers will exceed chance expectations we shall see (p > ·001).

We shall also be thinking back to our figures for parents in prison, and parents who had been in trouble with the Police, or just a dubious influence.

Of the 500 group, 12·6 per cent (sixty-three girls) were known to have one brother or sister, and 8·6 per cent (forty-three girls) more than one, who had been delinquent; it was not always clear, in the case of a delinquent sister that she had been before the Court, though recorded as having 'been in trouble'. (3·8 per cent more had a brother or sister who had been a dubious influence; this was recorded where, for instance, an older sister had been known to be promiscuous, but was not before the Court, for superior age or other reasons.) Of these 21·2 per cent, or 106 girls who had delinquent siblings, only twenty-six had a parent or parents recorded as in trouble. The total with delinquent parents or siblings was thus 156. This is shown in Table 43 based on Table 6 of Litauer's[3] I.S.T.D. study (1957). This latter is, of course, a younger group, with less time for delinquent histories. His figures are, however, entered for comparison, also Dr Epps'[1] results, and Dr Mannheims' (1948), despite age discrepancies.

The comparison with the I.S.T.D. sample is very interesting. While the Shaw sample probably suffers from the 'inadequate probing' suggested by Dr Litauer for other non-clinical samples, the low percentage of delinquent mothers in his sample is equally suspect, since mothers rather than fathers would be the informants at the Psychiatric Clinic, and his mothers rate surprisingly low! On the other hand, a delinquent mother may be a more serious handicap to a girl than to a boy, though some scanning of our present group suggested this was so only where the mother had been imprisoned.

105 girls came from homes described as having parents with *good moral standards*. Nineteen of these girls had no siblings, and seven were separated early from siblings; these last, if examined closely, were probably girls reared in morally good adoptive homes. Thirty-six—about one third—of these girls seemed to have reasonable

Table 43: Delinquency in Family

Delinquent Member of Family	Shaw Sample of 500 %	I.S.T.D.[8] whole sample %	Mannheim[6] (1948) %	Epps[1] (1951) %
1 Sibling	12·6	15·0	18·0 to 27·5 with one or more Sibling	
2 or more siblings	8·6	5·0		
Father	10·2	11·4		
Mother	5·0	1·0	—	
Total	36·4	32·4		
Both sibling(s) and parent(s) delinquent	5·2	—	—	
Percentage with one or more delinquent in immediate family	31·2	32·4	—	28·6*

* Dr Epps[1] *seems to have included some outside the immediate family.*

support from their siblings. But 9 of these 105—not a disproportionate number, but an unexpected number—had another sibling
who had been in trouble. (One recalls in this connection the girl who
resented bitterly when her twin brother left her side to team up with
the lads of the village in early adolescence; she went off the rails in
pique, and after she had been committed to Approved School he
began stealing.)

Twenty-two of these girls from 'good' homes were recorded
strongly jealous of a sibling or siblings, whereas records showed only
twice this total number as being excessively jealous at home. While
this supports my own hunch, that excessive sibling jealousy is more
a feature of protective homes (the kind which seek help at Child
Guidance Clinics) rather than where the struggle for existence
demands that all stick together, in however a rough-and-ready a
manner, yet there are arguments which make the figure unacceptable:

(a) The Social worker exploring the home situation for the pre-
committal inquiry did not need to look for sibling jealousy as a
motive in most home backgrounds—there was plenty of obvious
deprivation or insecurity or both.

(b) The writer in the same way, and other staff at the Classifying
School looked hard for sibling rivalry only when the home yielded
few other adverse factors.

Seventy-six girls were from homes with a parent or parents known to have been delinquent. Twelve of these had had one sibling in trouble, and fourteen had had two or more in trouble; this is a significant proportion, as we have seen.

Apart from delinquent records, there were twenty fathers and eighty-three mothers of 'doubtful morals'. The former had no apparent link with sibling complications, the latter did—14 of the 83 were separated early from brothers and sisters and ten had two or more siblings also in trouble.

Sixty-five girls were from homes where moral training seemed to have been neglected; this is obviously not an exclusive number, but cases where the more positive delinquent facts were absent. In these cases there was a significantly high number of dubious or delinquent siblings.

Some circular reasoning must be admitted where objective evidence was lacking, or had been deduced by the social worker visiting the home before Approved School committal (just as the writer tended to deduce it from what other evidence there was). Several siblings having been in trouble suggested inadequate moral training, though not always was there definite evidence of this; a mother's association with another man in her husband's absence suggested dubious moral standards, whereas dubious maternal standards would be a safer analysis; the last might lead to a break-up of the home and the dispersal of the children, hence the somewhat disproportionate number (fourteen), or a quarter of those separated early from sibs, who were said to have a less than moral mother.

Fathers in trouble with the police exceeded the score for mothers, but fathers of dubious morals scored much lower than dubious mothers. This speaks more, probably, of the dual standards for the sexes than for any very obvious finding, since unfaithfulness by the father would be less likely to leave evidence, or to be regarded as so 'unnatural'. The consequences of the mother's dubious standards (break-up of the home, or intermittent separations) may more often be the unsettling influence for the family than her morals in themselves. A girl was sometimes extremely attached to a mother who was spurned socially for her laxity of morals, and the same mother might be earnest and sincere in trying to help the girl to see straight. The 'nicest' girl in the 500 sample had a mother and other maternal relatives known as local prostitutes. Her half-sisters (older and younger) had proceeded or were proceeding in the same direction. She wept without bitterness, but great sorrow, when her mother was convicted for neglecting the younger children. Though she was the only one of the seven surviving children to be born of their mother's one brief and stormy marriage, and though the home was well known to the school attendance officer and the N.S.P.C.C., she wrote: 'Our family has not been one mass of trouble, we have had many happy times together,'—and described vividly the tableaux at the local festivals, and the rare outings to Blackpool and Southport. After succeeding at her Training School she was so home-sick that she ran away from a good residential post to be with her mother, still a marked woman locally, and so the girl had to play an evading game (within the law) to be near the mother, who, she wrote earlier 'loves us all'.

When we look closely at the families where two or more siblings of our girl delinquent have been in trouble, and where we find a startling link with the father's criminal history, the total being twice the proportional total, we must again be careful about influences; a girl might be devoted to her lax father, but the jibes of schoolmates at his Court appearances, or a neglected deprived home if he is imprisoned, will do little for her and her siblings' morale. Sometimes, for obvious reasons, the offending father was the missing link in a fatherless home, or a home with a rejecting step-father.

Briefly, of the 106 girls (21·2 per cent of our main sample) who had one or more siblings who, too, were delinquent:

21 seemed to be from morally neglectful homes
26 were from homes with one or more delinquent parents
22 seemed to be from homes with a morally dubious mother
9 were from good homes.

Of the 26 girls (5·2 per cent of the main sample) who had a delinquent parent or parents, *and* one or more delinquent siblings, a rough assessment of the girls' records and personalities suggests that

5 girls were very delinquent
10 girls were fairly delinquent
4 girls were mildly, or virtually non-delinquent
7 were more inadequate than delinquent.

9 of these 26 showed 'tough' characteristics which to us spelt either a tough exterior to a vulnerable child, or a rarely approachable being who constituted serious difficulties in the group. In the 100 sample, 20 per cent had delinquent parents or guardians, and 24 per cent had one or more delinquent siblings, i.e. considerably more of both.

Though the discussion has been mainly on environmental lines in this 'delinquent family' section, hereditary traits are by no means out of the writer's mind. Otherwise why did the 'nice' girl—nice by any standards—exist amid a depraved family? Or were they (the rest of the family) just as 'nice', but hounded by an uncharitable society, or by the whims of fortune?

Statistically there was a significant relationship ($p > \cdot001$) between sibling complications and delinquency in the home. 'Doubtful morals' tended strongly to lead to early separation from siblings, and all that this entailed. Moral neglect led significantly to sibling delinquency. But the circularity of the arguments regarding parental morals has been noted too.

Chapter Fourteen

STUDY OF HOME RELATIONSHIPS

199 of the 500 girls had no major detrimental home situation; both parents of the girl were living together. Of the 199, fifty-seven had even none of the listed minor problems of separation, as far as we knew. What sort of factors might have precipitated their maladjustment or delinquency?

Many writers on the broken home and delinquency have quoted opinions that serious quarrelling between the parents before the separation may have been the most destructive part. Of 100 girls who were recorded as having undergone the strain of serious parental discord in early or later childhood, about eighty had already separated when the girl came to us. Doubtless this was an underestimate, for a further sixty girls who were recorded as suffering nagging, bickering, and a feeling of unwantedness may have been observers as well as recipients of aggression. But we can by no means say that all 200 girls who lived with both parents had been enduring tension and underprivilege.

Although the home relationships recorded were deduced from remarks by the Probation Officer or other investigator in the precommittal inquiry, the relationships as felt by the girl herself were thought by the writer to be the potent factor in her adjustment then and later. These were expressed in her 'Life Story', or projective sentence or story techniques, in formal and informal discussion with staff at the C.S., or conveyed in letters to and from home. The fairly

Table 44: Home Relationships—Two Versions

Part 1	Recorded Officially %	Girl's Version %
Happy normal place in family	5·6	4·6
Happy—spoilt, indulged	16·2	10·4
Fairly happy. Discipline too slack, or no closeness to child	24·6	21·6
Nagging, bickering, felt unwanted	12·4	20·2

close comparison between the record and the girl's version is seen in part of the two tables which were not parallel throughout.

This part of the table can be compared as follows:

Naturally the girl is more likely to feel unwanted—'everyone on to me'—and to express this more easily when she looks back. She is less likely than the parents or outside observers to see herself as having been spoilt.

The other factors analysed in the girl's version of home relationships continue the above table (the officially recorded relationships could not include similar details):

Part 2	%
Felt rejected by mother (or step-mother, etc.)	9·2
Felt rejected, by father (or step-father, etc.)	16·6
'Put upon', rather than unhappy	2·6
Quite happy until adolescence, then troubled	3·0
Not enough said to deduce relationships	7·0
Variety of homes and relationships	4·8

Correlating home relationships with the detrimental situations so far discussed we found the following significant facts:

The twenty-three girls (only 4·6 per cent) recorded (from the girl's version) as having *normal home-relationships*, were as expected, drawn most from homes with no major detrimental situation—and even more disproportionately (disproportionately in this chapter refers to statistically significant differences) from homes without the minor breaks for illnesses, imprisonment, etc. Yet seven of the group had suffered major upsets. Lest the description 'normal' seems too easily attached, one or two examples may be called for: (a) A girl of very dull intellect but with a pretty face, whose mother, also not very bright, had a moral lapse and was in a 'Rescue Home' when about 20, but had lived a good, useful life since, and was an anxious, well-meaning, affectionate mother who had kept discreetly quiet about her lapse. None of the other children were difficult; the home was very well kept and the marriage seemed happy. (b) J's mother died of Bright's disease and a heart condition when J was three. She was tended by a neighbour for three years until the father married the neighbour's daughter, who looked after her very well indeed, and quite as well materially as her own two children. The home was clean and well furnished and the parents very concerned. J, a belligerent and vulnerable mixture, seemed equally attached to the step-mother.

The fifty-two (10·4 per cent, on the girls' version) happy but *petted, indulged* children were disproportionately from homes with no major break, but often a minor one; two examples were the child over-indulged during and after a severe or lengthy illness, and the only child petted by the mother and relatives in the grandparental home while the father was in the Forces. While these were predominantly spoilt, there had been the privation of the illness, or the reaction when she had to share her mother with the returned father. Few cases existed of indulgence all the way through; one feels, indeed, that much worse things can happen to a child than being petted and indulged. The question is also relative to the parental class and circumstances, to what parents think is due to their own children, and due to those of another stratum of society. 'You brought me to my sencus', wrote one 'normal' spoilt girl, who later did well.

The 108 girls recorded as being 'too slacky disciplined', and allowed to run wild—were almost normally distributed between whole and broken families—more from the latter because 60 per cent of families were broken. By 'too slacky disciplined' is meant something quite different from 'free discipline' as a progressive, usually professional class, line, where the child might seem to its aunts and uncles and neighbours to be 'running wild' in the home, but is unlikely to be running wild in the neighbourhood, and where there is no lack of moral principles in the home, whether acceptable or not to the average middle-class parent.

This kind of delinquent—the slackly disciplined and unsuper-vized—is well known to professional and lay people. Indeed to the popular mind this is THE delinquent. It is also the kind of delinquent Dr Gordon Trasler seems to have mainly in mind in *The Explanation of Criminality*[1], though his theory is extended to cover other classes of delinquents. In the book he links the mechanism of social learning —by conditioning through love-oriented discipline to acceptable social behaviour—with the studies by various sociologists (Sprott,[2] Mays[3] and others) of differing class methods of bringing up children. As the unskilled labouring class was 'considerably over-represented' in studies of Borstal boys by Ferguson[4] (1952), Morris[5] (1958), and Rose[6] (1954), the freer, less ordered pattern of the daily life of a typical child of this class should, he says, be studied against that of the typical child of the middle classes, who take a long-term view in their training (or conditioning). The fact that the middle classes, and the skilled and semi-skilled, who tend to emulate middle-class upbringings, are more efficient in the socializing processes, suggested that a process of conditioning to patterns of behaviour is the answer to at least one kind of delinquency.

As this slackly disciplined group comprises a fifth of both our samples, it has certainly to be considered as a possibly separate group. We recall that the girls are fairly evenly distributed between broken homes and homes with both the child's parents present. We find there is no significant relationship between serious illness in the home and slack discipline except when linked with very uncomfortable homes. There is a close relationship with slack maternal morals, and with lack of moral training. So far we see the easy-going mother giving little time (even when she is around) to avoidance conditioning of their behaviour; nor is she concerned with a long-term view of the child, more than of herself. Thus not only is our girl in trouble, but a disproportionate number of those who were under slack control had one or more siblings definitely in trouble, or acting as a dubious influence.

A factor not mentioned hitherto in the research now comes into the picture: the intellectual level of the girls too slackly disciplined tended to be definitely below average; 40 of the 101 with known Binet results had I.Q.'s of average or above, while sixty-one had I.Q.'s *below* 85, which was disproportionately many even for this sample. Here we can play with two theories: the parent of lower intellect could apply good training techniques less adequately, or—a more acceptable theory to the writer—the educationally subnormal child needs clear, firm lines of training, conditioning may take longer, but, other things being equal, is perhaps more lasting, as new mental influences are fewer and less disturbing. In the Classifying School, as we shall discuss later, we found it, on the whole, easy to keep the very dull girls happy and orderly, once they understood, through clear, patient instruction, what was expected. Without tram-lines to guide them they were soon lost. (We shall find their success subsequent to training even more interesting.)

The question of how far the unskilled workers, plus the dependent families, were the most prone to have slackly disciplined children leads us somewhat astray from Dr Trasler's[1] hypothesis. In fact the children from those backgrounds were distributed well through the home relationships column, and rather more of them than could be statistically expected were considered to have a happy and normal relationship in the home prior to the offence(s) bringing them to Court. Far fewer than expected were in the spoilt category, and fewer were rejected by the father, or suddenly became out of step at adolescence. There were, indeed, disproportionately more in the 'slackly disciplined' category; 65 of the 108 girls (more than half) who were allowed too much freedom were from the unskilled or dependent groups—but these also comprised more than half of the main sample (53 per cent).

This of course, may prove that the families in the other social categories whose children were allowed too loose a rein were un-representative of their own economic class; certainly one finds departures in all classes from a strictly defined pattern of upbringing. It may be, however, that the intelligence of the child is a more important factor.

A disproportionately high section of the under-disciplined were girls who apparently had suffered no major, nor one of the selected minor detrimental situations. Indeed they formed a third of that group of fifty-seven girls with more stable backgrounds and this included two or three exceptionally pleasant girls, who had given no trouble until adolescence, and gave no trouble once they accepted the plight into which they had landed. The fifty-seven with stable backgrounds socially also contained a few of the very spoilt girls. But about twenty of these last, whether feeling persecuted, or lacking fundamental training and example, were a peculiarly unlovable set, often unprepossessing in appearance. They tended to come into the 'rejected' categories. That they were rejected (sometimes as part of socially rejected families) showed in the distortion of the 'crushes' they formed, exclusively with one member of the staff (often a rather masculine person) and, while being frequently rude to her, were often totally objectionable to most others. These were not so much the child-like transferences that have been discussed in relation to the Institution child, indeed they were rather contorted adolescent fixations. They were inarticulate girls on the whole, who whined rather than cursed. Whether these girls were from homes incapable of giving sufficient warmth, or whether the whole family was the butt of the neighbourhood, or whether they were constitutionally handicapped (some were all three) they seemed to have great difficulty in working through their problems. We felt they needed, above all, tolerance, and were sent most frequently to a bluff, kind, rather mannish Headmistress with a great sense of humour. She wrote of one of these miseries two years after her admission: 'Not a fundamentally nice girl; was very spiteful and vindictive and jealous. Cordially disliked by the girls because of her acidulated tongue. A "creeper", who listened to other people's conversations and then passed on the information. . . . Made a great fuss of her mother when she visited, then gently relieved her of her bag to see what she had brought!'

Another of this less lovable group was one of three sisters committed in the Research periods. The parents, who had goodwill but indifferent capacity to exert it, could not understand why all their children (seven of them) hated each other so venomously.

The *unhappy* 101 girls (20·2 per cent by the girls' version) who felt 'everyone is on to me—nobody wants me'—were disproportionately from the broken homes. It was the step-daughter situation, as far as the girl herself saw it:

> This is my life story starting from when I was ten years old. My step-father was alive then and he used to hit me for the least little thing with his belt buckle such as taking along time to go an errand . . . but he started being ill . . . then he died . . . After his death I started to take advantage of my mother and going out at night when she had told me to stay in. . . . When I was thirteen I went in hospital . . . and I was in a month and when I came out I started to behave untill my Mam met this other chap and started going out with him and left me to look after the children . . .

However, a quarter of the unhappy ones were from homes with parents together; they might be the odd one out, or oldest sisters with a team of post-war siblings favoured by father. Or it might be just a cruelly rejecting family: L came to us seven and a half years after being committed to the care of the Local Authority, for running away from home. She was at two residential schools for Maladjusted Children (one a well known very 'progressive' one)—and failed. She was in three Children's Homes, but was violent and threw furniture around. She was remanded and committed to a Junior Approved School. She was very difficult there and unsettled other girls. She was in a well known psychiatric hospital but unsettled the patients and the hospital would not keep her. She was violent then in another hospital, where she kicked a nurse with shoes the latter gave her as a present the day before. She was moved to yet another mental hospital and was extremely difficult. (She was seen by another eminent Psychiatrist before each movement.) She was now transferred (under her original Approved School order) to the Girls' Classifying School for the South. She was so violent and disruptive that, on psychiatric advice, her Approved School order was discharged and she was sent home. Within a week or two she had run away. She came before a Midlands Court which decided she should have a new chance in the Approved Schools service; she came to us.

We did not ask L to write a Life Story, partly because her spelling was barely at the 7-year level; partly because we did not want to impinge on her in a personal way, especially during a very touchy beginning, when she was trying out her old brazenly disruptive tactics.

After respect had been won for stopping her (with a word) mid-way in a fight, she broached the subject of her life story. She was told that we knew she found spelling difficult. . . . She said it wasn't that, but such things had happened to her.... Her mother had always beaten her—she beat them all—'Beats little Mavis now'—and tears came to her eyes at this point. Her mother was just the image of *her* mother—'no wonder we all have tempers'. Father was all right —'I'm father's pet—but he's away such a lot and mother tells all about us when he gets back.... When other girls are depressed, they're depressed about letters, etc. I don't know what I'm depressed about....'

She came to talk about her troubles, between lesser difficulties, and softened a good deal. One evening when just a few girls were in the recreation room one of the staff went in and found L sitting on the mantelpiece. She did not chide her, but just held out her hands as to a little child, and L burst into tears.

Perhaps these last softer trends were the beginning of a new phase. In her Training School L was 'idle, uncooperative, and resentful of authority', but more the inadequate than the aggressive psychopath. On psychiatric advice she was placed out in a residential farm job in five months. Just over a year later she was in trouble and was recommitted to Approved School, spent another period in the Shaw Classifying School and was sent to a Senior Approved School for the older difficult girls. Nine months later she had absconded. The aggressive side had come more to the fore again but there had been some cooperation. No more was heard of L. The psychopath has been discussed elsewhere; at this point it is perhaps more salutary to see L as an unhappy girl, with 'everyone on to her', worst of all her mother.

The forty-six girls who felt 'rejected by mother' tended to be from homes which had split, for death or divorce. Often this was the over anxious or embittered mother whom we discussed previously, with two illustrative cases (Chapter XI).

The eighty-three girls who felt 'rejected by father' were disproportionately from homes with no major detrimental situation, but generally with a minor one—usually the father having been away in the Forces, or the father having been seriously ill.

More interesting still, the thirty-seven girls who felt rejected by father, but had suffered no major family break, formed the largest cluster of the 199 girls who had both parents together. Examining these cases, it was clear that the fathers tended to be restless, exacting people. A few were just bad-tempered, hostile individuals without much in the way of principles, but mainly they had standards, and pushed those mercilessly. Fairly often the mother indulged the child, to compensate. These girls seemed to have been drawn towards prostitution, rather than milder promiscuity. Here are some examples:

(a) A girl devoted to her father, who had a bad road accident when she was about 8, and became quite altered after it—less friendly, very hard to please.

(b) A father with many practical hobbies and interests who put tremendous pressure on to the daughter to achieve—at school, and in dancing classes. Before 12 she was slipping out unknown to her parents, late at night, and with a friend was associating with U.S. airmen. She was good at art; her father drove her to excel.... She was too dreamy at Art College, so was relegated to a job in Woolworths where she was also too dreamy ... She kept low company in her free time....

(c) An only child, very petted at home with her mother during the war years. Father returned, and more children were born, and he didn't seem to like her. (This story was repeated in several cases, with varying ethical ranges of father.)

(d) Child of an elderly, chronic sick and anxious father, and an anxious mother. The girl was fascinated by coloured babies, and helped some Indian mothers by taking their children to the park. On a call with a girl friend at the house of some chance Indian acquaintances she had sexual intercourse forced upon her. She was afraid to tell her father, who was 'in a temper' but this single episode came to light seven months later, when the girl friend appeared as the victim in another carnal knowledge case, and as our girl was still tense at the thought of facing her angry father and (by then) suicidal mother, she refused to live at home and was committed to Approved School.

(e) A typically educationally subnormal girl, pushed to scholastic success by her rigid father (more at some phases of the moon than at others, she said!) who continued in his letters to nag about her spelling, and about a career, and no efforts of Probation Officer and Headmistress of Classifying and Training School could stall his pressure on the poor girl. She decided not to return home—but did, and was soon in Court for larceny.

There were, of course, as many stories as girls, and not all were of ambitious fathers. Some were doubtless from fathers who, after absence in the Forces, were uncertain of being the girl's father; one girl tells of her father attacking her, and giving his rejection of paternity as the reason.

Obviously mistakes would be made in judging home relationships; sometimes the Classifying School, after seeing and hearing from parents and girl, would have a different opinion from the Social Workers concerned in pre-committal times; sometimes the opinion later of the Training School was different from either. On the other hand the classifying period was a kind of no-man's-land where the heat of home passions had cooled a little, and the girl was not yet facing a return there, even for holidays. Impressions gained of her reactions, and linked with earlier comments may be fairly accurate. If so, we know that more than half our Approved School girls were distinctly unhappy. One fifth felt generally unwanted, and about a quarter felt specific rejections. Another fifth had been on too loose a rein, or at too great an emotional distance from parents to feel sure of their identity. Another 10 per cent had probably been abnormally indulged. Links between these and more measurable circumstances (such as parental absences) have been traced, and the whole makes an unhappy picture.

But while links appear, each group has its mixture of 'types'. We seem to find little sub-categories, such as the very dull girls who had been cheated of the discipline they needed, sometimes with parental goodwill but misguidedness. There were happy, spoilt girls, who would probably have been happier if less indulged, though where the spoiling was as compensation for illness, perhaps the error was in degree rather than in kind. Then there were the little cinderellas with step-mothers and half-siblings, or the children of step-fathers whose attempts to control were resented. And there were the more 'normal' odd-ones-out, where they seemed to have been born at the wrong time.

The girls from reasonably happy homes were evenly distributed (by Approved School standards) among the I.Q. groupings; unhappy, neglected girls also appeared fairly evenly scattered. As we have seen, the uncontrolled girls, those who had run wild, were among those represented more in the below average and 'borderline' categories; most probably this was a two-way relationship, their lack of inner discipline preventing development of what natural resources they had. For similar reasons, but not wholly the same, girls with multiple homes and therefore multiple home relationships (or lack of) tended to appear among the dullards; emotional insecurity would often impair identification with teachers, or just prevent concentration, and abilities could tend to develop unevenly.

The definitely rejected girls, however, (149 of them) were distributed quite otherwise, with thirty-seven of good average intellect or above; sixty-nine low average, and this time less than a third dull or borderline. Two of our ex-Grammar School girls were severely rejected, and a number of our other 'good girls' had initially to be reassured that we accepted them. The statistical significance of home relationships linked with Binet I.Q. was at the ·001 level.

It is odd that at their earlier day schools, although more 'good' girls were from happy homes, the link with home unhappiness was not at significant level. This possibly shows how far school life can be complementary to a girl's home life—she may show her unhappiness in difficult behaviour, or she may make the most of her hours out of the home. Or in large secondary classes a vaguely unhappy girl's withholding of effort can pass unrecorded—sometimes.

Chapter Fifteen

THE INSTITUTION CHILD IN ADOLESCENCE

A special group of the separated, deprived children were our relatively small proportion of girls who had spent all, or very nearly all of their childhood in Children's Homes. Reference was made on the section on separations to Bowlby[1] and others who have dealt much with this problem, and while workers whose theories are less psychoanalytical would wish to modify the stress on separation as such, no one—especially those who have lived with the extreme manifestations of such conditions—would deny the peculiar personality difficulties that arise from children who have long lacked family life.

Although 29 girls in the 500 sample and 35 girls in the 100 sample had lived *mainly* in an Institution after the break up of the home, and though many more—about seventy-five—had been placed at an early stage of their difficulties, sometimes in the first few years of their life, in a Children's Home or Hostel, only about 10 of the 500 sample had spent most of their lives in Institutions from infancy or early childhood upwards. The impact made on the life of the Classifying School, and the attention they absorbed, was usually far out of proportion to their number.

Although the following case belongs to one of our sub-groups of the 1952–4 admissions, being under 14 on admission, she is such a classic example of early rejection that she cannot be ignored (indeed she never could!). She could also be placed in a group where brain-damage and/or psychopathy were queried.

L was admitted to the Classifying School as a special case, at the age of 12, because no school or institution could manage her, and fuller investigations were needed before a Junior Approved School was tried.

She was small, slightly built, and lean to the point of scragginess. Fair hair straggled round a small, ferrety face. There was something of the puppet about her angular body, stiff limbs, the lack of spring in her movements and the way her head and neck jerked out of her stiff, hunched shoulders. But all this tightness, hardness and lack of bounce did not incapacitate her physically; she was as restless and active, too, as a ferret, and scarcely noticed the knocks and bruises that followed her precipitate actions. She was ever on the look-out

172

for someone on whom to pounce—an adult on whom to make a demand, or a contemporary on whom to inflict some major or minor provocation. Her high-pitched, gloating, emotionless voice, with her native sing-song, whined on and on without mercy.

On admission, and at every serious crisis, she was a pathetic, white, nervous creature, weeping for her mummy, but her mood, like lightning, could change to callous, excited reactions to whatever was happening in the Classifying School—where, of course, so much was meantime happening. Normal kindness brought endless demands; absolute firmness, combined with the measure of gentleness her deprived nature called for, soon revealed her as barely past the social development of a difficult toddler.

Her contemporaries, who had begun by making this little shrewish scrap into the school mascot, were soon worn out by her inquisitiveness, her interference, her harping manner and her provocative actions. She turned them all against her, and was rescued one night from a dormitory, where the exasperated Prefect was literally sitting on her. The emotional breakdown which followed, though at a very childish level, did betray a rudimentary sort of feeling for others, and she became utterly dependent on staff for a time afterwards (assuming a stammer and an angelic politeness), until she came to lean first on an older girl who badly needed a child to mother, and much later on a contemporary in emotional development. She was in the Classifying School for six months before a Training School could or would accept her.

L was the second illegitimate child of a mother who fell down a tram-car stairway two weeks before the birth, and noticed no movement of the baby after that, and, though the birth was normal the baby was very blue. As an infant she seldom cried and took little notice of anyone. She was with the mother for sixteen months, by the end of which she was not attempting to walk or talk. She was in two Nurseries, in far-flung counties, in the next five years, and was 'something of a problem child'. She returned at $6\frac{1}{2}$ to her mother, who had married a farm servant, who lost his job within six months of having the child at home, because she chased the chickens and tormented everyone and everything. She went to school and her teacher had a nervous breakdown. She moved to a third school (having been 'terrible' at two by then) and stole other children's money and sweets. At home she tore sheets and blankets into ribbons. Soon after she pushed a little boy face-first into a 'swampy burn', and a fortnight later almost succeeded in sticking a knife into her younger brother's neck. Her step-father lost another job through her. She was taken into the Local Authority's care. For three years she was quarrelsome, domineering and cruel in the Children's Home. She returned home for three months until her step-father objected to the disruption caused. Returned to the Homes, she was psychiatrically examined, and found to have an abnormal E.E.G. A move to another home was recommended, to give other children a rest. Neither the new Homes nor the new Secondary School could manage her. She was committed to Approved School as a refractory child in the Local Authority's care.

However far this was a constitutional problem, each most dramatic moment of her behaviour at the Classifying School betokened more the rejected, deprived child, and when she was treated as such we saw traces of response. The predominance of older girls, some of whom were always happy to imitate Staff's sympathetic but firm approach, made it possible to tolerate and even enjoy her presence. She could never be a leader, only an irritant. Sometimes treating her as a tired child and tucking her into bed for a day or two was the only relief for everyone; she slept many extra hours and was more relaxed afterwards.

During the six months L was with us, the mother wrote to her only a very few times, as she was afraid to encourage the child in case she had to have her for home leave. Whenever we had persuaded the mother to write, L carried the letter round ostentatiously in her hand for days—and we carried a lump in our throats; she did not know the hard, rejecting sentences, for girls and staff read her only the kinder passages, and she herself could not read. In reply to one plea from the School the mother wrote, 'As far as homesickness is concerned she has never been at home for the past five years, except for a short holiday last year. As for her missing my letters is silly because I never wrote to her before she came to you and she had never been used to writing to me . . .'

After she had been three months at the Classifying School, and had formed a friendship typical of Infants School level (being by now aged 13, and her friend 14), the two girls and two other immature girls of 14 took the stage at an impromptu concert. The dramatic sequence (transcribed afterwards by one of the staff) was as follows:

Scene 1: Mrs Knight (L, the author of the play) is seated nursing her baby (the special friend) and rocking her to and fro and crooning a rhyme:

> My name is Mrs Knight,
>   Idi—idi—ido.
> I have my baby on my knee,
>   Idi—idi—ido.
> She's crying and she will not sleep,
>   Idi—idi—ido.
> So I stick a pen-knife in its heart,
>   Idi—idi—ido.

(She hides the stabbed baby behind the piano. There is a knock at the door, and two Policemen enter.)

Policeman—Have you a baby here?
Mrs Knight—I had a baby; but it died twelve months ago.
Policeman—Bring it to us, to let us see it. (The body is brought out).

With much scuffling the murderess (and author) is dragged from the room to the prison cell, where in Scene II she is begging for leave to go and bury her dead child. This is granted.

Scene III: The cemetery. Mrs Knight is digging with great gusto, while the Police stand watching. The body is carried in and placed in the 'grave'.
Mrs Knight—Now we'll kneel down and say a prayer: Dear God, keep this baby safe and sound, for Jesus Christ's sake.

Amen.

An observer reported that at this point our girl's face showed the strange mixture of ghoulishness and piety which only L could assume.

Scene IV: In the cell. Mrs Knight is sitting alone, hunched up, rocking herself backwards and forwards, and moaning, 'I want my baby'.
Then suddenly, 'I want my son, He's 15 years of age'.
Enter the Police.
Mrs Knight—What kind of food is this to give to me? I want some decent food, etc. . . . If you get my son he will bring them to me.

(Enter the murdered 'baby', still in baby clothes, now representing the son of 15).

Son—Mother, dear Mother what have they done to you? Look, I've brought you nice things to eat.
Mrs Knight—Oh my son, these two policemen have stabbed your baby sister in the heart with a pen-knife.
Son—(Punching the Policemen). How dare you kill my baby sister?
(A free-for-all follows. The Police are knocked out and Mrs Knight and son tie them to a chair and escape from the prison.)

There were other less dramatic enactions of similar kind by the two girls, but these aroused so much hysteria in the older girls in the Classifying School that they had to be discontinued; it gave a glimpse of what could be done in a less mobile population, and in smaller groups.

Meantime in our schoolroom little progress was made on L's illiteracy; here one could no more be dogmatic about her queried brain-damage than about her unstable, much-interrupted, early and later schooling. It must also be said that she required a specialist in remedial reading methods, which, with our girl population, we more rarely needed.

Our visiting Psychiatrist saw her at first as a 'child showing incomplete development of mind', and requiring ascertainment as a moral defective. A second opinion, a month later, stressed her low intelligence as a possible cause of her unstable temperament—though in fact her verbal reasoning could, by peculiar side-tracks, reach the conclusions normal to only slightly younger children. Her score in the Progressive Matrices did indeed remain at borderline level on much later retesting, but her Binet I.Q. was 85. She showed deftness in manipulative tests. In the community she could hold her own in far too many ways for us to think of her as mentally defective, and over the months we ceased to think of her as morally defective so much as morally (and emotionally) very retarded indeed, but showing some slight signs of growth.

She came to identify herself to some extent with adults who had never rejected her. She showed intense anxiety when a gang of tough older girls tried to upset her school, and asked the Headmistress one night at bedtime if she could help the staff in any way. By now she was doing her best to talk with the Headmistress's sweetness, and to walk with her grace—but could still ferret out every detail of community life without her old darting eye and head movements! And her childish development showed at Christmas when she and her friend trembled before a semi-familiar Father Christmas—like the keeper in another keeper's coat frightening one of Hebb's[2] apes.

Such a strong, concerted, loving approach to this child's problems was needed, even if within a perturbing group of contemporaries, for years. The few available steady older girls gave relief, and were like older sisters. At the Training School where she was received after six months, she was in a Cottage with two other girls and a House Matron, on all of whom a heavy load was laid. This was the kind of setting where she had failed in all her early years. Within twelve months L had been admitted to a State Institution. When seen there briefly by the writer a year later she appeared more institutionalized (less obtrusive; grumbling about the standard things). She was there for six years, and transferred to another hospital.

The above case has been painted as a classic rejected child. She had never fitted into institution (or other) life, and thus had not the classic institutionalized character. More often our institution reared girls, whom an emotional appeal rarely touched, fitted Dr Trasler's[3] analogy of the tone-deaf person. A charming looking, sweetly (but flatly) toned girl of nearly 17 had been a most acceptable child in the Children's Homes, but could not settle to work, or in foster-homes with relatives after 15, and proved sadly, frustratingly incapacitated for trust or normal response in the Classifying School, though an excellent practical worker, and when at her best even a good leader in organized and free time. She, too, had a prolonged stay with us, because, after repeated absconding, she guaranteed her settling on condition that she could work her passage to the outside world quickly. Attempts to pave the way, even to an early marriage, showed her still with far from a normal sense of responsibility, and she had to jump from a window, fracturing an arm and a leg, and undergo a tremendous amount of unrelenting challenge at a forceful Training School before she attained some measure of adulthood. This she seemed to do.

Some of these 'institution children' who made experiments with their own emotions and those of adults, like little children, reached out in each new environment, and selected some unfortunate adult, whom they pursued relentlessly, biting the hand which fed them. Briefly, the girl would be nice, telling her adult how much she loved her, and then a little torture would be tried out. We were accustomed to the 'playing up' routine, and tried hard not to reject (the result from the girl's side might be crazed hysteria) but the torture, alternating with sweet sentiment, could assume outrageous proportions, especially if the member of staff was young and vulnerable. This pattern was described in a report back from the Training School on another of our 500 sample: 'She cannot mix with people. She stares at them, is rude in her speech. Gauche. Has an annoying "crush" on a member of the Staff, and is a perfect nuisance—always grinning at her, and trying to touch her when she passes. We do understand her longing to belong to some one, but . . .' As there is no mention of the girl periodically 'rejecting' her favourite teacher (to test her out, as a token repayment for all adults who have rejected her— whatever the theory) one is hopeful that the battle for adulthood was then nearly won. Four years later the girl was a Nurse-trainee. Despite premonitions about her behaviour, on her return (twice) to the Training School for holidays, 'She behaved very well, dressed with taste, and was clean and smart'. Again emotional growth was slow and perverse, but came; she had nearly two years of early childhood with her mother before desertion, and proved unsuitable for boarding out to foster-homes from the local Children's Homes.

Some girls who went into Children's Homes over the age of 5 adjusted well to the companionable, organized life, and a return years later to a family was their great problem, especially to a family of strangers—step-mother, small siblings, and a barely known father. Perhaps the shock of return at any age would have proved too much, and it was better that she should adjust to the decisions and strains of family life before becoming a mother herself. Unfortunately she was due to have the adjustment to make all over again, after a year to two years in Approved School.

The size of the group spending their whole, or almost their whole lives in Institutions is too small for a link with other factors. The sample would, for relevance, have to be broken down further into age and reasons of institutionalizing, and then there would be the question of feelings of rejection before leaving home. Hereditary factors are here perhaps more important than in other groups.

Chapter Sixteen

RELATIONS WITH THE
OUTSIDE WORLD

In some detail we have explored the more intimate physical background of the Approved School girl's life. In many cases to say her 'home' is to oversimplify, because of the multiplicity of environments. Some even of the consistent backgrounds were not home in any cosy sense; it might be a two-parent establishment with inadequate supervision; or reeking of ill-health, poverty or low morality. Many lost a parent in childhood and failed in varying degrees to adjust to a change of mother or father-figure. Many spent interim periods in institutions; some returned to a changed home, some were given foster parents whom they rejected in some measure, some remained for long periods in an institution, or moved to strange new institutions for their own good or that of others.

However mediocre or bad the child's physical home, she did not spend all her time there: she went to school for the same duration as her contemporaries (true, sometimes as irregularly as she could manage); if old enough she had been to work—sometimes, again, with irregularity. She had played in the back-yard, in the parks and in the street. She had sat in the cinema, sometimes for large areas of her childhood. She had been, sometimes, for trial visits to Youth Clubs. Some had occasionally gone to Sunday School or Church, a few regularly. Most had been to dance halls, a good many had been in Public Houses. Some had been illicitly on board ships, and some had hung long hours round Camps and Air Bases, or been smuggled into the huts. Too many knew the worst aspects of houses of ill repute, even if they had gone there ostensibly to baby-sit. Some had lived intimately in over-populated slum houses with coloured immigrants. Some had slept in hotels with U.S. Servicemen. Wherever they went, they carried their basic insecurities, and often their chronic immaturity of outlook, and seldom did their life experiences outside the home do anything to heal the scars of earlier trauma. But the more glamorous pursuits did act as a drug, and so set them athirst for more.

Beginning with a provision made for all the girls, we shall examine their reactions to outside influences.

THE GIRL IN RELATION TO SCHOOL

Since the varying percentage of girls attending Grammar Schools in the mid-fifties was in all cases small, and since care is often taken to eject the anti-social in good time, the percentage of girls who had been or still were at Grammar Schools when committed was naturally small; it was 2·2 per cent of our 500 sample and 7 of the 11 had been to Girls' Grammar Schools, the remaining 4 to mixed.

Some of these had been expelled or quietly demoted when their work or conduct deteriorated badly. Most of these represented a section of the twenty girls in the sample with Binet I.Q.'s over 115; one or two were just outside this bracket. As these girls were more articulate, we hear something of their triumphs and their downfall:

In the March just before they (father and stepmother) married I had passed my Scholarship to go to a Grammar School. My aunties were delighted. So was I . . . It naturally fell to my father and mother now to buy my uniform. My aunties had very kindly helped but that wasn't enough for —— (step-mother) who kicked up the devil of a row. . . . I left school (i.e. at 15) as my step-mother kept nagging at me and when I had homework to do she would shout and tell me to hurry up and mind the babies while she did something or other and unfortunately my school work began to suffer so I agreed to leave school. . . .

Another:

Scholarship Day began badly . . . Mother (a divorcee) was by no means helpful for she threatened all sorts of horrible things if I didn't pass. [She passed]. Mother now began to worry about the clothes and things, and many times she practically blamed me for passing and incurring the expense. . . . At the end of my first day I hurried home full of news, and when I began to tell mother she said, 'I don't want to know, I'm not at all interested', so I went straight to bed to hide my tears of disappointment in case I should be punished for them. . . . I finally settled down to work for School Certificate and in the fourth and fifth forms was never lower than fifth out of forty in any subject. Half way through my fifth year, trouble at home began again. Trouble, with a capital T. Mother began to nag that I was not earning any money and she really didn't see why she should keep me in 'idle luxury' any more. (When the girl said she wanted to be a teacher, her mother retorted, 'Its not for the likes of we!' . . .)—Finally I got so desperate that I just left school and went job-hunting. I obtained a post as junior clerk . . .

Another told, more calmly of her friends going to the Secondary Modern, and her own failure to settle at Grammar School; 'I found my school mates of a much higher social position . . . People started to say I had taken up a place at that school of which I was not worthy. I gave up trying . . . I made my friends outside my school life. . . .'

An unhappy girl, second of a large family stemming from the father's periodic returns home from Prison or Mental Hospital, began stealing while at Grammar School, and her concentration failed. She too lacked adequate School uniform. The cycle of family scorn because of failure, then more stealing and more scorn, brought about her transfer to the Secondary Modern School—and more scorn at home. The failure by School to enlist or obtain Child Guidance help through all these desperate straits was hard to understand; eventually it was enlisted; the appointment was not kept and the matter was not pursued. Another Grammar School girl in the same county failed despite warm interest from the Grammar School, where they saw deterioration setting in after the girl heard from a school-mate that she was not the child of the adoptive mother, to whom, anyway, she had never related happily.

One, on the fringe of Grammar School success, wrote of the end of quite a happy childhood with her aunt:

I lived there until I was 8 years old, and it came as rather a shock to me when I found that it wasn't my home at all, and that my mother had been demobbed . . . and was getting married again . . . I am afraid I hated my step-father from the very first because he had no love or affection for me like my uncle had . . . I was literally afraid of him. . . . When he went back to sea my mother started letting me have much of my own way . . . Then came the time when I was ready to sit for the exam for the High School. I was coached by my dad for two hours every night and he paid a man to come in on a Sunday to learn me even more. On the night before the exam I was threatened by my father of what he would do if I did not pass, so the next day I set off to school feeling very nervous. About three weeks after the exam, we got to know the results and I had failed. I went home that night feeling very subdued and very frightened. After I told my father, he blew up in a fit of temper, and told me that I was hopeless and ignorant. I went to a Secondary School and I left when I was 15 . . .

Only 1·4 per cent had been to schools for Educationally Subnormal Children (though over 11 per cent had Binet I.Q.'s below 70) and only 2 per cent had been to Schools for Maladjusted (though 20 to 30 per cent were showing serious behavioural and/or emotional disturbances by the time they were 12). These ten girls will be discussed later.

Thus about 90 per cent had been at Secondary Modern or Unselected Schools; it was not always easy to judge which of these from the School report on the Record of Information, and difficult to know whether the Secondary Modern was mixed or one-sex. Sometimes the girl kept us right; 'Then I sat four the Gamer School but I binont pass. Sow I went to the Saning-Deremoden School'.

Girls who had moved around had, of course, many changes of school. This applied particularly to the 10 per cent who had experienced more than three living environments. When families were fairly united there were usually few changes of school, because—bar eviction, or removal to a Council estate from the City Centre—these were not very mobile families.

Only about 4 per cent of the official School Reports on the record failed to provide some indication of a girl's character or conduct. But these reports tended to be terse and no more informative than possible, partly because of fear of breach of confidence, and partly because—especially in Girls' Schools, where remands by a Court are relatively few—not enough was known of the people who would welcome information for the Court and later. Schools, especially if one can return to the Primary School, can be a rich source of information on children and their families, and it was a great pity that links were not forged—though to make preparative relations with Schools all over the northern half of England on the basis of our scattered admissions would have been a task for one member of Staff.

From the information in the files, one could, with the above reservations, venture the following:

Table 45: Level of Cooperation at School

	Sample of 500 %	Sample of 100 %
Cooperative and quite balanced	17	17
Vaguely unacceptable and considered less than reliable	42	40
Definitely unacceptable and considered less than reliable	32	34
Swung from one extreme to the other in the Secondary School	5	4

This provides a consistent but not a happy picture. When corroboration was sought from the girls' own impressions of school life there was a much larger gap in information. About 30 per cent of the 500 sample, and 66 per cent of the 100 sample, failed to talk of school, sometimes not even mentioning it by name in their Life Story. It was doubtful if this was avoidance of the subject of school so much as obsessive unhappiness or unrest about emotional life at home, so that school was barely real, and quickly forgotten.

However, one gathered from 22 per cent of the 500 sample, and

18 per cent of the 100 sample, that they liked school and felt they belonged there; this happened, as we can see, in some who were not so acceptable to the school. Some girls had been of exceptional helpfulness, and gloried in their school life, where they had been sustained in face of even severe personal unhappiness.

32 per cent of the 500 sample gave an impression of vague unhappiness at school, and a recurrent desire to be absent whenever possible. 11 per cent hated school, usually feeling unwanted and rejected. A further 5 per cent swung between liking and disliking in their secondary career.

Some girls had suffered bitter rejection at school; their behaviour may well have merited it, but not their past histories. A child, born illegitimately of a long co-habitation, was adopted by a middle-class couple, but heard, when 9, from a school-mate that she had been a 'dirty' and unwanted baby. This led to a period of withdrawal and depression, and later at the Secondary Modern School she pilfered, lied and caused great trouble. The Headmaster was reported as refusing to give her a reference, commenting that his Staff and he were delighted to see her go. She did not write or tell of this, instead expressing gratitude for all she had learned at school, especially the story of the Creation.

The occasional stories from girls of rejection and counter-rejection at school were outnumbered by those who were vague and uncertain about school life, which had been a misty period between an unhappy morning and an unhappy evening. On the other hand, writing bare outlines of schools attended, and the subjects studied, could be used for evasion of more intimate difficulties. Two-thirds of a Life Story ran as follows:

> I was born on —— in —— I went to —— School I went in the infants when I was 5 when I was 7 I went into the Juniors and when I was 10 I went upstairs in the Juniors I then went into the Senior School when I was 11 I was in the senior school for five years I left school on the 11 th of April and I got a good reference from Miss Brown our headmistress I went up to the bureau for my job. . . .

Thus she evaded talking of two grossly overcrowded rooms, in one of which the parents and two little girls shared a bed, and in the other—a damp, dilapidated room—our girl had sometimes shared a double bed with one adolescent and two pre-adolescent brothers; she could also evade the shameful matter of her incestual relationship with the eldest of the brothers. Her school attendance had, in fact been 'unsatisfactory'. She was found to be slightly spiteful, untruthful, and a keen smoker, but 'self-reliant and obedient'. Unsatisfactory health and lack of grooming would not breed popularity with others, hence the tendency to stay away.

About 9 per cent of the 500 sample had been addicted to truancy from school before the age of 12, and over 20 per cent were known to have truanted after the age of 12. However only 3 of the 500 were committed to Approved School for non-attendance at School; one of these, who was otherwise blameless, and a somewhat nervy, but mainly normal schoolgirl, soon became totally normal away from her neurotic but otherwise good mother.

Probably truancy was correctly named in most of the hundred recorded as having stayed away from school; often this symptom accompanied running away from home at an early age. These were defiant, escapist, avoidance gestures, or might be a means of drawing attention to unhappiness.

School refusal had not become well accepted as a symptom in the period concerned in this research, and the important distinction between truancy and neurotic conflict, which knotted the child to mother's apron, or at least made the confines of school unbearable, though school lessons might be pleasant to her when once there, was less recognized than now. Records where school phobia can be tentatively diagnosed after the event are the more interesting. M had been before the Court for non-attendance over four years before her committal to Approved School. Her only sibling, an older brother, was also under supervision for irregular attendance. The mother, described as weak and ineffectual, and (by her husband) as quite untrustworthy, concealed the fact of the Court appearance and Supervision Order from the father, who was tuberculous and in failing health, but a more intelligent and conscientious person. During the next years the girl had spells of frequent and often long absences from school without a doctor's certificate. She also disappeared from home on occasions. A reappearance at Court for Breach of Supervision was again concealed from her father, and it was learned how inadequate and deceptive was the mother's attitude. The father, his cooperation elicited, tried with all his failing strength to influence the girl, who seems to have been deeply attached to him. She continued to evade school, and after 15 evaded regular employment, and kept bad company. The father died in a sanatorium and the brother accused M of killing him.

M was found on psychiatric examination at the Classifying School, to be 'grossly maladjusted', and not only 'emotionally immature' but 'a warped personality'. She was 'so hostile and resentful that she might readily become mentally disturbed' and should therefore be in a school where a further psychiatric opinion was available, but also within reach of her mother. In fact she had to be sent to a Training School where little if any psychiatric guidance was sought, and at least a hundred miles from her mother. Six months later she was doing 'satisfactorily'. Eighteen months later she was 'helpful, kindly, greatly improved', and had excellent relations with home. At 21, when supervision ended, her social adjustment was 'excellent'. In a Sentence Completion Test at the Classifying School she responded to the stimulus 'mother' by writing 'is getting old'. When the mother, who looked unprepossessing and sickly, visited, M's attitude seemed to be compounded of pity, and a sense of obligation for her mother's past indulgence. That she probably did better with the hundred miles between (plus regular visits) was not surprising in view of the conflicting emotions which parents and brother had aroused. Indeed the history, though made more perverse by long delay before treatment away from home, answers the pattern of cure in many school phobic cases.

A similar case, again displaying a mixture of defiant running away, and fear of the daily fixed separation entailed by school, from—this time—a tuberculous mother who lived in a state of constant antipathy and spite with a non-working, debt-ridden but presentable husband. Away from the harrowing situation, the girl was gentle, biddable, acceptably schoolgirlish, and eventually was able to make a life of her own, with only a final burst of more seriously neurotic behaviour when her mother died. The pity is that these two anxiety torn schoolgirls could not have been treated in Boarding Schools within the Education Services before their symptoms were worsened by Court procedures. In fact Approved School treatment provided an equivalent régime, with more close and continued home links by Social Workers than might otherwise have been available, but this perhaps outlines the kind of controlled environment needed by older school-phobic girls. Indeed a good Children's Home and Day School would have sufficed in each of these, and in other cases, as long as the therapeutic effect of firmness was understood. These were by no means the only girls coming into our net for want of better facilities.

Scholastic Achievement

In the many uncorrected excerpts of girls' life stories the reader will have seen a wide variety of literacy and verbal comprehension. Because they were more facile with words, the average-to-bright girl has tended to be quoted more often than the very dull.

Measures of scholastic attainment are based on results of standardized attainment tests given soon after admission to the Classifying School. Attainment estimates in School reports on the Court record were too often non-standardized, and occasionally grossly misleading; one girl described as of 'average' attainment, had a reading age of about 9, and a spelling age of $8\frac{1}{2}$. Her arithmetic scores were more parallel to her mental age of $11\frac{1}{4}$, but certainly not 'average' at 16. Allowing for the tendency for school leavers either to drop in scholastic attainment in the first year or two, or to solidify their achievement if they have enough reading for it to be practised, these were serious inaccuracies, and not at all unique in our records. Intellectual assessments tended even more to unrealism. With the growth of knowledge in the field of educational measurement since then, such errors would now be less common in schools than in the period of this research.

We shall deal at a later stage with the problem of measuring the learning potential of our girls, through intelligence testing. We also gave scholastic attainment tests in a girl's first week or two at the Classifying School. During the period covered by this research we extracted information on reading and number ability by means of a large and unvarying battery of standardized tests. In 1952 these were Burt's Word Reading No. 1; Burt's Spelling, Ballard's Silent Reading, English Comprehension and English Construction, and Ballard's Mechanical Arithmetic and Reasoning Arithmetic. In 1953, Schonell's Mechanical Arithmetic was substituted for Ballard's. Unfortunately the standardization in most cases was pre-war (some doubtful then) and our generation of girls had their Infants and early Primary schooling from 1943 onwards, with all the disruptions and unwieldiness of school groups in that period of the war and post-war. Nor did we always use the best and most recent standardized tests; like boiled ham for Sunday tea, our scholastic test battery was built into the school's tradition. What we lacked in critical attitudes, however, we made up for in laboriousness and exactitude of administration and marking, and, judging by failures observed in other systems in the last two attributes, perhaps we just broke even. We had learned not to accept some of the standardized results at face value (for example in Ballard's English Comprehension Test) but entered the results on our assessment reports as if we did. We did not (as at Aycliffe[1]) set our test results against Approved School norms, but against outside norms. Though our scholastic findings were disturbing (but not so depressing as in the case of Approved School boys) it would not have occurred to us to spare the Training Schools from the shock of their backwardness. Perhaps because schoolroom facilities were a less prominent part of the Senior Girls' Schools, receiving teachers were more sensitive to a girl's behavioural upsets or to her manipulative difficulties in domestic training than to her degree of literacy.

Though much has been written about the scholastic backwardness of Approved School boys relative to the outside population, there is, as usual, little on record about girls, or about delinquent women. The Gluecks[2] record, of their *500 Delinquent Women*, that 93·5 per cent were literate, and 6·5 per cent were illiterate, but the standard for literacy is rather uncertain.

It is generally agreed, though in the absence of strong statistical evidence, that girls are more advanced in language development than are boys. Remedial reading groups tend to have a high representation of boys—generally 60 per cent or much higher. Educationists have attempted to explain this at various times as due, not so much to greater linguistic gifts in girls, but as due to the girl's greater social conformity, and to her sedentary interests, and therefore to more bookishness. Norms for Schonell's Test B were higher for girls than for boys. On the other hand, in the Ministry of Education's Pamphlet on Reading Ability, published in November 1950, and therefore chronologically suited for comparison with these research findings, girls at 15 were found to average about one point *lower* than boys, 'Evidence showed that very good readers among girls are as good as boys, average ones a little poorer, and very poor readers are somewhat less frequent. It will be seen indeed that there are about twice as many boys as girls in the lowest, illiterate, grade.'

Because the writer is aware of the limitations of the various scholastic tests used in the research period, she wishes to deal briefly with the results, and a comparison with Gittins'[1] findings on Burt's Word Reading Test will perhaps be the most valuable evidence, since both writers have the same doubts about findings from a word-reading test based on phonics, at a time when this method was less and less acceptable in schools.

In *Approved School Boys*[1] (Table XIX), Attainment Ages on Burt's Word Reading Test 1 are set against Chronological Ages for 762 cases. As the age range is from 10 to 15 plus, and as percentages of backward boys in each group varies, the writer has recalculated percentages for the age groups 14 and 15 upwards combined, and sets them below for comparison with the 14 and upwards Shaw girls.

These results are in the direction expected, but the results for the Approved School boys are less weighted towards illiteracy than

Table 46a: Reading Attainment (Compared with A.S. Boys)

	Shaw Girls Ages 14, 15+ %	Aycliffe Boys Ages 14, 15+ %
Normal	16·8	17·3
Backward by 1 to 2 years	43·6	36·0
Backward by 3 to 4 years	20·6	24·0
Backward by more than 4 years	19·0	22·7

expected compared with those of the girls, and indeed the 'good' boys are rather more in evidence than the 'good' girls.

When the figures are shown in a slightly different way, we have the slant noted in the Ministry of Education pamphlets noted above. The results from the Shaw girls and from the Aycliffe boys have been grouped as in the Ministry pamphlet (p. 34) thus:

(1) *Backward readers* are those whose reading ages are more than 20 per cent below their chronological ages, in the case of children i.e. those whose reading quotients are below 80. In the case of adults the expected average reading age may be taken as 15·0 years, hence backward readers are those with reading ages below 12·0 years. (The writer has taken a reading age of 11 years 2 months, as the cutting point for her 14-year-old girls, on the same basis. With the Aycliffe boys it was not possible to be more precise than taking eleven years as the margin.)

(2) *Illiterate readers* are those whose reading age (regardless of chronological age) is less than 7·0 years.

(3) *Semi-literate readers* are those whose reading age is 7·0 or greater, but less than 9·0 years.

All ranges of average and over have reading ages from 12 upwards, or from 11 upwards for our 14-year-olds.

Table 46b

	Shaw Girls Ages 14, 15+ %	Aycliffe Boys Ages 14, 15+ %
Low average to above average	62·8	54·0
Backward	26·8	24·0
Semi-literate	9·0	15·0
Illiterate	1·4	7·0

The greatest difference between the groups comes, in accord with the sex differences in reading in the Ministry pamphlets, in the Illiterate group, with, not twice as many, but *five* times as many boys as girls, and also a much greater percentage of semi-literate boys. Yet there are more 'backward' girls than there are boys.

Yet another comparison with Gittins' Approved School boys will also serve to link reading attainment with intelligence, without at this point going at length into intelligence test findings.

In *Approved School Boys*[1] (Table XXII), reading ages on Burt No. 1 (Word Reading Test) are set against Mental ages obtained from the Binet Test (Terman and Merrill) and a summary of results is given; the latter has been slightly elaborated for our use.

Nowadays Mental Ages are suspect as a statistical device, especially at the upper age groups with which we are dealing in this research; and likewise doubt has been thrown on the expectation that reading skill should correlate highly with intelligence. (See, for example, Pidgeon and Yates 'The Relationship between Ability and Attainment', *Bulletin, N.F.E.R.8* (1956).) Educational Psychologists and teachers still find the comparison temptingly useful. This said, we can proceed with the comparison of findings for Aycliffe boys (as above) and Shaw girls:

Table 46c

	Shaw Girls Chron. Ages 14 to 16 %	Aycliffe Boys Chron. Ages 10 to 17 %
Reading age more than 2 yrs greater than mental age	3·0	1·0
Reading age 1 to 2 yrs greater than mental age	24·0	12·0
Reading equal to mental age	31·0	29·0
Reading 1 to 2 yrs below mental age	36·0	37·0
Reading more than 2 yrs below mental age	6·0	21·0

According to these figures, on the usual assumption that over two years retardation in reading is critical, then a much higher percentage of the girls were fulfilling themselves than were the boys, where 21 per cent were outside this limit. The girls' reading results, at the middle and lower ranges of the table, were more closely associated with intellectual weakness; this would be in line with the earlier comment on the greater social conformity of the girls at school, and therefore greater attentiveness.

We used this last argument to account for our girls' straining (found in 27 per cent of cases, against 13 per cent of the boys) to reach a level well above their intellectual level in sheer parrot-reading of words, without comprehension. This argument can be taken only as far as can the water-tightness of the 'Mental Age' concept, especially for this age-group, and that is not a question to dwell on laboriously here, important though it is. Certainly a few of our duller girls achieved remarkably high standards of correctness in mechanical reading and spelling, matched by perfection of handwriting. This could be perplexing against a measured I.Q. perhaps between 60 and 65, until samples of the girls' naïve reasoning came our way from different members of staff, and other mental tests confirmed dull reasoning. Although we have no figures to prove it, these perfectionist trends in the schoolroom tended to go with very high perseveration. One case, already referred to as a perseverative thrower of faints, had for her first fortnight with us perseverated in absconding, until an accident led to the less active, still escapist, pattern of 'fading out'. When that was exploded, and she had been accepted again, she drove herself to perfectionist standards of housework and general helpfulness, on a par with her previous careful schoolwork. We were rarely without a few girls who chose to remain happily concentrated for an hour or more, copying poems or hymns or prayers in beautiful script. Had they been asked to translate the verses into words of their own, they would soon have betrayed their meagre verbal comprehension.

Confusions arose frequently from verbal difficulties. Not only did verbal usage vary by reason of social class and culture, as was illustrated by Gittins[1] with his Approved School boys, but our girls came from an even wider geographical area, comprising Lancashire, Yorkshire, Tyneside and Midland idioms, and a range of rustic as well as city usage. Areas even had superstitions about words which must not be used, so that the word 'pig' might send girls from an Eastern seaport into paroxysms of fear and rage. ('Cow' was a national rather than a regional slight!) Mainly, however, verbal confusion was due to plain simplicity of mind or to verbal impoverishment, but this was complicated by the earnest desire to identify with Staff thought—at least when in their presence. Thus 'menstruate' seemed grander than 'period', but could quickly become 'administrate'; and 'period' could be so loaded with emotion—not just a word to be smirked at as with normal contemporaries—that when a member of staff went away on leave of absence for study 'for a long period', the first batch of letters received from the girls were full of concern about her health.

If obsessed with a 'dirty' word, it was characteristically difficult for them to avoid it, and this was rarely to shock, as with the more sophisticated schoolgirl. In a diagnostic English test, 'VERDICT' was underlined with marked frequency as being 'a disease', because of the prominence (for them) of the letters V.D. Some hymns, usually the more rapturous ones about the love of God, were, for our girls, a matter of sensational excitement, and if a hymn concealed (by their rendering) the name of a special friend in its lines, ('Oh, give me Samuel's heart . . .') it would be chosen repeatedly for an evening rendering.

Living with the girls revealed, perhaps, more of these irregularities in their learned vocabulary than did their schooldays, with large classes in large departments, and the examples, in retrospect, may illustrate the confusions which must have arisen between them and their teachers and associates in the wider community.

One very borderline girl, eventually ascertained as mentally defective, was escorted to the Training School where an elder sister, Joyce, had gone some years before. The younger sister disliked the place and its Headmistress from the first moment, and said so, banging around hysterically in the meantime. The Headmistress, more accustomed to the dull-to-average girl's reactions said, 'But you're not Joyce's sister!' This was an insult never forgiven in our girl's unstretchable mind!

Number Ability

If our girls were (crudely speaking) less retarded in reading than expected from their mental ages, and not much more backward by chronological age than their contemporaries outside, their number work, by published norms, was more seriously below par. On a rough estimate, fully 70 per cent were backward in the subject, 15 per cent of whom were definitely average in reading. It was rare for a girl to be better at number than at reading. This is not a surprising finding with girls, but it would seem that the extent of backwardness in number was extreme even for the sex.

Since Schonell's Mechanical Arithmetic Test replaced Ballard's in our battery from 1953 onwards, the numbers and percentages of Arithmetic achievement for 1953 and 1954 respectively are given below:

Table 47: Mechanical Arithmetic Age (Schonell)

	1953 Girls No	1953 Girls %	1954 Girls No	1954 Girls %
14 years	14	7·4	9	5·8
12 and 13 years	31	16·5	33	21·1
9, 10 and 11 years	105	56·4	71	45·5
7 and 8 years	37	19·7	41	26·3
Under 7 years	—	—	2	1·3
Total	187	100	156	100

The percentages below 12 years Arithmetic Attainment Age are 76 and 73 in the two years. On a different test (Hill's Southend) Mr Gittins quotes 73 per cent of his boys (ages 10 to 14) as being backward by three to four years or more. The comparison is statistically very close.

Thus 39·6 per cent of our girls were more than two years backward in the mechanical processes of reading, and 73 per cent or more were backward to the same degree in mechanical number processes.

Their response to number teaching in the small classroom group at the Classifying School was very good indeed when given individual work, following on a diagnostic Arithmetic test. Then the perseverative trends, which had sometimes in their past schooling given a girl superficial skill in reading and spelling, came to the fore in number work, and, by choice, she would fill book after book with neatly arranged 'sums', which had to be ticked frequently. Whether she was wiser or even cleverer for the future was doubtful, but the sense of achievement in the present was worth much to her and to us. There was a degree of certitude about such results. We sensed that aggression was relieved in this way, as it was through repetitive cross-stitching, and—in some very aggressive girls—through scrubbing floors (if by choice). Not only the dull obsessional girl would choose mechanical number work, but a few ex-Grammar School girls are recalled as delightedly spending hour after hour on mastering what had been their weakest subject, given a sympathetic teacher and the minimum of competition for individual attention.

These glimpses of their prior attainment in the schoolroom, and their reactions to the Shaw Schoolroom, are intended more to fill gaps in our knowledge of their earlier life in one part of the community. One has no hesitation in saying that in some cases more understanding teachers and more skilful teaching could have provided a wind-break against home disasters or indifference; indeed many of us know girls who would have failed without this kind of help. Unfortunately there were many whose emotional problems had pushed them too far in upon themselves, or had unleashed too great resentment for any but superhuman efforts in the ordinary school to succeed.

Statistical comparisons show probabilities beyond the ·001 level that girls from the poorest homes, in the welfare and hygiene senses, were worst in reading and number attainment. The economic and material conditions were also linked with measurements on intelligence tests, verbal and non-verbal—a matter of circular reasoning which we had better leave in the air.

OUR GIRLS AT WORK

Fully 30 per cent of our Approved School girls were rated as still at school, mainly because they were aged 14, or very recently 15; or because, in the months from reaching school leaving age they had been on remand, and perhaps also in Probation Homes or in Children's Homes, and non-employed.

69 per cent had left school, but 7 per cent of the total worked so little as to be recorded in the research as 'unemployed'.

For a girl to have a good work record was rare. Of those who were of working age the following general assessment was made:

3 per cent were very regular, reliable workers, and further 12 per cent were regular workers, changing employment for legitimate reasons.

62 per cent had abnormal changes of job, through slackness, 'fed-upness', or doubtful redundancy.

8 per cent were dismissed (once or more) as recalcitrant, disobedient, quarrelsome employees.

11 per cent were dismissed (once or more) for dishonesty at work. Of the other 4 per cent not enough was known.

We are fortunate in being able to study these figures in more detail, since a girl's work history was carefully probed and recorded at the time of the Court inquiry, and often a Probation Officer had been much involved in the unsettled sequence of employment hitherto. Also this part of her story was more immediate to the girl herself, who often gave a reasonably accurate account in her life story.

We have a valuable comparison, for our purpose, in the Central Advisory Council for Education's Survey,[3] published in 1960—*15 to 18*. Our 500 girls were born between 1935 and 1940. The young people in the Central Advisory Council's study were born between 1935 and 1941, 68 per cent of them before 1940. Figures were given for subgroups of Modern School and All-Age School Leavers; this covers all but a very small percentage of our girls, especially as most of the ex-Grammar School girls in our study had been demoted (see last section). Thus we have a ready-made sample for comparison.

The number of jobs held by 786 Modern and All-Age School girls, in a period ranging from one and a half years to three and a quarter years, is given in Table 18 of the Council's Survey. On a rough and generous, underestimated average of two years since school-leaving, we can compare with our Approved School sample, whose number of jobs held had been calculated per year.

29 per cent of the 344 working girls in our main delinquent sample (and, indeed, 45 per cent of our later 100 sample) had held *five or more jobs per year*, whereas only 4 per cent of the national sample had held five or more jobs in one and a half to three and three quarter years. And indeed, for our least stable delinquent girls, a work record of five jobs per year would have been a very satisfactory one indeed.

There is a crude comparison of the two groups in Table 48, on page 194.

Table 48: *Jobs per Year (Comparison)*

Shaw Sample—344 working girls %		*National Sample—786 working girls* %	
One job per year	12	One job in 2 years	44
Two jobs per year	13	Two jobs in 2 years	31
Three jobs per year	18	Three jobs in 2 years	14
Four jobs per year	14	Four jobs in 2 years	7
Five jobs or more per year	29	Five jobs in 2 years	4
Not known	4		
Unemployed	10		
	100		100

A few examples will best illustrate the stormy (or sluggish) work-days of our girls admitted to Approved School.

P was a girl of poor social and health background, and had a Binet I.Q. of 69, and a reading age of 8 years 9 months. She attended ordinary School, Open-Air School, E.S.N. School, and a School for Physically Handicapped.

She left school soon after 16, and worked for three weeks in a clothing factory but was too slow for this job.

About a month later she was employed as a kennel maid, but found the work too hard.

She then worked for two days at a clothiers, but left of her own accord.

About August she got a job in a hairdressers. After two months she was off ill and was afraid to return as she had incurred debts at the place of work.

In October she worked for half a day in a biscuit factory, which she didn't like, and then for one week at a wholesale chemists, which she left of her own accord.

(She next refused to work, kept late hours and used obscene language to her mother, who complained to the Police. She was brought before Court as beyond control and in need of care or protection. After much debate and reappearance at Court, she returned home in December, promising to be good.)

She then worked of her own choice in a pet shop but was unreliable and lost her job. She made no effort to find another, until serious pressure was put upon her, when she got a job at Woolworth's which she kept for one day.

Under pressure she started work at a hairdressers, but was late in the morning and then tried to cover up further absences.

After threatening to stab her mother if she reported her, she was again remanded, and committed to Approved School.

This made, I believe, nine jobs, and much unemployment, in about eleven months' working life.

The next is an account from the girl concerned—a girl of a stable, rather old, middle-class home, but possibly a victim both of brain-damage from epidemic encephalitis, and of indulgence at home.

When I left school I started work as a Junior clark at the Railway in —— I stuck that job for about seven week then I throw it up, a few days later I get a job at a market garding place at ——, but got the sack after a fortnight, two days later I got a job at another marcket garding firm but that was over Christmas only lasting a fortnight. Then after a few mounths (during which the parents enrolled her at a business college, from which she just absented herself) I got a job at another ofice as junior clark, resepchinist, telephone, but I dident like it so I was always takeing days of so I got the sack after les than three week. (The record said at this point that the employer, when sacking her, told her not to go near the place again . . .). After a few more monthes I got another job as a cadet Nurce at —— and I lived in there but after about two and a half monthes I left. (The record says she resigned after being repri-manded for being out late, under the influence of drink). Then I dident work for several more monthes (she was a voluntary Mental Hospital patient) but then I got a job again at a cosmetick factory but only stuck it one day then I rang up to say I wasent going again. After that I had a few more months off . . .

This makes seven jobs and much unemployment in about seventeen months.

It will already be seen that cataloguing of jobs, and of reasons for changing jobs was almost impossible on the scatter of evidence. Here is a rough assessment of reasons for leaving employment:

No changes, or inevitable changes	14%
Left mainly because fed-up	44%
Dismissed as temperamentally unsuited	18%
Dismissed as dishonest	9%

A few left because their health suffered, a few were genuinely redundant, and some were never employed. But sometimes reasons were manifold. R left school in July and a few days later started work in a fish shop. In September she gave the job up as it was too cold. Four days later she was in a clothing factory. After about five weeks she left because she had hurt a foot. She went almost at once to a rope factory. After three or four months she left because the noise of the machines affected her. She then worked for some months in another clothing factory, but became entangled with a woman who left R baby-sitting for herself and friends while they went drinking. Through the N.S.P.C.C. she came to the notice of the Children's Department who helped her to find residential employment, but she stayed in it only two weeks saying it was too quiet. For the next few months she had no regular employment, and renewed her visits to the undesirable household. She was taken to Court as in need of care or protection, and was placed on Probation. She had a resident hospital job and stayed for two days, telling her employers that her mother was sick. She then disappeared, was arrested, remanded, and committed to Approved School.

Two main points stood out in this aspect of the present study. Firstly, the girls seemed almost totally without direction as to suitable jobs. The girl above who was a 'junior clark, resepchinist, telephone', was by no means the least qualified of those who tried office work. Some girls with I.Q.'s below 80 had been so placed or had placed themselves. One shudders more at the thought of the above girl being taken on as a student nurse, and wonders how the interview went, or who arranged the interview. Equally one grieves for the customers at the mercy of the girl above who twice worked as a hairdresser. The cases depicted were among the extremes, but there were worse instances; one of the 1957 group was so obnoxiously rude on entering the factory that the foreman reprimanded the Labour Exchange for sending her along. A girl outside both these samples put poison in her foreman's tea and regretted only that there was not a lethal dose in the bottle.

The second point is that our girls had reached the critical point in their maladjustment when out at employment, and their abnormality, their need for special treatment is glaringly clear. So rare, indeed, was a very good work record that we heaved a sigh of relief and foretold an easy case; whether our belief was statistically justified we shall see later.

In the work patterns, in so far as a job lasted long enough to assume any pattern, one could see the failure of early relationships. Being 'fed-up' doubtless covered a multitude of chivvyings and lesser reprimands, which, in their touchiness, they would find intolerable.

We also have, of course, the factors of dull intelligence (therefore need for initial patience) and poor muscular coordination, and indifferent health, not to mention parental example in maintaining a job. But mainly we had a group of girls who were in need of love and acceptance in the present, who could not easily win approval from fellow-employees, and would rather absent themselves from work and seek compensation elsewhere. Without repairing some of the gaps in their lives, the work patterns could be little different.

Let it also be said that there was the sub-group of underdisciplined girls simply without inner control, and lacking, in one category of cases, parental example of hard work.

That our sample's general restlessness at work was linked with other excitement is also suggested by the recent findings of Michael Schofield,[4] Research Director, Central Council for Health Education, that the more sexually experienced girls and boys tended to have had more jobs since leaving school; half the sexually experienced girls in his large sample had been in more than two jobs, and 25 per cent of the experienced girls had had four or more jobs, compared with 6 per cent of the non-experienced girls. The sexually experienced girls were also more likely to be unemployed.

The effect of Approved School training on work stability will be interesting to follow in a later section. Taking a brief preview now, we see some interesting results emerging.

School and Work Behaviour

Girls who behaved well at day school and were not suspected of being unreliable, were markedly more regular and dependable at work (p > ·001); it was rare for a good worker to have been a really difficult girl at school, but there were 'doubtful' schoolgirls with good work records.

Work Behaviour Compared with General Success within a Year after Licence

The time chosen on licence was six months to a year (because so many girls were married after that time and success would depend less on work reactions) and reports on that period of the already reduced sample who were in employment before committal amounted to only 128. These were scattered fairly evenly between the categories (p = about ·5).

To obtain a larger sample, but a less carefully timed one, the third report after Classifying School stage was chosen. (As we shall see, reports back might refer to whenever the last news came to the Training School from after-care agents, so inaccuracies for this calculation are inevitable. The sample was increased to 316.

There was still not a significantly uneven distribution (p = > ·05), but some tendency for the girls with few changes of jobs to be more successful, and for those mainly unemployed before committal to be serious failures.

With Borstal boys (Rose, 1956) their previous work records were found to be the most helpful predictor for later success. This is more difficult to study from a younger sample of adolescent girls, one third of whom had not worked previously, and whose working life outside the home became less relevant within perhaps a year of being licensed—because of marriage. Even before that the preoccupation of a 'good' girl with work was likely to be less intense than that of a 'good' young man at Borstal release age. As Michael Schofield's[4] study showed, instability at work level tended to be linked with personality factors in general. Likewise in *our* group, there was a significant link between later success and actual *behaviour* in employment—not number of jobs (see XV Appendix).

CONDITIONS OF RESIDENCE

Some girls had a taste of residential treatment before they reached us (i.e. apart from Remand Home or Children's Home). 27 of the 284 girls who had been on probation or supervision had a condition of residence combined with the order. They obeyed or rebelled, settled or absconded as anywhere else. A few had longer experiences of residence, as we shall see.

REACTION TO EARLIER APPROVED SCHOOL TRAINING

In the 500 sample we had a small percentage—only sixteen girls—who had previously been in Approved School, usually a Junior one. This is not the total of ex-Approved School girls who passed through the Classifying School in the years 1952-4. The separate group of fifty cases which were subtracted from the main sample as being under 14 years or as special cases in other ways, comprised a group of nine older girls from the southern half of England who were not fitting into the Training Schools where they had been allocated, mostly by the Southern Classifying School for Girls. Also seven of the twenty-three girls under 14 had previously been in Junior Approved Schools.

These sub-groups will be treated separately, so we must limit ourselves here to a brief resumé on the sixteen girls of the main sample who had been in Junior Schools.

Failure on licence and re-committal followed the usual pattern of committals in the first instance—an interweaving of personality and environmental breakdowns. The following examples may best show this:

An unprepossessing, masterful girl, who imposed herself on adults, and yet was acceptable as a willing member of the community. She was easily embittered if rejected, as she had been frequently by her father, and by her mother who followed his suit. Neither showed affection, or exercised supervision. The home was dirty and untidy. At 11 she was before the Court for giving false fire alarms, and at 12 was a truant, a heavy smoker, a bed-wetter, and she ran away from home at least three times. She was committed to Approved School and responded fairly well. She returned home fully three years later to similar home conditions, though licence had been delayed for this reason. She worked well for almost a year, then began to feel rejected at home, and by work-mates and others outside the home. She stayed off work frequently, and she stole from the girls. She deteriorated, left home, was immoral, and committed larceny, and was re-committed to Approved School.

The second example was the youngest of three children born to an elderly married man with whom the mother co-habited for twenty years. He died when this girl was 11. He had, when younger, had convictions for bigamy, assault, and murder (reduced to manslaughter), and for being drunk and disorderly. The mother had a conviction for larceny of a pram. When the girl was 5, a baby brother died, and some time later the broken-hearted parents legally adopted a little boy of very poor stock. About this stage the girl truanted from school, and she began (at 10) to steal money from children in the street, and fruit from the docks. At 11 she was brought before the Court by her mother as beyond her control; she was said to be corrupting her little adoptive brother. She was placed under Supervision, but continued to truant, and went to the cinema with an elderly tramp whom she 'picked up'. (Soon after this her own father, who had long been bed-ridden, and careless about personal habits, died.) As the girl was still not responding she was committed at 11 to Junior Approved School. After a bad start she made very good progress, becoming Head Girl. Before she returned home at 15, her mother had married a coloured seaman six years her junior. The girl found it difficult to settle, especially as her mother and stepfather were frequently quarrelling and contemplating separation, and the latter asked the girl to leave the house. She lived with a sister, and in residential posts, in one of which she stole a variety of articles, and was re-committed to Approved School, which she very much resented, having, as she put it, 'been someone' in another Approved School.

Both these girls learned to be ambitious and proud in Junior Schools, and could not settle to much worse than average home conditions. Each was rather robot-like in her social response, and cared terribly for the good opinion of others and failed to get it in home areas where the parents were looked down on, and the Approved School history known. Besides which, they had to make these desperate re-adjustments still at a difficult period of adolescence.

This tended to be one pattern of recommittal history—return from simulated middle-class family life to depraved and unloving home backgrounds, while social judgment was still very immature. The other main pattern (for this section of the 500, and for those in the little sub-group, as above) was of the constitutional problem, or sometimes the psychopath, whose early deprivations (and perhaps hereditary traits) had led to multiple attempts at remedial work. We shall see this in our example, pp. 207–8, of early treatment in a School for Maladjusted Children, followed by stays in three Junior Approved Schools—to be followed by one more, and two Senior Approved Schools, followed by Borstal. This group is the really crucial one, where the girl needed opportunities to live through the difficulties of her earliest years, rather than a pattern suited to the normal, the socially untutored, or perhaps the mildly neurotic. They were cushioned by the physical comforts and relative absence of emotional demands in the Approved School, but a return to the four walls of home and family emotions brought back the early conflicts, right at the most difficult period of adolescence. And then it was mostly years too late for such excessive early difficulties to be resolved, either in a Senior Approved School or elsewhere.

At the period of this research the younger girls admitted to Junior Approved Schools (i.e. under 14) were generally not classified, and assessment elsewhere was uncertain. A pre-committal psychiatric report to the Court on one case said: '*Her intelligence is below average—having an I.Q. of 98.*' At the Training School she was 'always treated as a border-line case' (from the Headmistress's report). Pressure was exerted on her there, without any allowance for the fact that she had learned during that Court appearance that her father was not dead, as she had always believed, but in Mental Hospital. As her mother had associated with men, the realization of the latter's unsatisfactory life also came to her as a shock—along with removal from home. Fortunately she was later treated with warmth, and as of normal intelligence, and she led a reasonably settled life on eventual release.

REACTION TO PREVIOUS REMANDS

This section will be very brief. Because the remand home's régime and purpose were nearest to our own, and were, indeed, often confused with it, it is most difficult to assess the setting and its success or otherwise.

The Remand Home is mainly a place of safety, where a delinquent is kept in storage, as it were, pending a Court appearance, or re-appearance for a decision to be reached. The Superintendent made a report to the Court, and generally a copy of this report (sometimes several reports) reached us, and often a specially written letter to the

Classifying School. We received such reports from six Remand Homes in the northern half of the country in the period of the research, and from two other Sheltering, or Refuge Homes. The reports were valuable because of their comments on the girls' reactions there, but often they were so coloured by personal feeling that we learned much more about the Homes and their personnel, and what they stood for, than about the girl herself. And they seemed from these personal feelings to differ very widely indeed. As we had not always kept a note of a girl's behaviour on remand, this had to be excluded from the research material.

Psychiatric reports obtained on remand (for the benefit of the Juvenile Courts) were carried out either in the Home, or at a Child Guidance or Hospital Clinic. In addition, with a view to reporting objectively to the Court, four of the Remand Homes used objective tests, mainly group intelligence and scholastic tests. The administration was not always under the direction of a trained tester, and the results were given without the qualifications necessary. The sort of duplication of effort involved was inherent in much criticism at this stage (and since) of having the dual system, rather than carrying out full-scale classification while in more adequately staffed and equipped Remand Homes. (Since then this pattern has indeed been developing, both for boys and girls.)

Since all our 500 girls (with one exception that the writer can recall) had been in a Remand Home for some part of her delinquent history, and some for a number of remands (usually seven days or fourteen days per time), the impact of that time inevitably had an effect on how a girl settled with us.

The least tension was usually felt in girls coming from a mixed-sex Home; if staff feelings about a girl's reactions there, *vis-à-vis* the boys, were expressed strongly in the reports, at least there tended to be less tension, and here the mixed-sex staffing probably helped as much. (We must not draw too much notice to this, however, for the proportion of older girls would be very small, and not comparable to a mixed Approved School.) On the other hand, girls from a very rigid, matron-dominated régime, if they arrived tense, soon showed such relief at 'softer' discipline that we again benefited. We suffered more from those institutions most like our own—all female, and fairly liberal, but sometimes the liberality had seemed to be more for one girl than another, and 'matron's pet' did not take kindly to being a new girl, especially if suppressed at her first presumption to special favour.

We also suffered from clannish friendships, and from anti-social ganging-up which dated from Remand Home friendships with other girls. These happened mainly, again, in those with régimes like our own—which is an interesting and sobering reflection. Possibly the all-female caste, and the rather warm individual handling (more so than ours, one would judge), with inevitable jealousies, were a major cause. Generally we accepted (at the Remand Home's suggestion) one girl of the alliance at a time, but she tended to remain unsettled until her confederate(s) came, and then they were once more as thick as thieves—only more often as thick as incipient prostitutes! Many window-breakings and group-abscondings followed such re-unions at the Classifying School. On the other hand, we were more often able to use a girl who had already settled well with us, to help a former friend to settle on admission. We looked usually for positive factors in our group manœuvres.

What we benefited from by the earlier remands were (a) the girl's experience of group living, and of a work and play régime rather like our own (as far as one could judge), and (b) the cleansing processes; series of girls who had arrived from their own very dirty homes, or from other people's (perhaps houses of ill-repute), or nobody's (from the streets or from lorries or camps) must have been a trying and sordid sight. We saw this aspect only when receiving girls from particularly depraved abscondings. Yet we lost something in the way of understanding her earlier plight though we still usually saw her arriving in her own clothing, cleaned up if necessary.

Without doubt a combination of the two systems—remand with classification is the right answer, with each streamlined to give the maximum information in the minimum time—and with the minimum personal involvement necessary for human understanding; when dealing with adolescents deep involvement may well be essential for adequate understanding, in which case resilience and a short memory may be the best qualifications for those assessing and observing. Our ideals at The Shaw were pitched as much at treatment level as assessment level, and some of our expertise could well have been used elsewhere.

Chapter Seventeen
MALADJUSTMENT

The term 'delinquent' covers a variety of symptoms. Indeed it has social rather than clinical applications; rarely is the word applied to a child or a young person until the point of Court procedure is reached, and, as we have seen, Court procedure begins at different points in different areas, and in different social classes, largely according to how much the environment tolerates before public sanctions are taken, or how soon Approved School training is seen as the constructive decision, and to what other facilities are available.

The delinquent girls who reached us were predominantly from unskilled, semi-skilled and dependent social gradings, and the parents tended to be inarticulate. They needed to be drawn into seeking and accepting help. Not only the girls themselves had suffered the kind of shocks and deprivations which set them aside from their contemporaries, but their parents (or remaining parent) had often suffered loss of partner, or much ill-health in the home, or the guilt and bewilderment of one or more children appearing before the Courts. This is not the setting from which many treatable cases come to Child Guidance Clinics, unless the latter are geared to this sort of problem. If an appointment with the Clinic is made for the delinquent and parent through the School it may not be kept, or may well lapse after the first interview. Travelling some distance to talk things over does not come easily to many mothers of delinquents—some one to drop in, and figuratively hold their hand would better fill the bill. In any case, an overworked service like Child Guidance has to put the child on a waiting list, and the speed with which things happened to our girls meant many new crises before even the beginning of treatment. Dr Ivy Bennett,[1] in *Delinquent and Neurotic Children*, says (p. 225):

> For fairly obvious reasons, many chronic delinquent children do not fall into the class of case suitable for child guidance treatment or even for individual psychotherapy. In a great many cases a distortion in character development has taken place very early in the child's life and a long-term programme of psychiatrically supervised emotional re-education (rather than intensive psychotherapy) is indicated. This tends both to be more difficult to put into practice and to take *very much longer* periods of time to carry out adequately than the so-called 'lengthy' transference

203

analysis of the neurotic. We know from our attempt to analyse those forces and conditions which go to the making of a delinquent child that it has taken a very long time for this emotional development to get set into its characteristic twisted and embittered course and we must expect it will also take us a long time to undo this faulty pattern and to transform the child into a happy and socially healthy being again. When normal home-life has for one reason or another failed to achieve its socializing functions, the substitutes we offer in the way of foster-homes, special hostels or institutions, etc., can only operate under a treble handicap; namely that their socializing and corrective influence, even when most wisely and kindly administered, comes after there has been a deeply inscarred, original failure, often publicly recognized; that these 'secondary homes' to which the child is transferred operate at best within a second-hand authority system which has weakened human attachments and diluted emotional meaning and is therefore a shallower soil for the child's roots than his own home; and thirdly that very often this 'second chance' in social adaptation is offered *so many years too late.*

While this statement emanates from a Child Guidance Clinic worker, the frustrations of not being able so very often to help delinquent children in the Clinics lead more often to impatient, sweeping statements, which suggest a hard and fast line between the delinquent and the neurotic, while the recognition that it is too late for treatment, is applied to what can be done by the Clinic, but not so leniently to homes and residential schools—least of all to Approved Schools. Yet we shall hope to see with our 500 sample of delinquent girls that very often it was not 'many years too late', and if we see this one hopes for due credit for the hard work of re-education by the Approved School staff concerned.

This project covers the early and middle 1950s. With the slow growth of the School Psychological Service, of Day Classes for Maladjusted Children, of improved psychological and psychiatric services working within Reception Centres and other Local Authority as well as Voluntary Homes and Hostels, one hopes that the mild and relatively unhurtful epithet 'maladjusted' can be applied to a proportion of disturbed and anti-social girls at the earlier stages; 15 per cent of our 500 sample (seventy-five girls) and 19 of the 100 sample had manifested their delinquency before the age of 12. But 30 per cent of each group had shown other serious behaviour difficulties by then. True that in a proportion of the delinquent cases their maladjustment was then well beyond the seriousness of what is treated 'normally' in Child Guidance Clinics, and too serious for Schools or Hostels for Maladjusted Children as they existed (or exist?).

Maladjustment

As far as could be judged from the Shaw records, 63 per cent of the 500 sample (but down to 46 in the 100 sample) had *not* been referred to a Child Guidance Clinic, nor to a Psychiatrist working in a Hospital, even for a pre-committal report. Of the 37 per cent who had been referred, 23 per cent were referred while on remand only, which means *one* interview. At least this service had been extended by 1957, so that 38 per cent were seen as remand cases. A report from this session was usually given to us by the Probation Officer, or Child Care Officer concerned. As it was a report specifically for lay Magistrates, its usefulness to us varied. Sometimes the reports were most helpful, but only a few seeing our admissions seemed to have specialized in the diagnosis and treatment of the adolescent girl, or of the delinquent of any age or sex. Some showed in their reports a sympathetic comprehension of the girls' problems. At the other extreme was one particular Psychiatrist who left the girls so perturbed that a similar situation (including cognitive testing, which this doctor had included in her session) brought out grave anxiety. 'I wouldn't answer these questions at ——, and that was to a doctor, so I'm not going to answer them for you!' And refusal in test sessions was as unusual with us as were tantrums with our own Visiting Psychiatrist.

Only 8 per cent of the 500 sample, and 7 per cent of the second, had been referred to a Child Guidance Clinic for diagnosis, other than when on remand. This was usually at the instigation of a Probation Officer, or Children's Officer (in the case of a child in care) and rarely by the day School. We sometimes then had a psychiatrist's report available. If other girls had been seen through the School Psychological Service, by an Educational Psychologist, reports never came to us from this source. Intelligence test results entered in the School Report section of the Record of Information were usually (one assumed in the absence of the relevant information) from group test results at school, or from individual testing by a School Medical Officer of Health. Without more information about the test the figures were useless to us. We accepted as valid test results known to have been carried out by a Psychologist, and retested only when our other test results were at wide variance, or if we knew that the girl had improved in cooperativeness since.

Further, 6 per cent (thirty girls) of the 500 sample, and none of the 100 sample had been treated at a Child Guidance Clinic. As elsewhere, we received those for whom the treatment had not sufficed. A sense of defeat could sometimes be read into the final reporting: S, with a long history of pilfering, and diurnal and nocturnal enuresis throughout a chequered home life, a Junior Approved School, a short-lived fostering and a couple of hostels, began, after intermittent Child Guidance treatment for three years, to respond to psychotherapy, and became more tidy and less inclined to 'borrow' possessions. When she added staying out all night with U.S. Servicemen to her repertoire of maladjustment, the psychiatrist concerned recommended Approved School 'as the only way of segregating her from males'. This spoke of ambivalence, from a profession that is usually so critical of the Approved School's segregatedness from males! Indeed the final report to the Court, on a girl well known to the Clinic, showed sometimes the same breakdown in hitherto liberal views of treatment as the rest of us are prone to; at the last ditch the girl had to be 'taught a lesson', and the Approved School would have to do it. Perhaps, as Approved School workers, we should be forgiven some annoyance at this typical attitude of Magistrates, Social Workers, and Psychologists and Psychiatrists who later did not rush to praise successes or to spare blame for failure, and tended then to ascribe punitive attitudes to us. Having wished them on the Approved School system, they then tend to wonder why they are not kept longer; their return to the community even on licence or under supervision could be inconvenient.

A reminder that these findings and comments relate to the early and mid-1950s must be repeated; psychiatric and psychological services have extended somewhat (but not nearly enough, of course) and more experience with the problem adolescent girl has been doubtless gained in more places, especially with slow development of Adolescent Units. But we received problems from the South too, who had been treated by acknowledged experts with the adolescent, and had not responded sufficiently. It is difficult for the expert working 'outside' to appreciate the views of Staff inside, as it is for the 'inside' expert to appreciate always the urges for 'new' methods and freedom by the outsider. A reconciliation of views has been eased within some Approved Schools in recent years, through extended psychiatric consultation, and one would hope that this is even more true in pre-committal establishments such as Remand Homes.

SCHOOLS FOR MALADJUSTED

A few had, quite early on in their history, been sent to schools or hostels for maladjusted children, and came our way as failures, as failures of all systems came our way. Often their stay at the Special School had been brief, and followed by numerous brief interim measures before they reached the Classifying School.

One such example was the girl of aggressive, rejecting parents, instanced as being in three Children's Homes, two Special Schools (plus two Approved Schools) and three Mental Hospitals before she reached us, and she subsequently attended two more Approved Schools before she disappeared. Three others of the eleven who had been to Schools or Hostels for Maladjusted fitted into a query-psychopathic category, and, like most of those who had been to Schools for Maladjusted were 'too maladjusted'. But four of these were less untouchable; the others ranged from the near-psychopath to the severely neurotic.

The most psychopathic, manifesting her non-conformity in sexual misdemeanours latterly, not in aggressiveness, was born of a most unsettled marriage, and reared—'a good child'—by grandparents. At 7, back with her parents and a baby born of a reconciliation, X began to wander from home, to steal dolls in prams, and then babies in prams. The Child Guidance Clinic took over. The parents again separated, a housekeeper failed to manage X and she was admitted to a local Children's Home which she left after a few months. At 8 she was sent to a hostel for maladjusted children. At 10 she was discharged as 'chronically unstable' and as 'incapable of benefitting from their treatment'. A year later she was wandering and began a series of bicycle thefts, which continued on multiple abscondings from *three* Junior Approved Schools over the next twelve months. She also stole from a Church offertory box, and cigarettes and sweets from a shop. Having again failed badly on a trial at home (and having, she says herself, had intercourse with a 'foriner') she was, at 12, admitted for the first time to the Shaw Classifying School. She was sturdy, healthy, and looked 14. She could sing like a linnet. Her eyes were secretive and her mouth tightly compressed. She was 'kept in order' by the older girls, who soon recognized the 5-year-old beneath the pseudo-composure. At her next Junior Approved School (about the only one she had not been to) she was a major problem, who 'electrified the air', and attracted men 'like a magnet'. When not luring other young girls to the house of a coloured man, she spent much time filling notebook after notebook with fantasy stories 'about men, etc.'. The School's Visiting Psychiatrist, asked if he could help said 'No thank you—she is a menace'. At that point some adults in charge of her diagnosed her ideal career as mistress to a rich man. The writer was inclined to agree; she had not coarsened; she was 'nice' in her unreliability; she looked attractive, and her voice and manners were good. Later, as we came to know only too well, she was to go well down the ladder, but remain a total prostitute. She had an interlude at home at 14, during which she associated freely with youths whom she picked up on the street. Of one she wrote 'he is a plecent love maker and I still love him to this day'.

This trial at home was such a clear failure that she came to us again, and the atmosphere at once seethed with her restlessness. She had no ill-will towards us (she wrote 'very nice beds, plenty to eat and lots of kind staff'. She also wrote: '*Grown ups* can help you when you are bad'; and '*My greatest worry* is that I have been bad too long.' She absconded again and again, unsettling others. She returned from a brothel in Manchester and needed treatment for venereal infections. She was re-transferred to a briskly tolerant and affectionate Headmistress of a Senior Approved School from which she again absconded frequently, and had relations with men of all kinds and conditions. The kindly influences made no impact whatsoever. When her full period of training, from the recommittal at 12 plus, had expired (at the age of 15 years 4 months) she returned home, but no one else had much hope of success, and X herself never thought into the future. Soon she had stolen from her parents' wardrobe, and was picked up badly needing treatment for venereal disease, of which she had now been cured repeatedly, and was committed for the third time to Approved School, against the advice of those who knew her best, for she was clearly incapable of normal social living and would unsettle and corrupt many girls. Her earlier leisure interests (games, dancing, singing, playing children's games) had been dissipated, and she was interested only in 'playing the fool'. After numerous abscondings she was committed to Borstal soon after she was 16—and wrote from there to her last Approved School happily. The sequel can with reasonable certainty be guessed. She had taken up an incalculable amount of time and energy, had upset many other girls, and had deteriorated herself. She had not even been contained.

Those girls who had been admitted to Schools or Hostels for Maladjusted Children tended, even when they admitted they were happy there, to talk of 'coming out' from them, as some would subsequently from Approved Schools and Borstal. Rarely did we receive a girl who was touched by the therapy given in the Schools; one was; she had been at a mixed School, but not sufficiently long when she had to leave because the School was forced to become one-sex. She attacked her adoptive parents physically. The softening process had, however, begun, and she responded well to Approved School training. (Unfortunately she was killed soon after in a road accident.) But another, at 14, was still at the 'messy play' and 'loud noises for effect' stage, that she had displayed in play therapy sessions at the age of 7. She was a subsequent Approved School failure.

Our perspective of the treatment of children as maladjusted rather than delinquent was damaged first, as has been said, by the fact that we received the failures; secondly because so few Schools for Maladjusted existed, and so few special classes, that only some of the most seriously disturbed could be admitted, and those who reached us were doomed to failure from the start. Once the majority of our girls manifested their emotional troubles, they were too old for the sparse vacancies and the kinds of régime existent in boarding schools other than those approved by the Secretary of State—which *had* to accept them, and on occasions be blamed for mishandling the failures of other systems.

SYMPTOMS OF MALADJUSTMENT

Most important still was the need to attune all these services to the often much more difficult girl who has not become delinquent before 12, but may at School, to the observant teacher, have signs of maladjustment. Not all girls aged 14 to 16 committed to Girls' Approved Schools in the 1950s required psychological or psychiatric treatment, but help in the form of a *full* diagnosis was required much more frequently than it was obtained.

There is little need to justify the belief that many of the girls were maladjusted, by referring to the symptom groupings 'which may be indicative of maladjustment', according to Appendix B of the *Report of the Committee on Maladjusted Children*[3] (The Underwood Report, 1955).

If we look first at the behaviour disorders, which we expect to stand out, we have the following table, giving the incidence *where recorded* only.

Table 49: Behaviour Disorders

	Sample of 500 known to have shown symptoms%	
	Up to age 12	Age 12 to committal
Unmanageableness—defiance, disobedience, refusal to go to school or work	19·6	42·2
Temper tantrums, aggressiveness (bullying, destructiveness, cruelty and jealous behaviour)	9·4	31·6
Demands for attention	—	38·6*
Stealing	17·8	43·2
Lying and romancing†	4·0	5·2
Truancy—wandering, staying out late	13·6	83·0
Sex difficulties—masturbation, sex-play, homosexuality	2·6	4·8

* *Figure at C.S., not pre-committal.*
† *Recorded here only if at pathological level.*

209

Nervous disorders were less consistently recorded; they were not exactly grist for the mill through which a delinquent girl must go. But fears, anxieties, depression, withdrawal appeared, and excitability (as various interludes show) was prevalent enough. Apathy and hysterical fits likewise.

Habit disorders. Speech disorders were not a feature, but night-terrors and sleep-walking or talking were so common at the Classifying School that one did not think of recording. (Sleep-walking was, needless to say, also claimed by night-prowlers.)

Nail-biting has been discussed.

Twitching was mildly represented.

Feeding difficulties occurred in the form of compensatory overeating.

Enuresis has been discussed.

Nine asthmatics were recorded in the 500 sample.

Organic disorders. 12 of the 500 sample were established or strongly suspected cases of early injury, encephalitis, cerebral tumours or epilepsy. More were queried.

Psychotic. Only 1 of the 500 sample was later diagnosed as psychotic, but within the three-year period five girls in the C.S. had well-defined symptoms of psychosis. These were admitted to Mental Hospital (one to Borstal), and not included in the sample though occasionally discussed.

Educational difficulties (backwardness not accounted for by dullness, for instance) and inability to keep jobs have been well discussed.

A few examples, all of the same initial, and admitted in one year, will illustrate that the girls' histories could vie with the most disturbed anywhere:

Case 1. Sixth of seven children of a semi-invalid, very difficult father. Of 'outstanding' ability at school, but of unsatisfactory achievement, and anti-social. At 15 she was a victim of carnal knowledge. She absconded repeatedly from hostels. Extremely obstinate and defiant, and negativistic; one scene lasted two days. Observation in Mental Hospital arranged but she absconded.

Case 2. Had meningitis at 3½. Was enuretic for a long time. Had two jobs in 9 months (with unemployment), then 'several different jobs' in the next six months, staying only a few days in each. She was associating with bargemen.

Case 3. A child of gipsy extraction, adopted by two intellectuals of little warmth. At 3 she was still not clean, and she continued to wet and soil. At 6 to 7 she was 'dishonest, disobedient and quarrelsome', especially with other children at school. (For the next six years she was taught at home.) At 12 she was behaving very badly, and was wandering from home. Allowed to go to school, she was found unreliable there, associating with girls of 'low mentality and doubtful morals'. At 15 she left school to work, but two months later left home. Returned next day, but missing again two days later. Threatened to repeat process. Remanded. Dirty in her personal habits and an absconder from the remand home. Next ran away repeatedly from a resident domestic post and had sexual relations with an older man.

Case 4. At 6 she was sent to a convent, after her father was killed through enemy action. At 14 she was sent home because of uncontrollable tempers. Did not settle at home. Sent to another convent. Within a few weeks her mother was asked to remove her. Advice sought, and she was believed to be in need of psychological treatment. In-patient for six months in well-known Mental Hospital. Discharged at 15 and went to a job. Much trouble in the home, and brought before the Court as beyond control. Placed in Approved Hostel, where the Warden could help her to control tempers, but this Warden left and the Deputy was unable to manage her. At this time she continued to be enuretic. Remanded (still very difficult) then sent to another well known Mental Hospital, from which she insisted on going home after a month. Quarrelsome and difficult. Again in Mental Hospital for three weeks. Admitted to a Training Home. Absconded. Remanded again. Serious temper outbursts. (After classification she remained subject to serious tempers, stabbing one girl at the Training School with a pair of scissors, and dragging another girl round the room by the hair. On psychiatric advice she was retained for a normal period of Training. By 21 was no longer having outbursts of violence. She had once attacked her husband but he retaliated, and she quietened down!)

Case 5. Saw her mother burned to death. She was then 3, and her father (a heavy drinker, with convictions) had already gone away to live with another woman. After two years in Cottage Homes, she was fostered out, then adopted. She was (from 6) said to be difficult, self-centred, aggressive and obstinate, and consequently had no playmates. Attended a Child Guidance Clinic for two years, but this not help relationships with home. At the Secondary Modern School she showed undue interest in the opposite sex. She spent four months in a School for Maladjusted Children, where she 'learned to consider others'. Only on her return from there was she told she was an adopted child; she felt 'uncomfortable'. On leaving school she made undesirable friendships and went to dance halls, and other places of doubtful repute, and was generally beyond control.

Case 6. Daughter of a couple who lived together unhappily, while the husband carried on associations with other women. Two boys were on probation. At 14 our girl was reported by her Head Teacher to the Probation Officer as a 'plausible liar' who needed constant supervision. Soon afterwards she was before the Court for making false telephone calls. At the Remand Home she seemed a maladjusted child, and was furtive, ill-mannered and a bad mixer. Child Guidance treatment was recommended (not, it seems, carried out). Within twenty-two months of leaving school, she had six jobs, from five of which she was dismissed, with long periods of unemployment between. She persisted in associating with a youth whose mother disapproved. She stole money from home, and stayed out late.

We must also remember that histories were of necessity far less carefully and fully documented than in Child Guidance files; yet our Classifying cases would generally more than hold their own for adverse symptoms, with samples from Clinics. To some extent the figures, when studied statistically, had a typical 'Approved School' trend; there was 100 to 1 chance that the dullards (I.Q. 84 and below) were those who were out late, while those average and above (having more initiative) were more likely to leave home for longish periods. But all groups could claim some maladjustment.

Chapter Eighteen

SEXUAL ABERRANCE

Although heterosexual behaviour has been a recurrent feature of our case histories, the extent of this problem has so far not been charted. It was often incidental to being unmanageable (beyond control) or to wandering impulses, and a fairly regular forerunner of a care-or-protection order.

The following information was gathered from the girls' files:

Table 50: First Heterosexual Experience (Up to time of Committal)

	Sample of 500 %	Sample of 100 %
None, as far as known	13·6	7·0
With a 'pick-up', usually on earliest acquaintance	48·8	54·0
Casual acquaintance, such as school-mate, work-mate or neighbour	13·4	8·0
Friend or fiancé	3·4	8·0
Own father, step- or foster-father, or adoptive father, or brother or other relative	3·4	3·0
Unknown (i.e. almost certainly had had sexual experience, but not established with whom)	17·4	20·0

The extent and the limitations of the experience was not so easy to record, and no attempt was made to do so. Some of the older, especially the more sophisticated, girls had had very extensive experience, and often with many men and youths. Others had had concentrated experience with one man, either in the home area, or after running away with him because she was unhappy at home. A few, though before the Court as in need of care or protection after a stated number of males had been convicted for offences against her, had not in fact had full sexual intercourse; one at 14 was said to have associated with men and youths between the ages of 69 and 13, and six were charged with indecent assault but when remanded she was found to be virgo intacta. Another, who was notorious to the Police in her home area and to the Military Police at a nearby large camp, claimed she was a virgin, and was delighted when this was established. However, these were fairly rare situations, and many of the dull girls delighted in giving the sum total of the times they had had intercourse—a word known to a group whose vocabulary would not have contained 'interrupt' or 'intersperse'.

In March 1954 the Technical Sub-Committee of the Association of Headmasters, Headmistresses and Matrons of Approved Schools produced Monograph 6 entitled *Girls in Approved Schools*. On page 6 were given figures for the sexual experience of 102 girls admitted to a Girls' Classifying School over a period of six months. (The number admitted in six months shows this was the other Girls' Classifying School.) Calculated in percentages, the following is deduced from the table:

73·5 per cent of the girls (aged 14 to 17) had had sexual intercourse.

11·8 per cent of the girls had indulged in sexual play, but intercourse was doubtful.

14·7 per cent of the girls were virgo intacta, except that for a third of these the finding was doubtful.

Rather more of the Shaw girls (13·6 per cent of the 500 sample) had almost certainly not had sexual intercourse, and a further percentage was doubtful; how many of these had had some experience was impossible to say.

In the same Monograph (above) it was shown that only 47 per cent of girls admitted to a Junior Girls' Approved School (i.e. aged 14 or under) had no sexual experience, as far as was known; 5 out of 27 girls aged up to 12 years were described as 'sexually experienced' or victims of incest; 12 out of 63 girls between 12 and 14 years old were similarly described. Seven men were in Court charged with offences against 1 of our 500 sample when she was 13; she had been seduced at 8 by an older man.

Until recently it was difficult to discuss these findings in terms of normality. However, with the publication in 1965 of Michael Schofield's[1] report *The Sexual Behaviour of Young People*, we can compare them with figures for a large representative sample of girls, from all levels of society and educational backgrounds. According to this (unlike the 70 per cent or more of the girls in the C.S. sample aged 14, 15 and 16 who were sexually experienced in the sense of having intercourse with one or more partners), only 6 and 7 per cent of those aged 15 and 16 respectively (from samples of 140 and 237 'normal' girls) were so experienced. Only 2·3 per cent of the total sample of over 900 girls had, on retrospective evidence, similar experience before the age of 15, and only 0·1 per cent (or 1 in a 1,000) before 14. (The word 'only' implies satisfaction in relation to the scare-mongers who feared for the sex morals of all young people, and in relation to the ultra broad-minded, who have implied in the writer's hearing that Approved School Girls' previous sexual misconduct was not out of the ordinary run.)

The correlations found in Michael Schofield's research between sexual experience and parental unhappiness, lack of parental supervision, unhappiness at school and unsettledness at work, all are reflected in the small section of his sample which would match our Approved School girls to some degree.

70 per cent of the Approved School girls were 'early starters' by Michael Schofield's definition (having had sexual intercourse at the age of 16 or younger); 5·4 per cent of his group were early starters. However only one of his early starters admitted that her first partner in intercourse was a pick-up, while well over half of his early starters had intercourse with a steady boy-friend. We have seen that about half our Approved School sample had their first experience with a pick-up, and only 4 per cent of the whole sample had their first experience with a fiancé or boy-friend.

The degree of promiscuity, implying lack of tenderness, and lack of respect for true personal relationships was part of the Classifying School group's excessive social immaturity; we recall, however, that there were indeed more ordinary 'boy and girl' sex relations, and some of the 4 per cent who were involved with boy-friends or fiancés probably needed (except where there was seriously maladjusted behaviour) guidance rather than such extreme measures.

The C.S. girls who had their early (usually their continued) sexual experience with 'pick-ups' gravitated to a few distinct groups— American Servicemen, seamen of various nationalities, and coloured immigrants in the over-crowded quarters of large cities, especially in Manchester and Leeds. By 1957 the Hungarian Revolution had sent a new group of uprooted males, this time to the East Midlands, and a number of girls had sought their company. There were of course, for both samples, other kinds of casual paramours, but the general pattern followed for half of both our groups was association with men far from home who, like the girls themselves, were without immediate loyalties and affectional bonds.

One of the most promiscuous of the group—a plump blonde, pleasant but pathetically weak—wrote at length of her experiences thus:

On the Saturday night I was just getting ready to go out with my friend Ann when a girl called P who lives just around the courner from us called for me and asked me if I would like to go to the town pictures, so I was in for 11 o'clock well P was 2 years older than me, and I was nearly

16 years, but she said she would come home with me, when we got in town it was about 8 o'clock, and she said let's go and play some records in the Arcade, so just as we entered the door we bumped into to American's and we stood talking to them and then went to the pictures, after the pictures we went in a cafe called the Holliewood cafe, anyway after they has seen us of home, we arranged a date for the following night but we did not go and meet them we starting hanging around the train station and cafes, and going with diffrent Americans, then she intrused me to some of the girls, which I knew by the look of them were prositutues, but they spoke alright with me, but all the time I was praying I would not turn out like them, so things started to go worse, my mother and father kept asking me were had I been and who I had been with but all I told them were lies, and then I started mixing deeper into the comany of the town girls, and going in pub's where the Americans hang out, then the girls told me I could have a smashing time without living at home and going to work, so I left home with a girl called G and that night we went to Blackpool with tow Americans, and every day and night for 9 days we were with Americans but the first time I got let of by the Police, and I promised I would not go of again, but next day I went into town to get a job, and when I was coming back I called the very same cafe which got me into trouble the first time and sat with two Americans I knew, and they asked me where I had been putting myself, so I told them and they said if I were you I go back home and leave these dives alone, because you are a good kid, and I would be lible to end up as the other girls I said I had to leave them because I had not been home all day, so just as I got out side I met T one of the lowest girls liven. I know I did wrong going with here she asked me not to go home but live with her, but I said the police would only fetch me back, but she said if you watch yourself you'll be alright, so I did not go home I lived with Americans in Manchester then I moved to Liverpool and lived with them there, then Warrington for 7 weeks I did it I was nearly droping I knew something was wrong with me, so on the following Saturday I moved back to Manchester where I got picked up and I was glad, and I wonderd why I ever got mixed up with such conmony for my mother and father had worked hard for me and to put me one the right road, so I went infront of the court and they sent me to a home for a medical report so I did 7 weeks at —— for I had 4 weeks longer because of a misscarrage so after that I went in a Hostel in —— to try and forget the past and start afresh for I was all set in taking up stage life for I am very interested in it and have always set my mind on it so they moved me to a hostel, I did not like it so me and a girl ran away we went up Londen and went with Americans and Cannadians for 4 weeks till we got picked up and they put me in a nother home in —— for 3 weeks, after that I went infront of the court and they said they were giving me a chance because of my good conduct and very good parents and a good home, and they asked me to leave Warrington alone and I promised, so I went back to Manchester on 2 years probation so I went home very happy knowing I

was going to keep my promise of stopping at home and starting work but I got a letter from one of my American friends asking me to meet him so on the Sunday I went down and met him when I met him of the train I knew he had been drinking so I ignord him and I went back down in the Holliewood and I met T the very same girl she asked me what I was doing and I told her so we both went for a drink and I no we mixed with the Americans for I could hardly stand up and we went to T's flat with 2 Americans into which they stayed all night, and I thought how I made that promise and I did not want to go on with that life again, but after I told her about what I was thinking she said if any thing whet wrong she would help me out, so I stayed with her for a week, as I would call it we were picking up diffrent Americans every night and takeing them back to the flat but I had just got rid of a dissis V.D., and I knew it was coming out on me again, I told T about it but she said it was just a rash with not being used to men, but I knew diffrent because I could not walk properly and I kept going dizzy, sometimes I thought I was going to drop on the floor, and I had a idea I was pregnat again, I told her about it and she said she would help me get rid of it but I would have to wait the following week till she got hold of some fellow called N so we both got ready to go out and she asked me to go with her to start picking coloured Americans up but I told her I would not lower myself to go with one and that I was to ill to go with one so she said you stop in and I'll bring you one back so when she went I got ready got my things together and went, so I went up town and phoned a American I knew up and told him I wanted to see him quick, so he said he would be up in a hour, so I sat in a cafe till then and the time would be 8.30 I told him all about it and what was wrong with me he said I knew you when you were a decent kid, I'll break her cheap ruddy neck he said and he asked me where I was going that night I told him I was going to walk around because I was no use to anybody while I was in this state, but he said I was and he would get me cleared up and start making a decent girl out of me, so he got me a room in the same Hotel as himself and as I went in my room he said good night kid, get all the sleep you want, in the morning I was awoke at 10 o'clock and I had Breadfast, then a bath then I got dressed I was ready dead on 12 noon and I felt alot better after one good nights rest, when we got out-side we sat in a cafe and he told me he could not stop with me long as he had to get the train and get to work, so I went with him to the station and he gave me £3 15 he said that would help me to get a room at night till he came down and pitched more money, so when he got on the train I went back to the Cosy kettle cafe as it was Sunday and the Pictures did not open untill 2 o'clock, so I sat there untill a girl I knew called B walked in and she sat down besides me, B was a nice girl very decent, but she told me she had run away from home, and she had been sleeping with diffrent Americans for 4 nights, and she was feeling ill so we planned to move right away from Manchester, so Sunday night we got a train into Carlise but we had not got enough money to carry on right through, so we started on the road and we got a Lorry into Scotland after a day and a half without sleep or food we walked around Glasgow, untill we got in with some hoys and they took us to there place and we stayed there 3 nights and we took another Lorry into Preswick and we started walking roung the American arodrome, and we got in with some American Air men, we stoped with them till 11.30. at night, and then we left them and took another lorry into London after 2 more shamefull nights we gladly arrived in Leister Square, so we went for a wash and we tided ourselves up and started walking around we no sooner got on the road when two American sailors stoped us so we told them our situation, so we stopped with them for two nights in a Hotel and all the time I was getting fed up worrying what was going to happen to me, and about my mother father what they were thinking to, if they ownly knew what there daughter was turning out to be, taking shameful Lorry rides wondering when your next meal is going to be and your next bed, and now I started to reilse it all why dident I take the right road and hold my head up instead of holding it down breaking my Parents hearts, them wondering what people were going to say when they went out, and now I reilised it to late, I had to take what was coming, so after we left the Americans, we went in a Arcade and hung around there till we got in with two more Americans called Lorry and Bob the time then was about 9.15 pm. so we told them what had happend and they said we could sit in the G.I. Bus till they came back form playing a match of Baseball, so we sat in but a coloured fellow started talking to us and gave us drinks, I told him about me being pregnant and he said he had the stuff to get rid of it so I drank 2 Bottles of wiskey $\frac{1}{2}$ bottle of Gin and a Bottle of Port, and I went flat out on the floor, when Lorry and Bob came back they started hitting this coloured man and he told them what he had give me and all I rememerd was waking up in a bed and finding Lorry with me I thought I had got every thing over but it did not work on me, I told him I did not no what I was going to do so he said I could stay here for 3 more days and nights till I felt alright, so I stopped there for 2 days and he was coming to see me and bringing me food but I kept thinking I was never going to get well and I wanted to be with my folks so we went but we could not get a lorry so we went dancing at a Night club where all sorts of people were there and plenty of drugs, we got in with some Greeks and they took us to there flat, and he told me he could get rid of the baby as he had done it before, he shown me how he was going to do it, it was like a long thin darning needle with a very fine point and he said he just had to stick it up and every-thing would be over, but I started crying said my inside might fall away, so he said he would not touch me if I did not want him to, so I sleeped with one of them and my friend sleeped with the other, and in the after noon when we were ready we whent back to the town on our own and met 2 English saliors, which they took us to the pictures, and after we came out at 9 o'clock we got picked up by the Police women, I sleeped in the police cell for 2 nights and then went in front of the court in —— after that I did 1 day at —— and 5$\frac{1}{2}$ weeks in —— General Hospital in ——. After having a miscarriage, then I went back to —— for 2 more weeks, after

I did my 2 weeks I went infront off the court to await my sentence the Judge spoke and said I have had alot of chances and I would have to go to Approve School and the time I did was entirly up to myself, so I left the court crying thinking how I could have had a good time without going the wrong-way, any how I brought it on myself and it is up to me to take the rightroad after, and be able to hold my head high not only for myself but for my parents to for it was them who did there best to put me on the right road.

This is admittedly an extreme case of promiscuity. Like most of the others she had only the occasional money gift, which she had not calculated as reward for services. Mainly it was only those under the 'protection' of older women or girls who practised prostitution, and these were few. There was one confirmed prostitute in each of the samples for the research. Some, both younger and older, had associated with older men for cigarettes or money. Others had made sure their services went not unrewarded, as when jewellery thefts were traced to a number of schoolgirls, 14 and younger, who had helped themselves whenever one of the group was upstairs with the jeweller. Two of the conspirators came to us.

Mainly the girls could be said to be emotionally little touched by their sexual experiences; it was a physical experience, simulating the adults. Some were in acute states of physical excitement, fed by everlasting reminiscences of other girls. Since as a group, their emotions were so immature or so confused, this was inevitable. However, we found girls with genuine affection for a boy-friend, often some nice lad who had watched her downward path, and waited. The occasional girl corresponded regularly with a boy throughout her Approved School career, and then married him. A dangerously aggressive girl had letters from a mild youth, who reminded her to clean her teeth. Others' emotions were, unfortunately, fixated in less helpful directions, or the lover's emotions were so fixated that she could not free herself without help. This could be particularly so where there had been an abduction, as of one 14-year-old girl who ran away twice with the father of five from the flat above her parental home. He persisted in his attentions after serving a prison sentence and jeopardized her successful training and subsequent release and marriage by again bearing her away.

Those who were hardly touched emotionally were often disturbed much by the aftermath, and doubtless the subsequent inquiries, physical examinations (often physical treatment) and Court evidence, served to magnify and distort experiences which were already so disproportionate for girls of their age. And few of the sexual aberrations had happened apart from other symptoms, such as wandering, petty theft or aggressiveness. For those who think of 'naughty girls', or of *Cider with Rosie*[2] it can be said that admission of cases on that level was rare enough to amuse us; when four younger girls came to us for more petty sexual misdemeanours, as part of a gang of twelve schoolgirls and seven boys, who had a not so unusual form of adolescent play in Air Raid shelters, we found longer-term problems in the girls' backgrounds as well, though mostly less acute than our average.

We have already discussed the incest group where the girl's father was involved; the eight girls concerned were prominent because of home disturbance and furore in the locality. Sexual assaults by brothers also formed a depressing background to treatment in five cases; the fixation did not always end with Approved School committal, and in one case there was a further Court case when sister and brother had each returned from Approved School.

Life seemed to conspire against girls who needed all the moral support possible. A rather dull but happy, friendly member of the 100 sample, was assaulted by an uncle when she was 5, and was just completing three or four years' treatment for a venereal disease as a result of this, when she was again sexually assaulted, this time by her paternal grandfather. Both relatives served terms of imprisonment. Her Headmaster was concerned about her gravitation from the age of 12 to the less desirable boys, but her mother was, if anything, over-optimistic and the reins were not tightened until she was being very precocious indeed, going off to stay with boy-friends at 15, and being irresponsible at places of work.

There were also many 'nice' girls, to whom the sexual part of an arrangement was (if existent) secondary to the material comforts, companionship and the sense of being needed, but one does not have to go to Approved School files only for these stories.

A stay in London 'on the run' was not always sweetness or elegance. The writer recalls spending her free day collecting from a Metropolitan Police Station an absconder who had been absent for a month. An hour or more was spent on tour with the Police, trying (with the girl's full cooperation) to find the dive behind the gay lights of Piccadilly where she had been locked up for most of the time by an Indian who had procured her for his friends' gratification, and beaten her if she tried to escape. The railway compartment on our return journey, while she told of the people she had met, reeked with every odour of corruption—physical and metaphorical. But for once the experience seemed to have been helpful—she had absconded as a tight little knot of hate and aggression; she returned a trusting child, and went to her Training School the following day in cooperative mood.

No, not *Cider with Rosie*. There was pathos and not much fun or humour in the premature sex life of most of these girls.

Chapter Nineteen

PSYCHOLOGICAL AND PSYCHIATRIC ASSESSMENTS AT THE CLASSIFYING SCHOOL

INTELLIGENCE TESTING

'How bright is she?' was the eager question asked often of the writer and subsequent testers of the girls at the Classifying School, by the Instructresses and other staff, who, in realistic terms, were in a better position to judge. The long sessions in the 'testing room' were held in considerable regard by the participants and non-participants. This was partly a result of the meticulous care taken over the arrangements; House Instructresses were briefed that girls doing housework near the room had to be quiet, and beds in the dormitory above would have to be moved before a session started. Access to the testing-room was taboo. These stringent precautions were taken largely because of the distractable, basically unwilling nature of the testee.

With the testing even greater care was taken. Until the 1957 period of this research, permission had not been granted for a Psychologist on the school's staff, and, whatever the qualifications of the person or persons administering psychological tests, her role was a mixed one; in the main period of the research she had an Honours Degree in Psychology plus a flair for taking team games in the afternoon, and was engaged as a teacher; or she was the Deputy Headmistress performing a multitude of administrative and assessment duties, with varied experience teaching non-delinquents, and completing a Second degree in Education embracing an Honours course in Psychology. Both met the girls in a variety of situations in the course of a day, so the normal process of forming rapport with a test subject was inverted; they started from a point of acquaintance, even *camaraderie* (though both, while being non-punitive, exercised controlling influences in the school) and had to be concerned to gain the essentially neutralized atmosphere for good cognitive testing, while being totally reassuring and unperturbable. Few psychologists would probably regard the difficult teenage girl as an ideal testee, and the writer has little doubt, from reflection and subsequent experience,

221

that the scene-setting and eliciting of cooperation were well and wisely tackled.

A refusal to be tested and to give apparent cooperation was almost unknown, and if this did happen with a subject, or if the pattern of response showed her cooperation was far from real, re-testing was possible with some of the tests.

The writer subsequently, for the 1957 sample, was working as a part-time external member of the Classifying team as Psychologist, and, despite the earlier years of intensive experience, found rapport harder to gain from girls who had not seen her hourly about the building and so often talked to her in other connections.

In retrospect one is disturbed that so much time and effort were spent to far less purpose than was believed at the time. The elaborate test procedure was intellectually satisfying to the psychologists involved, and gave a kind of academic aura to the work of the community which was, of its nature, mainly the practical field of domesticity, child care and teaching. Most of the workers believed that the test results told a great deal about each girl, and the intensity of our belief was conveyed as far as possible to the receiving Training Schools; they, who did not live with the mysteries of psychology at work, remained—fortunately—more sceptical, though the cynicism of a few was far more dangerous than our blind (or partially sighted) faith, for they lost the benefit of the glimmerings of knowledge that had been gained.

Where did the Classifying School fail? Mainly in using methods suited to research purposes and in expecting to gain invaluable insight into each girl's potential and real abilities; that they did gain a great deal of insight thereby is part of the writer's own faith, which might be unwarranted. Gittins,[2] in his chapter on 'Psychometric Investigation' of his *Approved School Boys* explains the then general lack of knowledge concerning the reliability and validity of tests when applied in an Approved School, and describes the procedure adopted within an early year of Aycliffe's existence as a Classifying School, when, as a systematic experiment, each boy was given a selection of seventeen tests, including attainment tests, and also two subjective assessments. The results of the experiment are given in his book but the subsequent programme of psychological investigation at Aycliffe is not known to the writer. At the Shaw Classifying School a battery of eleven tests (seven of them attainment) was given during most of the research period (which was not planned as such) and projective techniques were added in *most* cases. The battery was reduced then by three attainment tests, subsequently by four, and by a group intelligence test, and then in 1957 was given new blood by the addition of the Rorschach test, and by the Porteus Mazes, both carried out as consistently and conscientiously as the rest. Yet most of the observations of the value of each test (discussed already in connection with scholastic attainment) which we made at any early stage were valid enough for some useful modifications, and a request for outside advice from a University Psychology Department could well have been made in order to vet our system thoroughly. As with much of our work we were, as a team, too close to it, and were working far too hard and too diffusely for us to see the important issues. Regular oversight by a well qualified Psychologist not involved in the work of the School would have helped us to ask the relevant questions in each particular case, whereas the allround knowledge of the less detached tester on the resident staff would have prevented the imposition of testing procedure which might have disturbed the comparative equilibrium of the School and its Staff.

There were many cases where the cognitive and attainment test results were a vital part of the girl's assessment. Instances have been quoted of girls who by sheer perfectionism had achieved scholastic and practical standards well in advance of their expected level. The strain of maintaining this was great, and the relief when some strain was quietly removed helped a girl greatly. Others, suffering set-backs in schooling and deciding they 'weren't much good', were braced by a reassurance of being 'quite ordinary' and being helped then in the schoolroom to catch up in basic subjects. There were other cases where interesting patterns of success and failure showed up. But in probably at least one third of the admissions one reliable group intelligence test result, taken not too literally, and comparing well with staff observations and with comments in the girl's record was quite ample evidence on the subject of intelligence; it happened that the group test used (the Simplex) had a high degree of validity with all of our population except those with I.Q.'s over 100 (only 16 per cent of the total) and with the illiterate and semi-literate minority, who could not read the instructions. With simplified testing of the less complicated minority, more time should have been left for treating each really problematic case as a challenge to tests (including many we never used) as well as to the tester (who should therefore have been adequately qualified for the job).

Early in the chapter it was suggested that the Instructresses and other staff were often in a better position to judge a girl's brightness than were those with psychological qualifications, except in so far as the latter observed girls, too, in other group and individual situations. Yet there was a tendency to take the test results as nine-tenths gospel, and to regard commonsense observations as suspect. An example was a 16-year-old girl who remained for a long period of observation and finally was licensed home from the Classifying

School. She seemed simple and impressionable on admission and had barely any conversation though the writer recalls asking her if she knew a certain old girl of the school from her home area. She replied, simply and adequately, 'Yes, but I'm not as bad as her'. She gradually became acceptable to girls and staff. Her I.Q. on the Binet was 53 when first tested, a week or two after admission (the mental age being computed as 8 years), and her I.Q. on the Simplex was 63; her reading age (Burt) was only 8 years. All objective measures were comparable. On Raven's Matrices she made a score initially of 19, which placed her conceptual reasoning still in the defective range. On the Alexander's Passalong she scored a test age of nearly 11. The visiting Psychiatrist reported: 'Her ability to benefit from training is so doubtful that it is recommended that she should remain at The Shaw for further observation.'

As a few months passed the girl's simple smile became one of serene confidence (she had also stopped wanting to run away). She spoke a little more, and her communications to other girls often contained shrewd advice. Her domestic work became satisfactory; she was particularly helpful on personal tasks, not only remembering always which staff had sugar in tea or coffee, but foreseeing other people's needs. When almost stable enough for returning home she was re-tested. Her Binet I.Q. had gone up only to 61, and her reading age only to 8 years 9 months; her Matrices score rose, however, from the total of 19 eight months before to 31—only into the 'dull' category, but much more like our subjective image of the girl, which was, indeed, the correct one. We had, for instance, not ascribed much academic importance to the fact that her contribution to entertainments in the school was singing her National Anthem in Welsh, and that the family was mainly Welsh-speaking, as well as being unstimulated and unstimulating socially. The girl's dullness was important to know, but with reservations about the so-called objective measurements on the tests regularly used. Had we had real doubts about our subjective assessment then what was necessary was, of course, further non-verbal and performance tests, until a hypothesis of higher potential learning ability was either proved or disproved. She had a shorter Approved School training than the average, behaved and worked well on her return home, and her marriage—up to the point of discharge of the Approved School order—was satisfactory.

However the test batteries for various reasons prevailed. One reason was an expressed wish by the Home Office that certain tests (including the Stanford-Binet) be given to all admissions (unless recently reliably tested thereon) so that comparisons could be made over the whole Approved School population. Representation during these discussions was by the Classifying School Principals. The

Psychologists did not, anyway, demur, for reasons already discussed, but they lost much in scientific interest through their conformity.

For the purpose of the present research the material which accumulated may well prove of some interest and value, especially for comparison with that from parallel fields. It may be possible also to align aspects of the individual girl's test findings with her subsequent response or failure.

At the same time it should be stressed that the nature of the link between intelligence and delinquency had been much questioned since the period fifty years ago when, particularly in America, low intelligence was considered the most important single cause of crime. Dr Mary Woodward's study of 1955[5] (published by the Institute for the Study and Treatment of Delinquency) goes carefully into the evidence published in the preceding forty years, by Burt[3] (1925), Norwood East[27] (1949), Stott[28] (1952), Sheldon and Eleanor Glueck[29] (1950), and others, and concludes that 'the question of the relation or not of low intelligence to delinquency has not been settled'. 'The same cultural factors which depress the intelligence test score are also associated with delinquency.' At the period dealt with in the present research the tendency of the Classifying team was still to question how far the non-conforming dull girls had failed to understand social demands—and indeed they often had, but more because of conflicting standards in their unsettled lives. We were just beginning to see how far under-motivation, especially through poor or everchanging personal relationships, had stunted their mental and social capacities. Without considering all the other adverse factors, we can appreciate slowness of mental development, especially in verbal communication, in a young population of which 20 per cent had experienced more than one major change of environment, and many of whom never knew a satisfyingly stimulating milieu.

Presumably such effects would be comparable in other studies of the intelligence of institutionalized delinquents, though, as we have seen, our female population may have been particularly hard hit.

Test Used from 1952 to 1954

The Scholastic attainment tests used during the research period have already been discussed, and the results compared with those obtained by boys in Approved Schools.

The intelligence tests used, in practically every case, were the Stanford-Binet (Terman and Merrill revision, 1937),[1] mainly Form L but Form M for checking in doubtful cases; the Simplex (Senior) Group Intelligence Test and Raven's[8] Progressive Matrices (1938). We used as a Performance Test the Alexander's Passalong and we also applied a battery of Projective or Personality Tests. For results of cognitive and other tests and various comparisons, see Appendix.

The Stanford-Binet (Terman and Merrill Revision[1]). To those who know the Stanford-Binet, or know of the test, repetition of the usual criticisms would be tiresome. To those who do not know it they would be meaningless.

I.Q.'s or intelligence quotients are by now meaningful to most likely readers; the scepticism necessary has already been dwelt on above. The following table (51) will thus be of some value, as we have compared scores for two large samples from the Classifying School with samples from three other sources, and with the distribution for the general population.

The one Shaw sample (column 1) is our research group of 500, minus 19 girls for whom we had no Stanford-Binet test result. For 129 of the remainder the result recorded was for testing before admission, if known to be by a qualified psychologist.

The second Shaw sample (column 2) is of 1,000 girls tested consecutively *at* the Shaw Classifying School only, between 1950 and early 1958, by six testers, whose separate samples varied from about 500 to 38.

Some comments need to be made:

The two Shaw samples can be seen to be further removed from the general population distribution even than the Aycliffe sample of Approved School boys, aged 10 to 16, where the mean I.Q. is

Table 51

I.Q.	Shaw C.S. 1952–4 %	Shaw C.S. 1950–8 %	Aycliffe C.S. Boys* 1950 %	Burt 1925† %	I.S.T.D. Boys‡ 1952–3 %	Distribution General Population %
130 plus	0·6	0·7	1·55	1·0	10·5	2
115–129	3·5	2·6	4·27	1·5	11·5	14
85–114	49·1	47·4	56·67	62·0	61·5	68
70–84	34·9	36·0	29·64	27·9	12·5	14
Under 70	11·9	13·3	7·87	7·6	4·0	2
No. tested	481	1000	327	197	200	—
Mean I.Q.	86	86	89·5	89	—	100
S.d.	—	15			—	About 17

* On Terman-Merrill Revision of Binet, like The Shaw.
† On Burt Revision of Binet.
‡ On various individual and, presumably, group intelligence tests.

226

fully three points higher. The trend on the two samples is, however, similar. This may be due partly to age factor, with cultural and emotional effects less hardened in the younger delinquents. Also we can affirm (more than speculate, because of personal experience) that intermediate and senior Approved School girls are more disturbed emotionally than boys, more resistant, and more likely to function unevenly in an individual test situation.

While in a complete delinquent sample (as quoted by Woodward[5]) no sex differences in intelligence were found, C. W. and H. P. Mann[6] found that particular groups of girls, such as adolescent sex delinquents, have lower I.Q.'s on average than boy delinquents. Merrill[7] also found that lower intelligence in juveniles was associated with sex offences, truancy, vagrancy and assault. All but the last misconduct were truly represented in the Shaw sample.

The Portman Clinic Sample (I.S.T.D.) is naturally nearer to the average population figures; the disproportionate number at the upper and lower extremes is as now expected in Clinic referrals—the good verbalizer who responds better to classic therapy, and at the other extreme those referred because of marked backwardness. Also removal from home has not yet placed a further barrier between adult and child, selection having been made partly because cultural or emotional factors are not conducive to further probation, supervision or fit person orders.

The Simplex Group Intelligence Test. This was usually given as a preliminary (as mentioned earlier in this chapter). As a group 'I.Q. test' it had all the faults one needs to recognize, and as a *verbal* group test, with a group where 10·4 per cent had a reading age below 9 years, one knew its limitations.

Raven's Progressive Matrices (1938). The Matrix test,[8] with its book of sixty sets of 'patterns with a piece missing', is well known for its very wide use in H.M. Forces during the last war, and a casual comment to this effect, inferring that the test was not 'babyish', helped to put our girls in the right frame of mind. Generally they enjoyed the test, and much interest could be gained from observing a small group tackling the sixty problems, from the dull or easygoing girl who romped through the first very easy few and seemed not to notice the growing difficulty, to the effortful concentration of the more intelligent or more obsessional testee.

During the 1952-4 research period the test was administered in small groups (usually about six) but in 1957 it was given as an individual self-administered test. At neither of the research periods was it given with a time limit, but the time taken was recorded.

Table 52 gives the results from the three intelligence tests regularly used with the 500 Shaw sample, graded according to Raven's five categories in his guide,[8] and matching the previous Binet and Simplex categories—albeit roughly.

Table 52

	Stanford-Binet %	Simplex %	Matrices %
Superior	0·6	—	1
Above average	3·5	—	8·2
Average	49·1	44	38·6
Below average	34·9 } 46·8	39·8 } 56	39·4 } 52·2
Below the 5th percentile of the population	11·9	16·2	12·8
No. tested	481	420	500
Mean	I.Q. 86	—	Mean score 36, or rather below average

Comments. For the reasons mentioned above, namely our batch of poor readers facing a verbal group test, we find 56 per cent of the girls scored below I.Q. 85 on the Simplex, as against 46·8 per cent on the Binet. Yet a correlation of ·89 was found between results on the two tests, which was higher than the Aycliffe[2] finding of ·755 in their research; 22 per cent of the Approved School boys had reading ages below 9 years.

The Simplex I.Q.'s could have stood the girls' Classifying School in quite good stead as a verbal intelligence measure, but we should have learned less about the girl as a person than in the face-to-face Stanford-Binet test situation, and made more misjudgments of some, for it proved insensitive above the I.Q. 100 level.

Dr Epps'[9] sample of 300 Borstal girls had an average score of 34·87 on Raven's Matrices, very close to the average for our sample. In both those groups of delinquent girls, therefore, half of them fall into the least equipped quartile of the total population. On the other hand, nine or more of our girls could have taken their place—other things being equal to intelligence—in the professions.

This is a higher 'above average' section than was found by the Binet test, while, interestingly enough, more girls were assessed as below average on the Matrices.

The correlation found between Binet and Matrices results for the Shaw population was, in fact, found to be ·63, which is rather higher than that quoted by Gittins[2] for Senior A.S. boys (·539). Raven[8] gives a figure of ·86 in his guide, but in an experiment described in *Standardisation of Progressive Matrices*[10] dealing with 301 children

Psychological and Psychiatric Assessments at the Classifying School

and adults attending London Psychiatric Clinics, the correlation seems nearer to ours.

In the above table 47 per cent of the 500 sample scored below average in the Binet, compared with 52 per cent in the Matrices; in an experiment by Walton[11] the situation was reversed—68 per cent of Approved School boys were below average in Matrices, against 52 per cent in the Binet, and he used this as an argument for unsatisfactory testing in a Classifying School.

The writer has found indications that the discrepancies for these test results at the Girls' C.S. group may instead be related to different personality types, as discussed by Raven[10] (1941). In a group of clinical cases, where there was a group scoring two 'classes' higher on the Terman-Merrill than on Matrices, and vice versa, he showed the former to have been, as a group, 'talkative, superficially intelligent, but excitable, unstable, lacking in self-control'. They were at a disadvantage on logical problems of the Matrix type.

His other clinical set, for whom the Matrices were much easier than the Binet, had emotional disturbances which 'frequently existed in the form of deep anxieties, fears or night terrors'. They felt more confident with tests of the Matrix type.

This use of intelligence test deviations to unveil emotional differences ties up in an interesting way with two 'Shaw' experiments which may prove of considerable interest. As it is hoped to publish these at length, they will be outlined only very briefly.

Experiment I. For this we introduce a further test, given to 100 girls in 1957—the Porteus Mazes,[12] which yields Test Quotients (a quantitative measure of 'foresight') and Q-scores, or qualitative scores, which are postulated as measuring degrees of carelessness and impulsiveness.

(a) *Test Quotients.* As with other ability tests at the C.S., the distribution was skewed, with a mean of 88·5 (s.d. 16·45). 48 girls scored below this mean, and would be predicted as poor social planners. The following table will interest those who wish to compare populations and tests:

Test Quotients on Porteus Mazes	Girls with Matrix grades higher than Terman grades		Girls with Matrix grades lower than Terman grades	
	No.	%	No.	%
89 to 126	19	63·3	6	30
88 and below	11	36·7	14	70
Total	30	100	20	100

The more excitable and unstable (Raven, above) seem also to be the poor 'planners', perhaps more psychopathic.

(b) *Q-Scores.* The higher the Q-scores, the more typically delinquent (careless, impulsive) is the subject likely to be. Eysenck[13] quotes high Q-scores of Gibbens' Borstal lads[14] to support his typically-extraverted-delinquent theory. The Shaw group had a mean Q-score of 28·6 (Gibbens' mean was 35, supporting theories of less extraverted girl delinquents, though Porteus[15] quotes 32 as the critical scoring point for delinquent females).

Again readers interested in statistical comparisons of populations and tests will be interested in the following table:

Q-scores on Porteus Mazes	*Girls with Matrix grades* higher than *Terman grades*		*Girls with Matrix grades* lower than *Terman grades*	
	No.	%	*No.*	%
0–29	24	80	8	40
30 +	6	20	12	60
Total	30	100	20	100

The more anxious, fearful types (Raven, above) seem also to be less impulsive, less extraverted, perhaps further from the psychopathic, according to Porteus Maze Tests.

Experiment II. The other indication of marked test deviations being linked with special personality features in this Approved School sample was again referred to by Raven, though Vernon and Parry[16] say 'no evidence could be obtained—that men with scores which Raven called unreliable, i.e. irregular patterns of scores on the five sections of the test, were more neurotic or in any other way different from men with "reliable" scores'.

The Headmistress of the Shaw Classifying School at the time of the research, Miss Wannop, regularly drew attention to a section of girls who found Set D, intentionally the second hardest set of the Matrices, to be easier than Set C by a number of points. They seemed to be anxious girls, who could not take pressure but identified with kindly authority.

Two criteria were selected for the present research: (a) Raven's criterion of a deviation of more than 2 on the score in one of the sets from that normally expected from his total score; this occurred with 142 of the 500 Shaw sample; (b) The 'Shaw' criterion—the score on Set D more than 2 points greater than the score on Set C.

This occurred with 17·8 per cent, or 89 of the 500 girls.

As regards (a) no significant link was found with prevailing mood, expression of feeling, or with future success.

But as regards (b)—the Shaw criterion—the probability was between ·05 and ·02 that the discrepancy was related to the girl's prevailing mood, and on inspection it was seen that the cheerful, serious and anxious all tended to have the 'pattern', while the resentful, the regardless and the apathetic tended definitely not to. Generally speaking, the more neurotic, and sometimes the 'normal' showed the 'D−C>2' pattern of scoring, but not the more anti-social, or the psychopathic. In Chapter XXI we shall see hints of a relationship with later success.

To illustrate these deviations, which were far from atypical of the C.S. population, and a source of much puzzlement to Training Schools receiving our assessments, here are two examples of cases from opposite categories:

Case 1. F (aged 14) had a Binet I.Q. of 91, but scored only 22 in Matrices, and only 2 more on re-testing; this placed her in the very dull to defective range in that test. It was inferred as due to inability to concentrate without close individual attention. Her reading and spelling were about normal, but her number work poor.

The Test Quotient on Porteus Mazes was average, but the Q-score was 52, i.e. very high, even for our delinquent group; she was regardless of minor rules, even when reminded, and tended to repeat mistakes. The matrices scatter was 'normal'.

In the Rorschach, unlike the usual emotionally constricted, but power-seeking personality patterns in the school, she seemed to be seeking an escape from her feelings, through excitement. She was finding satisfaction, too, in a rich fantasy life.

The School's visiting Psychiatrist found her a cheerful dullard, who showed little emotional disturbance.

In day-to-day Classifying School life she fitted in very well, and tried to do all that was asked of her; her shortcomings were due to 'her immaturity and her tendency to day-dream'.

F had perhaps more than the average Approved School girl's run of difficulties. At 4 she and her little sister were removed from a dirty, verminous room, and their mother was sent to prison for neglect; father was already in prison. At 5 they returned to the parents on trial, and the latter disappeared with the children, having taken to the road. The children were again placed in a Children's Home, but F after a time 'felt lost' without her mother and took to running home. She stole, and was moved, to save her sister from her influence, but they were reunited two or three years later, by which time she seemed to be settled. When F was 13, both sisters were allowed home, where the father had a regular job, but he lost this a year later, and home conditions deteriorated again. Father had an accident, and while he was in hospital the family was given notice to quit their house. There was a lodger in the home. Much disquiet was felt about home morality, and eventually F was removed in her own interests. She was very difficult at first at the Remand Home, and remained evasive and unreliable.

At her Training School she was most uncooperative at first, and absconded several times. Once she found where her father was (in prison) she settled down, and was helpful still when last heard of (aged 15½).

Her personality was indeed in keeping with Raven's definition, but fortunately seems to have been modifiable in the right atmosphere.

Case 2. Matrices scores at least a grade higher than Binet: Q-score below 10. C (aged 16) had a Binet I.Q. of 96, but her Matrices Score was 50, which placed her in the 'above average' category. That she had not been stimulated enough intellectually showed in her vocabulary deficiencies on the Binet.

On the Porteus Mazes her Test Quotient was 121 (i.e. foresight well above average). Her Q-score was exactly one. This meticulousness for detail showed in the Rorschach, where she was driven compulsively to search for reality in all the more shaded parts of the card. In the achromatic cards she saw lambs sucking bottles, and birds on nest, and searched for comfort in all sorts of ways—despondently often. On the coloured cards she saw pictures of war and destruction.

Her father was killed on active service when she was 3, with two older siblings, to one of whom (her brother) she was attached. He was killed, while a National Serviceman, when C was 15.

At the Junior School C truanted. By 14 she was a lonely, difficult child at school, given to truanting. At home she stole from her mother's purse. Her mother who had never been able to give affection, tried, in desperation, to take her own life and C's.

At work C had six different Mill jobs in six months. She stayed out late, and cheated to get more pocket money. At 15 she planned to run away with a young man with whom she had had intercourse, but was apprehended. She was kept under supervision, but ran away with a girl, and stole. Eventually they lived immorally, and also stole a fair sum of money.

At the Classifying School she was at first very withdrawn, but gradually livened up a little, and became 'a contributing member of the group'. She was considered by the Visiting Psychiatrist to have improved so much in two months at the Classifying School that she would manage with periodic psychiatric supervision at her Training School.

There was difficulty for a long time, partly because her mother was trying to win her affection by giving gifts that were contrary to school rules. Eventually the school gained the mother's confidence, but the latter never achieved a really helpful relationship with her daughter, who was, however, doing fairly well at 18 in a job away from home.

PERFORMANCE TESTING

In the last pages we have examined what was for long a hunch shared by a few staff at The Shaw, and seems now to have scientific value. Many scientific eyebrows were raised by visitors to the Classifying School when they heard of the theory!

Likewise eyebrows were raised on hearing that the only performance test used was the Alexander's Passalong.[18, 19] (It has already been mentioned in connection with our observation of left-handedness.) It has not over the years been a highly regarded test in clinical use. It may be that the test's diagnostic value increased for the sex and age group. Certainly we looked at the results when considering girls for schools where practical initiative was especially valued—and we shall see (Chapter XXI) that test scores linked with success in training at ·05 level.

The test is made up of a series of nine graded 'puzzles', where square wooden blocks—red and blue—are converted within the space of a standard box to another arrangement shown in a diagram on a card. The performance was timed, and test ages calculated.

Roughly 24·2 per cent of the 500 Shaw sample were above average, and 32·6 per cent below average.

The scores correlated more highly with the three intelligence tests discussed than in the case of the Aycliffe testees (·398 correlation with the Binet, against Aycliffe's ·284; ·412 with the Simplex against ·276; ·540 with Raven's Matrices against ·382).

PROJECTIVE TECHNIQUES

The above has, in recent years, been not quite a respectable topic of discussion in wider psychological circles. To lend projective techniques a better aura, statistical measurements have been applied occasionally, even by enthusiasts. The writer's efforts to do so have been rewarding, but none the less this section will be abbreviated, lest delinquent girls should be contaminated by the company they keep.

Over the years Murray's *Thematic Apperception Test*[20] was administered, until the clothing of the humans in the set of pictures about which stories were invited seemed hopelessly old-fashioned to the teenage jivers of the mid-fifties. Similar tests soon acquired the same deficiency.

A simple but productive technique was a Sentence Completion Test—an adaptation of that used by Himmelweit and Petrie.[22]

Administered by someone who understood adolescent girls, this test brought out less resistance or antagonism than most.

One completed example will best illustrate the release given to emotions. This was by an intelligent and apparently hard-boiled 16-year-old, who revealed the hurt child beneath. She managed to start off in a matter-of-fact vein, and was briefly facetious in Sentence 2:

1. *I like* English lessons, far more than Arithmetic.
2. *Father* Christmas visits all good children.
3. *I fear* that I am rather backward in Arithmetic.
4. *When I am older* I want to take up Mental Nursing.
5. *My school work* hasn't been so good lately as it used to be.
6. *I hate* people who tell tales of people for the sake of being better thought of.
7. *I dream that* my mother is coming to see me every night.
8. *I become embarrassed when* folks discuss my singing voice or my hair.
9. *I am very sorry when* I have been in a temper.
10. *Other children* don't seem glued to trouble like myself.
11. *The teachers* in this school are very understanding.
12. *I try to get* better at Maths, but I just can't.
13. *In the dark* I am always frightened.
14. *What annoys me* most is to see one person cling to another as if they will never let them go.
15. *My brothers and sisters* are all at home and happy.
16. *School* days are the happiest of one's life.
17. *Grown-ups* always seem to speak of 'When I was your age'.
18. *I need* a father. That's what the judge said.
19. *Mother* is something that I wish my mother would be to me.
20. *I can't* control my temper.
21. *The only trouble is that* I haven't really tried very hard.
22. *Most girls* of my age seem to wish they were a lot older.
23. *I hope* that my mother will write this week.
24. *My greatest worry* is my mother.
25. *I secretly* wish that I was nine again.

The writer made her statistical study of this technique in 1954, matching forty-four of the Classifying School testees for age and intelligence (on Matrices) with forty-four girls from City Youth Clubs, who were non-delinquent, later introducing a third, very small sample of eight girls who were on probation.

The sentence completions were scored according to Murray's[21] 'needs and presses'. After a statistical procedure blessed by the University department concerned (this small piece of research formed an unpublished B.Ed. thesis at Edinburgh University) the following needs or presses differentiated significantly between the forty-four Approved School girls and the forty-four Youth Club girls:

Table 53: Significant Scores on Need or Press

(a) With delinquents scoring significantly higher need or press

Need or Press	Abbreviation of Murray's Definition	Significance
N. affiliation	Need to form friendships and association	P·001
N. Counteraction	Need to overcome defeat proudly by restriving and retaliating	P·001
N. Similance	Need to imitate or emulate or identify oneself with others	P·001
N. abasement	Need to comply and accept punishment	P·001
N. blame-avoidance	Need to avoid blame, ostracism or punishment by inhibiting asocial or unconventional impulses	P·001
N. defendence	Need to defend oneself against blame or belittlement	P·02
N. succorance	Need to seek aid, protection or sympathy	P·01
N. cognizance	Need to know facts	P·01
Press family insupport	(Unnecessary to define)	P·01

(b) With Youth Club girls scoring significantly higher

N. acquisition	Need to gain possessions and property	P·001
N. achievement	Need to overcome obstacles, to exercise power	P·05
N. sentience	The need for sensuous gratification	P·05
N. aggression	No definition needed	P·05

Some of the needs and presses gave surprising findings (e.g. need acquisition). There was also the question how far the 'put away' factor was being measured, rather than traits of the delinquents themselves.

The introduction of the third small group (eight) who were on probation but not removed from home, made it easy to sum up the findings:

(1) *Need affiliation*—the need to make friends or form associations —still stood out. The Classifying School group seemed to have had this

need intensified by removal from home, but the delinquent girls on probation still expressed the need about five times as often as the Youth Club girls.

After all we have read of the backgrounds and behaviour before committal to Approved School, we need not dwell further on this.

(2) A similar statistical pattern was followed by need succorance, and for press family insupport.

(3) *Needs acquisition and sentience* seemed to be very much dependent on the environment and its opportunities; both were expressed about equally by the girls out in the world, within reach of cinemas and shops, but much less by the Classifying School girls, whose current material and sentient needs seemed at least to be supplied; the world was not so much with them.

(4) *Needs defendence, counteraction, abasement and blame avoidance* appeared rarely in the Youth Club responses, but built up in the girls on probation, and were intensified by removal from home or by further Court procedure. They had to find excuses, had to make up for the past, and to build up resistance against anti-social conduct in the future.

(5) *Need achievement* showed a pattern of its own. The delinquents on probation and in the world barely expressed the need; they lived in the present, as expected. It seemed as if the shock of committal and concentrated interest by others in their future awakened a little ambition, so the C.S. group expressed the need about twice as often as the girls on probation, but only with about one-third of the frequency of the non-delinquent adolescent girls in the Youth Clubs.

The motivational lack in delinquents explains to a great extent their failure to settle in a job.

In our regular use of the Sentence Completion test, such scoring was not used. One is, however, relieved to find that it was a technique yielding data which seemed able to stand up to scientific scrutiny.

RORSCHACH TESTING

Presenting the well known and sometimes lampooned set of ten standard photographs of ink blots to difficult adolescent girls took about the same courage as examining their bodies for vermin, except that in the latter case the object of the search could be explained.

Rorschach[23] testing 'Look at this ink blot . . . Tell me what you see' was the kind of challenge which was generally avoided in the Classifying School. Typically they reacted to challenge by negativism, or by very superficial, measured response. In other projective tests, where a greater degree of persuasion or humouring could be used, the girls were often expansive.

Again a statistical comparison[24] was used, by scoring the quantitative data from the tests only, but this time the comparison was with *results* from a published sample, of the same age limits but not of the same intellectual range. Fifty C.S. girls of each age group (14, 15 and 16) were compared with Ames's[25] samples of the same age.

The median and mean scores were found to differ very markedly, and yet no typical delinquent girl could be traced by matching girls and Rorschach records. Extreme values were typical of the population.

Further respectability was lent to a rejected test procedure by Josef Schubert,[26] who studied the statistical assessments by Richardson[24] and arranged for the testing of twenty adolescent girls from a Secondary Modern School, thus amending the intellectual discrepancy as between the Shaw sample and Ames's[25] sample.

Using non-parametric tests and avoiding 'capitalization on chance', he showed that

The records of the delinquent group are characterized by: (a) paucity of response, (b) a tendency to give extreme reactions . . . A comparison of the 15-year-old group with the dull-normal control group (as above) showed that the dull-normals differed significantly from the delinquents in variables purported to be related to personality adjustment; they differed significantly from Ames' bright-normals in variables related to intellectual functioning.

Mr Schubert confirmed, without seeing the Shaw Rorschach records in words (only the quantitative scoring) what the writer has taken many pages to sum up from her experience of living with the female adolescent delinquents.

General Comment on Test Findings at Classifying Approved School for Girls

The figures on the cognitive tests speak for themselves. Much has been published, critically and comparatively on the various tests, and psychologists of all shades of opinion sometimes use them; the Porteus Mazes are less in use, but fortunately Dr Gibbens[14] has published some very comparable recent material.

Through the Porteus Mazes we have a carry-through to personality measurements, for the Q-scores are a device for measuring certain qualitative differences in people. It also provides a theoretical link; we have, for instance, Professor Eysenck[13] using Dr Gibbens' figures on the Q-scores of his Borstal Lads to substantiate theories on extraversion in criminal populations.

The Rorschach, T.A.T. and Sentence Completions, as used, were techniques and scoring methods which are the prerogative more of psychoanalytically orientated workers, than of an educationist and eclectic psychologist. Educationists must keep faith in their skills and in their methods, and respect the skills of social science and psychiatry without handing over. It is not always easy to justify one's consumer attitudes, and these methods seemed to suit psychologist and subjects.

The Classifying School was dependent on and grateful to its Visiting Psychiatrists with their Clinical approach; the Headmistress at the Research period was sympathetically inclined to the psycho-analytical approach to delinquency. It was inevitable that our jargon and our attempts at aiding in diagnostic work were couched in the language of most clinical workers in the mid-1950s. By applying statistical measurements to the findings for the Rorschach and the Sentence Completion Tests, and by other comparative assessment, the digested results may be of some interest and value to workers of varying theoretical standpoints, and to those who, like the writer, uses the tools at hand, even if they need to adjust them a little. With so many roles to play in the life of the Classifying School there was sometimes no time even for adjustment.

PSYCHIATRIC ASSESSMENT

As well as the contributions to the assessment report by resident staff in all departments, including the psychologist, there was a report by the Visiting Psychiatrist on many girls. During the main research period this was a well-known woman psychiatrist, whose contribution was much respected by staff. Four or five girls were seen during a Saturday morning each fortnight, specifically for diagnosis, but the psychiatric interview was structured so as to release tension and also to restore equilibrium as far as possible. Lay staff appreciated this concern for the peace of the community.

Our consultant was often unnecessarily pessimistic about those very dull girls who were then described as 'borderline defectives'. She would have been very gratified to know of the later 'success' of some of these educationally subnormal girls, with I.Q.'s in the low 60 regions, but her surprise would have been shared by many people, professional and lay. Her judgment was otherwise very valuable, and probably the judgment of relatively untrained staff was reciprocally valuable.

We trusted her judgment also because she was a woman, and we agreed with Allport (*Personality*—p. 519): 'If the male student of personality is able to free himself of his own self-consciousness in relation to the opposite sex, if he discounts his own idealistic or cynical bias and is able to escape from his "mother image", if he has no preconceptions of the proper social and economic role which women should play, he will achieve a certain objectivity and will improve his judgments of women. . . .' And one of the features of our male psychiatrists at a later stage seemed to be that they had to see our adolescents as women, not as children (mostly) with a physical component of woman thrown in as extra, and the certain knowledge of how to disconcert the male.

The Visiting Psychiatrist was in a better position than the very involved residential staff to assess the girls' attitude to the future.

This was of immediate importance, needless to say. A negative attitude could be wrapped up with deep resentment towards her home and other adults, but at this stage the here and now mattered more than cause and effect.

The following scores (on a scale chosen by the writer) were reached, for the two samples, by selecting from the psychiatric reports where available, and judging as far as possible from the whole assessment otherwise.

Table 54: Attitude to Future

	Sample of 500 %	Sample of 100 %
Constructive Attitude	36·8	31
Vaguely means well	42·8	39
Negative attitude	18·2	17
Variable	2·2	13

Comment. We see the two groups as comparable. The more variable attitudes in the 1957 could be partly due to the non-representative group, but also to the many changes in their lives, shaky relations with substitute homes, and therefore perhaps fewer visits and letters to sustain morale.

We shall see in the next chapter how far attitudes at this stage had good prognostic value.

The Visiting Psychiatrist was also in a good position to judge *Acceptance of Committal*, and this was again calculated from her comments, or the C.S. report.

Even though a girl aimed at doing well, this was not the same thing as genuine acceptance of having been committed to Approved School, though related.

We see that about 20 per cent of both groups had failed, after perhaps three to four weeks at the Classifying School, to accept their committal. We shall see in the next chapter whether this carried through to their Training School record, and later. These would tend to be the most resentful girls, often those pushed from pillar to post in

Table 55: *Acceptance of Committal*

	Sample of 500 %	Sample of 100 %
Has accepted	43·0	31·0
Has partially accepted	34·4	50·0
Has not accepted	22·6	19·0

childhood and adolescence. Indeed they were the girls who, on objective measures of difficult and disturbed behaviour, most needed strong measures, but also were justifiably resentful. The less disturbed girls were readier to listen to our rationalizations of their plight. The third estimate, sometimes included in the psychiatric report, and of value here, was of *strong or weak character*. It was something that could otherwise be sifted from the files, together with the writer's long-term recall of the girls. Used here (perhaps rather loosely) it rescues us from the conflict between psychoanalytical usage and that of behaviour therapists, bringing us somewhere on the borderland of psychology.

Though much space has been given to the environmental difficulties of our two samples of Approved School girls, we know that others of their age were leading seemingly normal lives after similar difficulties. This may be due to the interweaving of natural toughness with external circumstances, producing a character stronger than all but a few of our girls had; a few of ours were indeed amazingly strong, but manifold detrimental situations had linked up with adolescent instability to constitute a failure while in some cases quite good parents and teachers and others had lost faith too soon.

Comment. On the scale used, the two groups vary considerably, and the increase in those who seemed seriously warped in character is nearly 100 per cent. It is worth once more recalling that there was

Table 56: *Estimate of Character Strength*

	Sample of 500 %	Sample of 100 %
Strong	24·4	16·0
Indecisive—can sway either way	42·2	53·0
Weak—immature, or with marked defects	20·6	8·0
Warped—seriously damaged	12·8	23·0

also an increase of nearly 100 per cent in the proportion of the 1957 sample who had more than three different home environments, or who left home for the first time at 4 or under.

These attributes did not belong to particular ages or intellectual sets. One can recall a plump and placid owner of a 66 I.Q. who might be fetched by the prefect of another dormitory to quell anxious or aggressive behaviour late at night.

This strength or lack was an important component of our life together, but the correlation between cooperativeness and strength was far from complete; some girls of strength were far from cooperative, and some were far too critical of our weaknesses (some very real) to be helpful to the community.

One stalwart, whose respect we had just managed to keep—more because none of us were afraid of her strong influence and of her violent temper than because all of us exceeded her in strength of character—created havoc at her first Training School, though qualifying for its favours had been our principal challenge to her. She was transferred to a 'tough' school with a challenging and fearless Headmistress, and responded so well that she was successfully at home in record time.

Chapter Twenty

ALLOCATION TO TRAINING SCHOOLS

The Classifying School existed for allocation of girls to suitable Training Approved Schools, after a period of residence during which each girl was observed and assessed, both in daily leisure and work situations—at bed-time and meal-times and even at bath-times as well—and by the reputedly more objective procedures of intelligence, performance and personality testing. The classifying report produced in each case was intended as a practical as well as a descriptive document, and comments from a Head Teacher that a report proved helpful were always welcome. Comments were in fact mixed; according to one school of thought the assessment records were too wordy, and depicted girls' responses to a particular school, namely the Classifying School. Doubtless there were occasional murmurs on reading of difficult behaviour: 'We'll cure that...' The sheet of psychological and educational test measures was naturally puzzling on many occasions, with such widely discrepant results sometimes as to be meaningless even to the partially initiated. The fact that some 'average' girls were proved in everyday situations to have the common sense of an 8-year-old was (as can happen in Day Schools) taken as nullifying the intelligence test's reliability.

With all the mass of assessment material, how was the training school allocation reached? This is more difficult to explain than perhaps any aspect of the School's work, though it was our *raison d'être*!

If we think back to the early chapter on classification, we mentioned, I believe, that at an early stage classification was by religion and by age. We shall deal with these two first.

RELIGION

Any girls in the Classifying School who were Roman Catholic had been admitted as special problems, usually after failing at a Roman Catholic Training School, and generally they were allocated to another.

The Protestant, or nominally Protestant girls, were not often classified by denomination, but a parent's or girl's choice would be respected. One school in our northern area was run by the Salvation Army, and we 'fed' two Church Army Schools.

127 of the 500 girls were aged 14 to 14 years 11 months, and these could be allocated to four schools in our northern area, and occasionally to two others in the Midlands and the South. In fact most were allocated to the Intermediate School for the area, receiving girls aged 14 or 15, while 21 of the 500, who were 'younger', suitable 14's, or whose homes were in the North-East were allocated to a larger Junior School run on Cottage lines. Emotional considerations could rarely outweigh age, but they determined the allocation of this age group to a considerable extent. The 'Cottage Homes' school had a schoolroom of its own, as well as sending the more adequate to outside school. The atmosphere was very much as in Children's Homes, except for being single-sexed and having older age groups, being fairly homely, and later in the research period it had its own pre-release hostel from which girls learned gradually to return to working life. A few 'younger' 14's in the research period who went to a Junior School in the Midlands, from which they had then to attend outside School, fared badly, for their sex experiences pre-committal, and their more precocious sex conversation simulated from older girls at the Classifying School made them unwelcome at Secondary Schools in the town; when one ponders the problem of a 'normal' new girl coming into a school in the final year, it is not surprising that these abnormal girls made the only sensational approach within their power.

Overlapping with a few 'younger' 15-year-olds, seventy-eight girls were allocated in the three years to the Intermediate School mentioned above. This school had shortly before organized itself on more full-time classroom lines, with especial emphasis on domestic science teaching. Cookery, needlework and housewifery reached good proficiency levels. Drama, dancing and games were taught in a business-like way. Girls gave the impression of outward control and poise; discipline was very firm and expectations high, but we knew from sharing their psychiatrist that girls were aware of individual understanding, and a feeling of just treatment, if they were not too disturbed to await the point when the help was given; at the Classifying School we had to excel or fail in making quick relationships, and this impact was missed by girls who wanted least of all to be unobtrusive.

The 16-year-old girls, and most of the 15's—about 70 per cent of the 500 sample—were allocated mainly between nine different Senior Training Schools, mostly in the northern half of England. A small additional percentage were allocated to schools in the South normally receiving girls only from the other Girls' Classifying School, and a very few, admitted as special problems, were allocated to Roman Catholic Approved Schools in the North or South.

As regards the 350 or so girls sent to the nine regular schools, there was a degree of specialization in most cases, but in so far as they catered for different emotional, and even physical needs, and only to a minimal extent on a vocational basis.

VOCATIONAL

The short-term training Approved School for girls from the whole of England and Wales, from which they could be licenced from nine months after transfer there, received the most cooperative and most stable girls, but also, as far as possible, girls who had enough intelligence (I.Q. 85 upwards, preferably well upwards) and manipulative ability to profit from a good domestic science training. The social and cultural aims were high, and by the time the girls had been working in posts in the market town itself (after perhaps six months in the School) and sharing the leisure activities of the community, they were more typically middle-class products, some of whom married respectably in the town, lived in owner-occupied houses, and brought the 'grandchildren' back to see their motherly Headmistress.

Another school which shared its facilities with both Classifying Schools was run on hostel lines, in a terraced City street, and the girls, after a few months of stabilization, went to work, mostly in factories, but were under close discipline throughout. While there was privilege in the going to work, the régime was exacting, and we had to consider emotional toughness as well as vocational aspects.

One northern school at the time of the 500 sample was able to offer some secretarial training to a few girls, first in the school and then at outside classes; again stability and ambition came into this, but the decision about her readiness could be reached at the school itself, which also gave domestic training, and catered for a wide range of emotional conditions which could respond to a sound lay approach; accessibility to psychiatric advice was poor. Control was quiet and persuasive, and also suited the girl of limited, but not borderline intelligence, who required social training.

One school then (a different one for the 1957 sample) was vocational in the sense that it trained the very dull girl, from I.Q. 75 downwards, and an occasional brighter girl, who needed the reassurance of not being overtly challenged where she felt inferior. We shall see that this was generally a responsive group, mainly stable, but able to absorb a few very disturbed subnormal girls. One failed to settle in two Junior Schools, achieved control and some skills in this Senior School, but could not manage outside, and was eventually ascertained as Mentally Defective (the term used at the time). Mainly their intellectual disabilities proved less crippling than most would have predicted in the research period. The girls were trained in routine domestic procedure, and enjoyed the training.

PHYSICAL NEEDS

While several schools accepted a few girls requiring treatment for venereal infections or other medical conditions, two schools received most of those who still required, on transfer, concentrated treatment for venereal infections, or other chronic health conditions such as eczema or asthma. The choice between the two schools was in emotional terms. One, run by a religious organization, had a highly-charged atmosphere. The initial impact was by long and concentrated interviewing by the Headmistress. This degree of emotional challenge, spun out sometimes over two years or even more, wore down many tough but permeable spirits. The other 'treatment' school also received tough spirits, but the less permeable endured best, as far as our research would indicate. Life was very active, and classes and outdoor activities were being developed as a feature. Yet in the 'treatment schools', as stressed in Monograph 6 of the Headmasters, Headmistresses and Matrons of Approved Schools Association, 'the fact of treatment tends to keep the sexual side of the problem in the foreground'.

EMOTIONAL, OR PERSONALITY NEEDS

This is the most difficult classification to explain, partly because it overlapped with the other categorizations. We have seen, for instance, that the least mature 14's emotionally or socially were generally allocated to a particular school, and the 'tougher' 14's to another.

In staff discussion on a girl's allocation we might pronounce: 'She needs —— School', or we might say: 'She needs Miss ——'. This can best be illustrated by a few descriptions or régimes (just as we have done for the two kinds of girls needing treatment for venereal disease).

In the North-East was a unique school, with just over twenty girls in a rather small, shabby and not very tidy old house. It was run almost single-handed by a woman of tremendous humour and courage, whose greatest misfortune was that she had belonged to another era of training, and could not catch up on the modern trends in treatment which would have suited her temperament. Yet she kept a gay little community, full of affection and fun, but oozing with the anxieties of some very troubled girls whom we sent there, along with a proportion who were more robust. There were then no outside specialist facilities for resolving the anxieties, but they were given the courage to live with them as long as they had this superb mother-figure. Most of the girls sent should have had regular psychiatric treatment, but the one school ear-marked for that was ever full of the even more needful from both Girls' Classifying Schools. When psychiatric advice was sought at a nearby psychiatric unit, the Head-mistress was puzzled by the communications—not surprisingly on an occasion when Borstal was recommended for a girl whose psychopathic urges had been miraculously under control, and had given no sufficient cause for being brought before the Court again.

The Training School with regular psychiatric facilities, managed by the National Association for Mental Health, received only thirteen of our girls in the main research period. The girls were discreetly selected by the School's Managers (officially), after perusals of her file and classifying report by the Headmistress and visiting Psychiatrist(s), and if a girl was found not to respond to the psychoanalytically orientated treatment she had to be re-allocated later. The intellectual level was from good average upwards, with an occasional 'just average'. Activities within the school at that period were very similar to those in most of the girls' Schools—domestic and school-room, and the usual leisure activities. The régime was perhaps more elastic to accommodate the regressive behaviour of girls receiving psychiatric treatment, and staff were more adequately trained, for enlightened staff were attracted by the facilities. But it must not be forgotten that these were carefully selected cases, and their régime could be regulated differently.

Of the regular nine there remains the most challenging School of the northern area, where we sent aggressive older girls, some with propensities for physical violence; we sent persistent absconders, for it was a more 'closed' school than the others, though with an 'open' section to which the girls might graduate; we also sent a few more 'average' delinquent girls, and, like all the schools, some very dull girls who could not be more suitably housed. Discipline was hearty. To some it seemed on the raucous side. It was less inhibiting emotionally than some other schools, and the success rate can be seen partly against this feature, but mainly against the preponderance of coarse, obscene, rebellious and often grossly disturbed girls admitted there, not least the aggressively psychopathic minority.

Sometimes it was so difficult to allocate a girl that the opinion of the Home Office Inspectorate was sought; this would be particularly so of a girl from the southern area transferred to us as a special case, but it also happened with the most colourful problems, especially those who had required an interval in Mental Hospital. Occasionally a call on the Home Office Children's Department Inspectorate would be made by the Head (usually in her own time) about particularly difficult cases; such was the easy and not too formal access to the top advisory level.

Where decisions about Training Schools were made through the normal channels, we were often by no means in the clear about a girl's future; we might well find from the Training School of our choice that no vacancy existed, and would not exist for several weeks. Then we could decide (contrary to official guidance) to await what seemed *the* suitable vacancy, or we could reconsider the transfer; with one girl it might be possible to picture her in more than one setting, while another had seemed tailor-made for one school and it was disturbing to have to fit her to another pattern. Some girls could not be cast (by our imaginings) for *any* existing Approved School, and if, after much thought, we had seen that she might be suitable for one place, it was then particularly frustrating to find there was no vacancy, or that the Headmistress and Managers of the Training School objected to her as an unsuitable case for them; this was excusable where too many absconders, for instance, or too many hysterics had been received within a short interval. (Anyone who has tried to place a child in a School for Maladjusted Children, where it is commonplace to have ten applications for one vacancy, knows what this sort of set-back means. Our difficult cases were the queens of maladjusted children, and had to be lived with as amicably and constructively as possible pending another decision.)

The consequence for some of the girls in not having the right treatment (where we knew her needs, and the right school was there, but not a place in it) does not bear thought. Love and bonhomie were not enough for the neurotically disturbed girls who were not accepted (for reasons of vacancy, too low I.Q. or propensity for frequent absconding) at the one School then supplying regular psychiatric treatment. Occasionally a girl with severe disturbance but leaning in the psychopathic direction had to be allocated to a 'tough' school (i.e. a school for tough girls) because the habit of absconding had become so strong, and containment had been, after all, a condition of Approved School committal.

Frequently girls were retained at the Classifying School to await a place at a suitable school. The most difficult girls were on occasion retained even, in a few cases, for the whole training period, but more often the 'cream' was kept to await a place for short-term training. This laid a stable layer over the restless currents of the community, but did not endear us to the Home Office and sometimes not to the Training Schools.

There was criticism too that the Classifying School did more than classify—that it attempted training, and that during the long interim period—perhaps up to three months while awaiting a scarce best placement, then failing that a second-best placement, or during prolonged medical treatment—the girl's attachment to the Classifying staff made settling-in difficult at the next stage. Figures on prediction of later success may indicate how far long stays at the Classifying School were ever necessary or good—if vacancy for training was available in a few weeks.

Chapter Twenty-one

TRAINING, LICENCE, SUPERVISION AND SUCCESS AND FAILURE

The question of suitability of Training School leads us to the issue of *successful* placing. Not only should the new Headmistress and her Staff have a picture of a girl's personality and potential, but the new régime should provide the best recipe for rehabilitation. For it was neither a training for girls eager to be equipped for a certain job, nor was it a Finishing School for girls whose parents asked for talents and graces to be polished up for the marriage market. In most cases the girls were itching to be at home, or in a flat, or with a lover; and parents wanted at best their company and at worst their wages.

Society expects delinquent young people, like maladjusted, and unlike physically handicapped or educationally subnormal, to be cured by the Residential School of their handicap, not just taught to live with it. Whether or not this is a reasonable expectation, especially in cases where symptoms had been present since early years, and where many people had previously acknowledged defeat, this book will betray the same expectations as elsewhere, and will even presume to criticize the Training Schools for not fulfilling expectations, regardless of inadequate or unequal provision of Staffing, buildings, equipment and many other deficiencies which varied from school to school.

MEASUREMENT OF SUCCESS

Home Office statistics for success of Approved School boys and girls is a very simple one—not being found guilty of an offence after leaving. With ex-Approved School boys this criterion can just about hold water, but in the case of girls, of whom about 36 per cent had been committed as being in need of care or protection (even if a further 3 or 4 per cent of these have been offenders technically before), the criterion of reappearance in Court is a useful but very inadequate one. A girl could thus be classed as a success if she had produced one illegitimate child per year, or co-habited with a series of men, and had mental breakdowns at intervals, while the girl who stole the ball-point pen from the hospital supervisor would be recorded a failure.

249

At the same time, by giving figures covering an inclusive period, allowance is not made for continued improvement after leaving the Approved School. Guilt for a petty theft in the first month after would affect the statistics over the three year period normally studied.

The Eighth and subsequent Reports on the work of the Children's Department of the Home Office give, as we have seen in the Introduction, from 82 per cent to 88 per cent as the level for 'satisfactory' cases placed out in the years between 1952–9, and found guilty of an offence.

That alternative figures can be given in the present research is due to the cooperation of all the Training Schools to which girls were allocated during the research periods, and up to 1960. The promotion of this follow-up scheme was supported by the Home Office.

Figures were prepared previously by the writer in 1958 for a Review Meeting held at the Classifying School, and were subsequently published in the *Approved Schools' Gazette*. Though the methods used for the alternative findings to be given here differ from that used in 1958, statistics will be seen to be confirmatory.

The first forms sent by the Shaw Classifying School to the Training Schools in 1952, called for a report back in three months after transfer, and each twelve months subsequently, during training and while on licence from the Training School. This could cover a total period of six years (according to the legislation still in force during the period under study) with our population, but for various reasons to be explored rarely did.

The initial report back from the School was the following year and onwards requested at a six-month interval from admission, and still annually thereafter. The supervisory agent and the School might lose contact with a girl well before the end of the supervision period (three years after licence, or up to age 21) or supervision might be terminated by the Training School Managers. On the other hand contact might continue unofficially for years afterwards, through warm and helpful relationships between girl and Head Teacher or Staff. In a few cases later information came from newspaper headlines or Police inquiries. Even at the Classifying School the odd call was made by young wives and mothers, known many years back, and more frequently by girls (not always successful ones) who had been briefly out in the world.

THE REPORT FORM

The format of the report form used is shown here along with a complete write-up of one case, not a spectacular case, but a girl of 15, of low average intelligence, and some scholastic retardation, from a poor social background. She was transferred in 1953 to a Senior School run by a religious organization, catering for a wide range of intelligence and trainability.

1st Report on S, aged 15 (six months after transfer from C.S.)
(1) *Health:* Good.
(2) *Reaction to Training:*
    (a) Practical Work: S works well and willingly, accepting instruction cheerfully.
    (b) Classroom Instruction: Does her best but has no special aptitude for classroom work.
    (c) Leisure Pursuits: Fond of swimming and games generally; knits, reads light literature.
    (d) Social adjustment: Accepted in a group, probably because she lends herself to the atmosphere of the group: if the group is quiet, she too is quiet; if the group is noisy then she becomes a noisy member and often behaves foolishly, becoming a nuisance.

(3) *Relationship with Home and Home Situation:*
    Mother writes regularly and S appears dependent on these letters and the visits of her Mother, but the woman is not helpful, and usually visits the public house on her way here, arriving late. The parents have separated since S came to the School.

Second Year Report on S—dated 1955
(1) *Health:* Very good.
(2) *Reaction to training:*
    (a) Practical Work: Pleasant and willing worker. Works well under supervision but shows little initiative.
    (b) Classroom Instruction: Not very outstanding in any subjects, but appears to enjoy housewifery class.
    (c) Leisure Pursuits: Knits or reads, or just sits. Quite fond of games.
    (d) Social adjustment: Has tended to withdraw from groups and sits alone or with one special friend. Has recently developed a silly friendship with ——

(3) *Relationship with Home and Home Situation:*
    Parents still separated. Both write and visit infrequently. S is very fond of her mother, though increasingly aware of her weaknesses. The Mother drinks too much and is co-habiting.
General Comment: S absconded on September (with —— and ——), but while the other two went Eastward, she made straight for home.

Third Report on S—dated 1956
(1) *Health:* Good.
(2) *Reaction to training:*
    (a) Practical work: Quite good.
    (b) Classroom Instruction: Worked hard, interested.
    (c) Leisure pursuits: Very fond of sport—Netball and Swimming.
    (d) Social adjustment: Pleasant and fitted in well.

(3) *Relationship with Home and Home Situation:* Worried a good deal about her Mother who is very unsteady.

Fourth Report on S also dated 1956
After Care Report: Had a difficult time at first due to adverse home circumstances. Is now married very happily and obviously gets real satisfaction out of her life as a housewife. She and her husband have recently got a house to themselves and reports state that she continues to do very well.

Fifth Report dated 1957
After Care Report.
Employment: Housewife.
Wages: ——
Relationship with Home:
Social Adjustment: S was married on ——. Her husband is a steady, dependable man who is determined that S shall have a settled and secure existence. S is very happy and keeps her home beautifully clean, obviously getting real satisfaction out of her life as a housewife. Application was made for the discharge of her Approved School Order and it was granted on ——.

These, then, are the reports on our first case, a rather homely person, whose disturbed phases in the Training School could have been described more objectively and in more technical terms. We should have been none the wiser for that and are freer to make our own diagnosis. Can we doubt that S was helped to live through her difficulties, both in Training and in her own marriage? The calm, tolerant phraseology is perhaps the best key to how her emotions were educated in the Training School.

This one report makes it clear that the headings could stimulate verbalization, or terse remarks. Research was in mind, but the forms were not prepared by research workers, and would have required much more itemization, and more pursuit of nil returns in any section. Dates would especially have been required against news received from the after-care agent; sometimes the complete report was undated. At the time the pleasure felt at the launching of such a valuable scheme would have made such precision seem niggling— and indeed the lengthy information often received was impressive, when one knew the long hours worked already by some of the Headmistresses concerned.

STATISTICAL MEASUREMENT OF SUCCESS RATES

For those who knew the cases individually, each report was of interest throughout. As far as extracting research data was concerned, the task was more difficult. What the writer felt justified in drawing from all but a few of the reports submitted, whether very discursive or terse, was the general fact whether a girl has done very well, satisfactorily, indifferently or badly. This estimate is partly related to her own social surroundings (e.g. S would not be considered highly successful if her parents were doctors or business directors), but partly to commonly accepted social standards of that time. It may well be that a scorer to whom the girls were just names would doubt the objectivity of her judgment and it may be that many readers will be sceptical about the rating method used. In fact a large section of the writer's scoring was checked by a Social Science degree student on a residential visit of observation to the Classifying School, and agreement was usually very close, although the latter did not know the girls personally. One school which received 79 of the 500 girls, in fact, responded mainly with 'satisfactory', 'unsatisfactory', etc.

Again, doubt might be thrown on the Training School's judgment of a girl's progress, or on the meaning of the words used to describe her behaviour. But after all, the girl has been committed to Approved School on the verbal description of her past conduct by social workers, parents and teachers.

Some examples of scoring may best illumine the discussion.

Examples of Scoring Success

A report on A, aged 18, two years after her transfer from Classifying School reads:

A was admitted to the Mother and Baby Home —— but she absconded the next day. After three days she was apprehended and returned to the Mother and Baby Home, but stayed only half an hour, and Matron refused to have her back again. We decided to licence her to her mother and she apparently settled for the time being, reasonably well. In February it was reported that she was beyond her mother's control; she had been admitted to hospital in false labour. In March it was reported that she was not living at home, but with Italians. A daughter was born in March. Report in June tells the same story of violent quarrels with her mother. A still not married. In July A left the child in her mother's care and disappeared. In September she was charged with theft of clothing from her mother and remanded on bail for one week to find employment. She returned to Court on —— and after Court was taken to the Probation Officer's Office whilst that Officer went to get her car. A has not been seen since.

A is hardly a stabilized girl, meriting a high rating for socialization. Both on absolute social standards, and in relation to the unruly conduct which brought her into Approved School, A was a failure at the time of this report.

253

The following is a more indeterminate story. This time the report was written in the third year after transfer from Classifying School, and the girl was then 19.

D had a splendid job when she left School in April last year. Her employers were paragons of consideration and generosity; they also had a really good standard. Amongst other things, they took her with them to Scotland. However, she could not play straight, and showed herself to be a terror with the local boys, so that her name became a legend. She was dismissed. She got herself work in a Hotel in ——. She also became engaged to a weedy youth with whom I had an interview one memorable Sunday afternoon. D terminated the engagement, but remained friendly with this boy.

D was dismissed from the Hotel as unsatisfactory. She had grown to look very 'common', plastering make-up on her face in a most inartistic manner. She lost weight, interest, vitality, became nervy and bad-tempered. I urged her to go to the Doctor, which she said she would do. She did not return and at the present, I am sorry to say, I do not know where she is. I am trying to find her and hope to be successful. I feel that, if and when she needs help, she will get into touch with me. It is more than likely that, having made a mess of two jobs, she is determined to do better before she visits us again. I am very disappointed indeed not to be able to give a more satisfactory report on her progress.

While one warms to poor lonely D and while one doubts the rosy prognosis in the second last sentence, one feels justified in labelling the success level 'indifferent'.

An example of a glowing report may seem an extreme after these, but in the files there are a good many which rank with it:

Has never caused a moment's trouble. Is very happily and comfortably established in her own home. Her husband has his own business. J continues to work as Secretary to a large Company. She has been a member of the local Operatic Society for the past three years and has this year been given one of the principal parts in a Gilbert & Sullivan production. She has been having voice training for some time. J is Godmother to ——'s oldest son and fulfils her duties very faithfully. She visits the School regularly.

There are instances when it is very difficult to think in 'success' terms. One of these was a schizoid girl of charming disposition who was living, two years after the end of Classification, and after a period in the Approved School with special psychiatric facilities, as mistress of the son of a well-to-do London Club owner. In relation to her difficulties, one had to steel oneself to rate her below the success line. (She would certainly have been rated 'Satisfactory' by the Home Office method, as she had been guilty of no offence.) She was committed to Approved School as in need of care and protection, for wandering and for irregular relationships of the kind—if not the quality—of her post-training years. In such cases it was necessary to think of the strictures of Society which brought her into the delinquent category—and also of the possibly short-term solution she had found.

Finally four ratings were decided on, namely: 'Good', 'Satisfactory', 'Indifferent' and 'Poor'. A 'Good' rating was given only for those who had excelled in several behavioural aspects, and showed no serious regressive trends. An example is J above, who appears to be socially acceptable, a good employee, a happily married, respectable housewife, and to have a sense of responsibility towards a former old girl of the Approved School (the mother of the Godchild mentioned). It was possible to graduate to the 'Good' group without being such a paragon as J.

The 'Satisfactory' rating belonged to those who, in the Training School, were reasonably cooperative and industrious; who were not absconders; who showed some awareness of social responsibility and some thought for the future. A 'Satisfactory' rating in the licence period would require a fairly steady attitude towards employment, to home relationships (or substitute relationships); at worst there would be no further offences, no drunken brawls and no illegitimate babies, though a total recovery of self-respect after a lapse could bring her back into 'Satisfactory' grace.

These two categories of 'Good' and 'Satisfactory' held the girls who, for that particular year, were in approximate terms above the success line. They might maintain this place, or have to be added to the less than successful later.

The Follow-up report on D given earlier, the girl who left two jobs, had an unsatisfactory boy-friend, and was the scandal of the village, is a fair example of the 'indifferent' group. There is a good chance of recovery, for one senses that her feeble adventures are an attempt of a lonely girl to affiliate herself, and the next chapter could contain a healthy-minded swain to whom she is devoted. But she is far from adjusted, far from happy at this particular stage.

A, the girl who played ructions in the Mother and Baby Home, and absconded from the Probation Office and eluded official After-Care from then on, is an example of the 'Poor' group. There are fewer of these, and care was taken not to move a girl into this category unless she was seriously asocial or anti-social, whether in Training School, on licence or under supervision.

Subsequently the first two categories ('good' and 'satisfactory') and the other two ('indifferent' and 'poor') were combined for statistical purposes, there being too few of the extremes. This is a pity, as we lose something of the quality of the 'Indifferent' group, wavering often on the way to recovery—or to failure.

Rating 500 girls in each of our four successive years from the time of transfer from the Classifying School was not an easy labour. The writer was protected from ennui or a sense of futility by her abiding interest in the cases, whose history and—above all—whose personality was clearly alive to her. It was like renewing acquaintance with hundreds of friends; that, as we all know, would be very exhausting.

SUCCESS AT TRAINING SCHOOL

The training period not only represented an earlier period in the girl's adolescence, in her re-education, in her enforced further separation from the world where she wanted to be, but it represented the stage where environmental influences on her, however varied they might be from school to school, were more inter-related than the later post-licence influences of 500 different home environments would be. The Training Schools were sufficiently comparable to the Classifying School for us to wonder how far behaviour at both would be correlated, and different enough to make one inquire how relevant the observations and assessments made at the latter mattered in the new setting. One would ask inevitably too whether the period of classification was necessary at all, or whether aspects of the girl's pre-committal relationships and conduct were sufficient to mark her as suitable for certain training or treatment.

While some of the girls, especially some of the duller ones, seemed to regard the Classifying School as an island of experience, and would make stodgy parting comments such as, 'Ah well, miss, I suppose the sooner I go to my school the sooner I go back home', to others it was either the end of a hard-fought battle for promotion to a 'good school', or the end of a frustrating patch where one hadn't been able to do as one pleased and yet hadn't been held in check harshly; indeed the failures were of a nature felt so often before, and success was so remote that one felt (as with so many contacts in the past) 'They'll be glad to see the back of me'.

For these girls the move was often an irritating continuation. It might well be that those who went into a very firm régime were relieved even temporarily by the checks on unruliness, by the barriers against 'playing-up'. Yet mainly they would have a long way to go before 'being good' was more than an exercise in unnatural restraint.

For those who had been stable enough to conform genuinely or even superficially at the Classifying School, and who had after a month or six weeks been given responsibilities which would come

256

after six months or more at the Training School, the new beginning was sometimes hard, though this very inhibiting experience could itself be a source of new insight into her own personal limitations.

Under Rule 40(1) of the Approved School Rules, 1933, and as amended in 1949, Approved School Managers had a duty to release a boy or girl on licence as soon as he or she had made sufficient progress. The maximum period of detention (including the classifying period) for the girls of the age group in this research was three years, or (in the case of girls over 16 on committal) until the 19th birthday. In exceptional cases the Secretary of State could be asked to consent to a further period not exceeding six months for additional training. Detention could also be lengthened by periods spent in unauthorized absence from the School, but in all cases to cease by the age of 19. The Secretary of State's consent was required also for the release of a girl on licence within twelve months of committal.

The length of training (i.e. actual detention within the Training School, apart from the Classifying period) varied for the research group from nine months to just over three years. This included any periods when recalled from licence for further training. The average length of training was fully eighteen months, with a scatter as follows:

Table 57(a): Period of Training

Detained for	No. of Girls	%
Less than a year	33	6·6
1 year up to 15 months	41	8·2
15 months up to 18 months	58	11·6
18 months up to 21 months	127	25·4
21 months up to 2 years	109	21·8
2 years up to 27 months	65	13·0
27 months up to 2½ years	22	4·4
2½ years up to 3 years	25	5·0
Fully 3 years	3	0·6
Total	483	96·6

The remaining seventeen girls (3·4 per cent) were either very briefly in Training Schools, and then admitted to Borstal or Mental Hospital or ascertained as Mentally Defective, or their time of licence was not clearly given.

We shall later see what relation existed statistically between success and length of training. Meantime the summary is given to justify the choice of interval at which success in the Training School was measured—namely from twelve months up to eighteen months. None had then been long away from the institution, and roughly half were in the later phases of training.

For 476 of the 500 girls there was an adequate follow-up report, which, within the limits stated for the material, gave an indication of her relative success or failure at that period. 17 of the 500 were, as we have seen, not long enough under training, and for the further seven reports were too sporadic for the timing of events to be acceptable.

This method of assessment required a good deal more work than the earlier one, as published in the Approved Schools' Gazette (see above), but was more accurate, since, as we have seen, the intervals of reporting changed in 1953. In addition the follow-up forms were by no means punctiliously returned, as is usual with such systems.

When the ratings at this period were tabulated, the distribution was as follows:

Table 57(b): Success Percentages in T.S.

	No. of Girls	%
Good	49	9·8
Satisfactory	234	46·8
Indifferent	151	30·2
Poor	42	8·4
Not known, or not in training	24	4·8
Total	500	100

As the first two categories, and also the poor and indifferent groups have had to be combined for subsequent correlations, and since the final thirty-four girls are not part of this estimate, we can re-group as follows:

Table 57(c): Success Percentages in T.S.

	No. of Girls	%
Reasonably Successful	283	59
Doubtfully Successful	193	41
Total	476	100

This is a useful stage for correlation with prior figures, both of social conditions and behaviour pre-committal, and with estimates at the Classifying School.

The following list shows columns which were found to be linked significantly, and some which were not:

Table 58: Factors correlated with Success after 12 to 17 months at Training School

	See Table*	Prob.	
Conduct at the Classifying School	8	·001	Highly Significant
Prevailing Mood at the Classifying School	7	·001	,, ,,
Expression of feeling at the Classifying School	6	·001	,, ,,
Estimate of character strength	56	·001	,, ,,
Acceptance of committal	55	·001	,, ,,
Age when girl first left home	39	·001	,, ,,
Concentration and persistence in work at Classifying School	p. 25	·01	Significant
Relationship with (day) Schools	45	·01	,,
Passalong Test Results	p. 233	·05	Barely Significant
Number of detrimental situations	37	·05	,, ,,
Adults girl mainly lived with	30	·05	,, ,,
Binet I.Q.	51	·1	Not statistically significant
Relationships in the home	44	·1	,, ,,
Economic Status of Parents	22	·1	,, ,,
Supervision Order before Committal	—	·1	,, ,,
Abnormal Matrices Scatter (D − C > 2)	p. 230	·1	,, ,,
Material Condition of the Home	21	·7	,, ,,
Probation Order before Committal	—	·5	,, ,,
Matrices grading	52	·8	,, ,,
Physical Type	13	·7	,, ,,
Age on Committal	15	·7	,, ,,
Age at first known delinquency	p. 91	·2	,, ,,

* Tables usually regrouped for statistical purposes.

DISCUSSION

Conduct at the Classifying School. Table 8 was more descriptive of behaviour than the ratings for success in training. Behaviour at the Classifying School is seen as a highly significant predictor. Only seven of the sixty-three girls (11 per cent) judged as cooperative there were in the unsatisfactory 41 per cent at the Training Schools. Of the childish girls (the socially very immature) about 40 per cent were above the success line, instead of below it. Those who had childish tantrums had about a 45 per cent chance of doing reasonably well, the openly uncooperative rather better (about 50 per cent).

Prevailing Mood at the Classifying School. Table 7, though a crude list of personality descriptions, proves generally a good predictor. The cheerful, the serious and the anxious had 74 per cent, 86 per cent and 63 per cent chances of success respectively in training. It may be that the serious and anxious belonged to a graduating scale of anxious girls, with a degree of anxiety (somewhere in the 'serious' group) which was optimal for success, and with a goodly number of over-anxious individuals who would tend to fail; the cutting-off point would, of course, vary much with the type of environment.

Meantime the depressed had only a one-third chance, and the sullen, the 'couldn't-care-less' and the apathetic all were about as likely to fail as to succeed.

Expression of feeling. Estimate of Character Strength. Acceptance of Committal. In a sense these could have been deduced from the moods; for instance an apathetic girl was not oozing emotion or strength of character, nor was she likely to be very constructive about her training. But all three tables gave highly significant findings, and deserve to stand on their own. A girl who had accepted her committal at Classifying stage had three times the chance of doing well. Indecisive characters came out quite well, along with the strong, while those classed as weak and warped more often did badly. Feelings had to be easily expressed *and* under control.

Age when girl first left home. This, of the earlier life factors correlated with good response to training, alone had a highly significant probability score. According to Table 39 a parting from home in the 5 to 8 year era gave the worst chance (only 35 per cent) of settling in at this later adolescent stage. Those who had been separated from home before the age of 5 had a 50 per cent chance. Doubtless, apart from possible lasting damage, the early feelings of rejection or neglect were reawakened, especially when the earlier dispersal had been to an institution of some sort.

Concentration and Persistence in Work at the Classifying School. Apart from a spell at the Remand Homes, girls had often done little serious domestic work of the kind provided at the Classifying School. Even if they had helped at home, the size of the school altered the scale. Generally, therefore, factors from the working life were not used for correlations, but this one more general table (which might include school work for the 14-year-old section) predicts at the 1 per cent level.

Relationship with (day) Schools. Here we have a significant relationship (less than 1 per cent chance) with a directly reported observational fact. Though the school report section of the Court's record was, as we have seen, often thin in information, what we could deduce suggests that fuller reports might be even more usefully predictive. Even so, those who were depicted as cooperative throughout had a 70 per cent success distribution at the Approved Training School.

Results of doubtful significance, (less than 5 per cent chance) included *the results in the Passalong Test,* while the Binet Test I.Q.'s were very doubtful predictors (between 5 and 10 per cent) and the Matrices Test Gradings even less (80 per cent). The emphasis on practical skills at the Training Schools will doubtless account for the greater usefulness of the Passalong; it may be useful knowledge to those who deny the Passalong validity.

The number of detrimental situations in the early life may again have some significance. If so, those with *no* recorded major or minor detrimental situation in their earlier life (no longer or shorter separations through death, divorce, hospitalization, etc.) seemed, oddly enough to do worst, along with those who had an accumulation of major and minor. This odd finding may be caused by a tendency to commit only extremely difficult cases if the home was intact. We must also, however, remember such factors as rejection by father, which occurred in 37 of the 199 cases with no major break.

The Adult(s) mainly lived with—Again the probability is only about the ·05 level, but inspection shows that the girls who had responded best (with a 70 per cent chance of success) were those who, for much of their lives, had been without their mother. Thus the all-female staff at the schools fulfilled an important role. At the Classifying School these motherless girls had been disproportionately subject to childish outbursts; this regression may have been an important part of their later success. They were less directly aggressive, while girls whose fathers were absent erred in the opposite direction. At both Classifying and Training Schools those who had mainly had neither parent tended to be less cooperative (about 40 per cent success at the Training School).

Despite the doubtful significance, we again have the trends expected from classical work on early childhood deprivation, with the recurring significance of paternal deprivation, already highlighted in this research.

Not Statistically Significant

Relations in the Home. Only 10 per cent significance, but an interesting point was that the least successful group (40 per cent successful) was of those who revealed little of their attitudes to home in speech or writing. Perhaps this contained some of the most seriously rejected girls, and indicates the need for skilled interviewing of girl and parents at this stage.

Supervision or Probation Order before Committal. Neither of those has much relation to responding to training, which is surprising, in that the Probation Officer, Child Care Officer or other person responsible would be likely to have been the appointed After-Care agent (ideally in touch throughout training) and contacts between home and school might be expected to be softened, and therefore helpful. In fact those who had previously been under supervision tended to do *less* well at this stage—which is probably just a measure of excessive personality disturbance and earlier Fit Person Orders which failed.

Matrices Scatter. We have seen that the 'Shaw' criterion of uneven scatter (score on set D exceeding score on set C by 2 or more) applied with some significance ($p < \cdot 05$) to girls' prevalent moods, the serious and anxious tending to show this 'pattern'. Again there was a tendency (but slighter—barely 5 per cent) for girls *with* the pattern to do better at the Training School. Thus 68 per cent of these were satisfactory, against 59 per cent of the whole group. We have already seen that the serious and anxious girls tended to do better—the girls who most often had this Matrices scatter. This correlation may be worth pursuing in further research.

Economic Status of Parents. The slightly most responsive category, both at the Classifying School and at the Training School, were those whose parents were dependent on Welfare Services, or on Old Age or Widow's Pension. Doubtless the contrast of plenty after poverty had some effect here. 74 per cent of this group of seventy-three girls were satisfactorily responsive to training.

Not significant. The material condition of the home, the girl's age on committal, and her age when first reported delinquent did not prove to be significant, nor did her physical appearance (as related to physical types in Table 13 regrouped).

General Deductions. What kind of girl, then, was likely to respond at the Training School? The answer seems to be the responsive girl. If she cooperated with teachers at day school, or with staff at the Classifying School, there was a good chance she would at the Approved Training School. She tended to be a cheerful extravert with some control, or a more serious introverted girl, who perhaps appreciated the strong minded female figures on whom she could lean. Sometimes she enjoyed food, comfort and clothing which a family dependent on social welfare had sadly lacked. She would tend to have fairly good practical ability, but overall did not need more bookish intelligence, or even the capacity to think abstractly, for more than one school was attuned to dull serious girls.

Feelings of rejection or neglect at early separations might be re-awakened, but we cannot assume at this stage that lasting damage had been done. Indeed girls with no serious early losses had a slight tendency to do badly, as if delinquency through some basic character failure was less treatable in the schools than impairment through neglect and deprivation, even when piled on top of each other. Yet personality types as linked with physical types seem to give us no lead (P = ·7). Ectomorphs, endomorphs and mesomorphs seem to be doing alike at this stage.

But we have been studying types of trainees rather than types of Training Schools. We should wish to claim that each girl was selected for a certain 'best' school for her, or diverted to a second or third best, according to our discrimination of her needs, or to the need to send her somewhere. How far can we discriminate which type of girl went to which school? This involves studying 'school types' in a way we did not attempt to do in the chapter on allocation. And since we have success measures at hand, we had best compare the success of different schools, though in fact such a direct comparison is unfair, since (as we shall see) the types admitted varied from one to another.

We must also recall that, for several of the Training Schools, Shaw girls were only a proportion of their intake, and may have been an untypical minority in a few. Eleven schools received ten or more transfers from the Shaw Classifying School during the three years under review. Two years from transfer from the Classifying School the success ratio for these eleven schools was calculated on their admissions. *Percentage of good and satisfactory response ranged from 85 to 29.* (Two years later still the success rate was from 95 to 40; this was partly because some of the worst failures were lost.) The list was as follows:

Table 59: Success rates in terms of different schools

School	No. Transferred in 3 years	2 years after transfer % success	4 years after transfer % success
A	53	66	72
B	62	29	40
C	49	80	60
D	33	45	47
E	42	57	46
F	25	64	57
G	39	85	95
H	80	73	58
I	39	44	47
J	10	40	67
L	24	75	70

Five schools had success rates of 65 per cent or over, six had rates below 65. This somewhat arbitrary *pass* line was drawn as a result of earlier figures.

The writer and other members of staff, from visits as escorts to the Training Schools, as well as from other sources, had opinions of the disciplinary lines, and of the pervading atmosphere. From these an admittedly subjective three-point grading was made, thus:

1. *Somewhat rigid*—Schools D and I.
2. *Calm, controlled, medium strict*—Schools A, C, G, J and L.
3. *Relatively permissive and ebullient*—School B and School E.

The estimates had nothing to do with doors being locked, or with checking of linen, or even with walking in crocodiles, but refer to the give-and-take between girls and staff. Actual régimes within groups might differ vastly. Thus School B was hearty and tough, with plenty of 'talking back'. The staff would hate to think they seemed permissive and they would have had little in common with staff in 'free discipline' schools.

School E was brimming over with the milk of human kindness; and even their tougher element found little in the environment to rebel against. The conflicts were in the girls themselves, for the neurotics who found no place in School J tended to find their way there.

Schools A, C, G and L, all rated as having calm, controlled, medium strict discipline, have the four highest success rates. School J, which at that time in history, was rated similarly for control, received a third or a quarter of the Shaw girls admitted to the other four, so results must be dubious statistically; it had in fact facilities for regular psychiatric treatment, and drew from both Girls' Classifying Schools.

School H, with a success rate over 70, was by no means permissive. The age group (14 usually on admission) may have favoured the tighter system, the orderliness of the activities. It must be remembered that this group on licence still had the middle years of adolescence to live through. This may partly be the cause of a drop to 58 per cent success after two years from licence.

FURTHER LOOK AT ALLOCATION

Let us now look back at the process of allocation to Training Schools. Relying on memory alone, one recalls the reviews of progress, formal and informal, and the casual or heated inter-staff discussions about the kind of régime needed for response and rehabilitation. M was arrogant, domineering, emotional, and quite bright, with a mother who secreted cigarettes in parcels of 'love books', and wanted M to marry a boy-friend who stole cars. M also needed regular treatment for venereal disease. She required (we felt), someone very strong-minded to redeem her, someone prepared to work on M and on her mother. Nearness to home could be useful. Absconding needed at the same time to be difficult, for M had by no means accepted her committal. (Her career at the 'closed' treatment school was very mixed.)

V had been a 'good girl' since admitted, apart from tearful episodes if other girls tried to undermine her determination to do well. She was of average intelligence, but socially retarded, and emotionally disturbed by past and present quarrels and separations at home. Her domestic work was messy, but she was eager to please. Contrary to the advice of about three quarters of the staff V was sent for short-term training. The strong practical bias, and the maturity of most of the girls nonplussed V. She absconded occasionally, and her practical ability was poor. Scholastic difficulties ruled out examinational work in domestic science. But she still was anxious to please, and the school had a degree of trust in her placement there. She eventually did well, responding to the emotional warmth she needed—but not in a short term.

Statistical Evaluation of Allocation

Turning to a more objective study of which girls went to which schools, we have Table 19. As above, schools were grouped into those with a 65 per cent or over success rating (Schools A, C, G, H and L) and those below. A variety of factors in girls' lives and personalities were correlated with the 'successful' (group I) and 'unsuccessful' (group II). Results of the Chi-square calculations are as shown in Table 60 overleaf.

Factors not related significantly were delinquency in the home ($P = \cdot1$), the number of detrimental situations in life ($P = \cdot5$) and concentration and persistence in work at the Classifying School ($P = \cdot5$).

But what come out as 'good' schools had received 65 per cent of those with constructive attitudes to the future, and only 28 per cent of those with negative outlooks. They had 74 per cent of the socially positive, and only 38 per cent of the disruptive. They had 80 per cent of those who identified with the best of the group, and only 30 per cent of those who identified with the worst. 64 per cent of the good mixers went to 'successful' schools, only 28 per cent of the isolates, and only 10 per cent of the very changeable. They had 67 per cent of the socially controlled extraverts, but only 43 per cent of the wildly impulsive extraverts.

Table 60: Factors Related to Allocation to Schools I or II

	See Table*	Chi-sq.	D of F	P
Attitude to Future at Classifying School	54	26·136	2	·001
Contribution to Group at Classifying School	4	28·619	2	·001
Identification with Contemporaries	5	59·391	4	·001
Group participation	4	34·706	3	·001
Expression of feeling	6	17·027	3	·001
Prevalent mood	7	23·506	7	·01
Binet I.Q.	51	14·931	4	·01
Conduct at work pre-committal	p. 193	18·062	4	·01
Chief misbehaviour from age 12 to committal	p. 49	33·022	4	·001
Relationship with (day) Schools	45	6·321	2	·05

* *Table usually regrouped for statistical purposes.*

The girls allocated to the 'picked' schools had changed jobs less, and been far less dishonest and quarrelsome as employees in the past. They stayed out late, and were dishonest in proportion to their numbers, and had been excessively prone to truancy from school, but they were much less likely to have left home completely. One reason for the truancy, and for the fact that they often had immature companions at the Classifying School, was that, far from being the brighter girls, they were predominantly dull, and very dull at that. 77 per cent of the forty-eight girls of I.Q. 60 to 69 on the Binet who were allocated to these eleven schools did well. Only 29 of those 69 with I.Q.'s over 100 were in the prize schools. But those very dull 'good' girls we expected to be good, because they had proved stable at the Classifying School; the very dull who were bad were a different sort of problem—and they went into the rag-bag. We were much too nice a staff to talk in that way, and, like many who were involved in difficult social work, we were afraid to face such unpleasant facts, as, to some extent, the receiving schools were.

But in fact one half of the schools were receiving an undue proportion of the population which (generally speaking) were already conditioned to doing reasonably well, and which in the past tended to be less extreme. The remaining six schools, two of which anyway had success rates over 50 per cent, received a larger proportion of those who were not tuned in to the social wave-length, and were often raucously—occasionally even joyfully out of tune with all but their own section of society.

When they absconded from the Classifying or Training Schools they could usually find a place in a degraded quarter of a large city, and when they were tracked down and returned, they could generally find a clique who were impressed by how they had spent their stolen time. And the near tragedy is that good, capable adults were working very hard with inadequate tools, methods and colleagues for an exceptional population.

While we vaguely thought of three or four schools as places for the most awkward girls, there was no spoken or written agreement that they would not be expected to stabilize them. Nor were they given higher staff ratios, nor were recommendations made (to my knowledge) that specialist trained staff should be appointed, so that pioneer work could be done on the psychopath, the sexually aberrant, the near-psychotic delinquent or very unstable E.S.N. girls. The need for such or similar provision was reiterated at almost every review meeting of Heads, Managers and Home Office representatives at the Classifying School, but always in a way that inferred 'somewhere else' rather than in some of the schools represented there.

The tendency in the schools receiving the worst of the resentful, apathetic, regardless fringe was to lack detachment about the girls' misbehaviour—to wax indignant—and yet be far too great a distance from their deep-rooted emotional problems, or even their social conditioning in the past. A comment in a follow-up report reads: 'E is staggering sometimes in her simplicity! Her attitude is that she has really accomplished something great in having an illegitimate half-caste baby!!' And then a comment on home relationships: '—— Biased by her extreme simplicity which apparently is shared by mother who proudly tells you that she is a divorced woman with an "intended"!! Mother is also illiterate so that really the only bond between them is "family love" '—and then the truth dawns—'which perhaps, after all, is all that is necessary'. At least there was puzzlement in this report, a sense of groping into the unknown. From one Training School came reports which smacked of moral superiority; the success rate there was 45 per cent.

Probably infallible tolerance and love—charity or compassion, what the reader will—was the main ingredient for success, and even more with the most intractable. But highest educational skills, personality strength and tact, combined with intellectual awareness, could be in a prescription for the ideal (and rarely obtainable) staff.

SUCCESS AND FAILURE ON LICENCE OR UNDER SUPERVISION

399 girls were followed up for four years from transfer from the Classifying School. This involved rating them for success at a stage

two years up to two years eleven months from being licenced from the Training Schools. Some were still on licence during this later period of assessment—but only the youngest of the girls, for all those 16 on admission would be 17+ on release from detention, and would therefore be at most two years on licence, and thereafter under supervision. It is good to have an estimate after the period when a lapse could mean being brought back to the Training School.

Briefly we might trace at this stage the whereabouts of the remaining 101 girls.

Of these twenty-five had by then been committed for Borstal training, three having been brought back before the Court and charged with an offence, or with persistent absconding from Approved School. These were included in the failures in the year of the lapse, but after that were officially out of the ken of the Approved Schools, and might well have been responsive to training.

Ten had been certified under the Mental Deficiency Act. Again these were recorded as failures in the year concerned, but as they might have proved trainable in the more suitable environment of a Mental Deficiency Hospital, they were not included in later figures. (Eight girls had already been dropped from the research sample because they were ascertained from the Shaw.)

One had been found to be too sick mentally to benefit from Approved School treatment. (This does not, of course, include all who at some point required Mental Hospital treatment. Five others were excluded from the research sample because of prolonged Mental Hospital stays at the Classifying stage, and eventual discharge of the Approved School Order.)

Three girls had died—one from a known heart condition while in Approved School, one in a scooter accident when going to work, and one from an unstated health condition while on licence.

Of the remainder about sixteen were missing. While some of these were likely to be living in dubious circumstances a few were simply sick of being watched, especially if by a Local Authority which had seemed to hound them and their family for ever.

The others had genuinely been discharged from supervision, either because they were over 21, or because the Approved School Managers in question felt supervision was no longer serving a useful purpose; this did not always betoken success, so they could not be graded automatically.

We follow up, then, 399 girls from two to two years eleven months after licence, and find the figures shown in Table 61(*a*) opposite.

Again we combine into two groups and find percentages of the 399 known cases. This gives us the figures shown in Table 61(*b*) opposite.

Table 61(a): Success Percentages 2 to 3 years after licence

	No. of Girls
Good	7
Satisfactory	241
Indifferent	94
Poor	57
Not known	101

Total 500

Table 61(b): Success Percentages 2 to 3 years after licence

	No. of Girls	%
Reasonably successful	248	62
Doubtfully successful	151	38

Total 399

While the percentage of success is three points higher than after twelve to seventeen months training, the number of untabulated cases must be borne in mind. It is unlikely, however, that failures among these would far outweigh successes, so we may fairly assume that *around 60 per cent* is the standard success rate on these gradings, at both intervals.

In fact 60 per cent 'satisfactory', just within three years of placing out, coincided with the figure calculated for boys placed out in the combined three years (Eighth Report of the Children's Department (1961)), 1953, 1954 and 1955—roughly the years in which these girls were licenced.

OBJECTIVE MEASURES

If there is doubt about accepting a success figure based on loosely constructed verbal information, to which has been given a female judgment in vaguely defined terms, let us turn to objective measures of a kind which match reasons for girls having committed to Approved School in the first place. Extracted from the same 500 follow-up reports, covering the period up to two years eleven months after training, we have the facts recorded overleaf.

Objective marks of Non-success in Licence and Supervision Periods
Charged in Court with:

(a) *Offences and found guilty.*
  25 girls had been committed to Borstal
  33 girls had been placed on probation
  7 girls had been fined
  6 girls had been given other judgments
  2 girls had been discharged
  4 girls had been sent to prison
  Total 77 Court Cases.

Note. This would leave a total of 423 'satisfactory' follow-ups, or 84 per cent; the Home Office combined figures for girls placed out in 1953, 1954 and 1955 is 85 per cent satisfactory, but covers the whole country.

(b) *Moral Danger* indications. *Out of Control* behaviour (as judged pre-committal). *In Need of Care or Protection.*
  57 girls had had one illegitimate child
  8 girls had had two illegitimate children
  19 girls were uncommonly promiscuous
  4 not included in (a) were recognized as being prostitutes (i.e. by other prostitutes or by Police, as a rule)
  5 were cohabiting with undesirable partners
  10 had been certified as mentally Defective (though they had not been considered so at the Classifying School, and were nearer usually to moral defective)
  1 was mentally too unstable for normal life.

Total failing for moral and emotional reasons which could have necessitated committal if under age 17 = 105.

Combined totals of (a) and (b) = 184.

Success rate is thus 316 out of 500, or *63 per cent* which is 1 per cent more than the figure for the later follow-up period. This, allowing for errors, including reporting errors, seems satisfactory.

Having argued the case for a truer estimate of success, let us now look at factors which seem clearly related to these estimates, as we did for the period following training, or late during training. We may in this way find how far some later improvements were due to belated effects of the training, or how far later deterioration might be traced, for instance, to inadequate supervision—or how far both were due to the real girl's reactions to freedom.

Comments

The first generalized comment that one can make is that, if the girls who did well at Training Schools were those who were conditioned

Table 62: *Factors Correlated with Success 2 to 2 years 11 months after Licence*

Highly Significant, or Significant	See Table*	Probability
Success after 12 to 17 months training	58	·001
Conduct at the Classifying School	8	·001
Prevailing Mood at the Classifying School	7	·001
Character Strength	66	·01
Appearance (physical type)	13	·01
Contribution to the group at C.S.	4	·01
Time spent in Training School	57a	·01
No. of detrimental situations in early life	37	·01
Concentration and persistence in work at C.S.	(p. 25)	·02
Possibly significant:		
Relationship with (day) Schools	45	·05
Not statistically significant:		
Abnormal Matrices Scatter ('Shaw' criterion)	(p. 230)	·1
Age when first left home	39	·2
Expression of feelings	6	·3
First known delinquency	—	·5
Number of home environments	29	·8
Delinquency in the home	43	·7
Relationships in the home	44	·7
Passalong Test Score	(p. 233)	·7
Matrices Test grade	52	·8
Binet Test I.Q.	51	·7
Economic Status of Parents	22	·9
Material Condition of Home	21	·8
Been under Supervision before Committal	—	·7
Been on Probation before Committal	—	·9

*Table usually regrouped for statistical purposes.

to doing well—those who wanted to do well—then the same holds in the main after they have been out in the world for up to nearly three years, during which a considerable number are married and running homes of their own. Both conduct at the Classifying Stage and responsiveness to training predict very well. The second assumption is that, whatever shaped the girl herself at some time in the past, launched her into the relevant stream at this later stage. Closer examination of some of the particular findings may help here.

Success after 12 to 17 months training

73 per cent of those who did well at the one stage did well at the other. There was doubtless a follow-through, in that good relationships during training inspired confidence all round. Expectation by others often plays a major role, but *character strength* again scores.

Concentration and persistence at work in the C.S., and earlier *relationship with the day school*, again are significant pointers.

Conduct at the Classifying School

About 80 per cent of those who were cooperative, or even just toed the line, at the Classifying School were doing well two up to three years after licence from Training School; that is four or more years after classification. Only 40 per cent of the openly uncooperative and childish were doing well. Observation, even in the lay terms as depicted, seems to have justified itself. At this later stage the factors in the home background (apart, possibly, from early feelings of rejection) would be less help for prediction.

Prevailing Mood at the Classifying School

The serious had an 80 per cent chance of doing well, the cheerful a 71 per cent, and the anxious a 68 per cent. Only 1 out of 3 of the apathetic did well, but the depressed (perhaps no longer so depressed) had a 50 : 50 chance.

Whether these moods, so-called, could have been measured in similar terms in a different setting than the residential one described would require much thought; how far, for instance, was the seriousness a positive response to anxiety engendered by Court appearances? Yet one feels that training in observation at day schools could refine the instruments of earlier prediction. 'Character strength' might be deduced as successfully there—and probably is done.

Contribution to group at Classifying School

Again we find positive out-going behaviour towards contemporaries acting as a predictor, this time for behaviour which may be centred within a family group rather than among workmates and leisure companions.

Time spent in Training School

Here the prediction was in inverse ratio—the long terms of training were not conducive to later success. 80 per cent of those trained for a year to eighteen months subsequently did well; only 52 per cent of those trained for two and three quarter years or more did reasonably well. Of course far more of the latter might otherwise have failed— they were retained because of their needs. On the other hand we do not know how far some of the failures would have been 'helped' by release earlier.

Appearance (*physical type*)

This column for the first time comes into its own. The precise finding is that 70 per cent of the stalwart and sturdy succeeded out in the world, while only 52 per cent of the slim and lanky did. One wonders if this is sheer physical success—advantage to the strong, who are quickly accepted for the kind of jobs (or marriages) most of the Approved School population was mentally attuned to. Whether the lesser degree of sensitivity linked with the mesomorphic physiques is the important lead, one cannot do more than conjecture, without further research.

What this finding does not do is to answer an earlier prediction that the mesomorphs might contain most recidivists.

Number of Detrimental Situations in Early Life

Again the distinguishing link is between *no* known early separations, through major or minor losses, and failure. Only 35 per cent of this group followed through to this stage did well. In view of a similar finding earlier, this small section could well do with further study. For those who did have separations, the timing of the first seems more vital (*v.* age when first left home).

Matrices Scatter

Again we find a slight tendency for those with a score in set D more than 2 points higher than in set C to do better—enough tendency for this tentatively suggested measure of anxiety to be explored further.

Age when first left home

The very fact that less significance (if any) attached at this later stage to traces of rejection or neglect from early separation from home is important; the training response was conjectured as triggering off such earlier feelings. At this later stage, those who did not leave home prior to the events leading to Approved School committal were 70 per cent successful. Others were more or less true to statistical expectations—though only half of those who left home before the age of 5 did well in the late teens; this was as for response to training, and may reflect lasting affect. The figure of 35 per cent for those who were separated between 5 and 8 (due, we conjectured, to old feelings of neglect being aroused) has now improved to 56 per cent.

Intelligence and Performance Test Results

These, most interestingly, now have no significant link with success. Nor do material and economic or moral conditions. Again being on probation before committal, and the opportunity of a well-forged relationship with the subsequent after-care officer, does not tangibly affect results.

Chapter Twenty-two

OUTLOOK

The writer has had decreasing contact with Girls' Approved Schools since 1958. Some of the success/failure figures for this research extend beyond this point. News also filters through, and certain evidence presents itself in the form of posts advertised in the service. The following table has been compiled for six complete years of posts for Headmistresses and Deputy Headmistresses, advertised in the *Approved Schools Gazette* which is a monthly publication. This may not be a complete list; on the other hand there may be over-estimates if the same vacancy was advertised after a considerable gap, without meantime being filled.

Table 63: Advertising for Head Posts

Year	Headmistress		Deputy Headmistress	
	No. of Advts	No. of Posts	No. of Advts	No. of Posts
1959 (10 mths)	7	6	11	7
1960	5	4	6	4
1961	6	4	6	4
1962	9	2	10	7
1963	4	3	11	4
1964	6	4	7	6
1965 (2 mths)	1	1	1	1
Total	38	24	52	33
Mean No. Adverts per post	1·6		1·6	
Mean No. Posts per year	4·		5·5	

At the end of 1960 there were thirty-five Approved Schools for Girls, so about one school in nine was needing a new Headmistress each year. This allows for one new school opened in that time.

Further study shows, in fact, that the twenty-four posts were for about seventeen schools, for the others had made new appointments within the six-year period. This suggests more unrest still. One school, for instance, had a vacancy in November 1959, and again in December 1961; another (an older school reorganized) had a vacancy in

274

April 1959, and was again advertising for a Headmistress in August 1961, and in June, July, October and November of 1962; a vacancy in March 1960 was followed by a vacancy in March 1962, and was then advertised in October and November 1963 and in January 1964.

In the older pattern for Girls' Approved Schools, especially the Senior Schools, the Headmistress was an all-prevailing influence. At her best she was a beloved matriarch, at her worst an iron-willed tyrant—but there were fortunately few of the latter, and most came between—good, effectual mother-figures, reacting to the challenge of their calling in the pattern of their own upbringing and schooling (both usually nice and orderly, but rarely culminating in University, and sometimes not in any Training College).

One has heard rumours of a new look to the work in recent years, the main solutions being a house-system and a married Headmistress, or even a Headmaster. When we look at the advertisements we should, then, sense the new stimulus, in the form of highly enlightened wording.

The following appeared, as late as 1964, for a Junior Approved School where 'teaching and training facilities are provided on the premises for the very disturbed or backward girls' aged 10½ to 15 years on admission: 'Executive and administrative abilities are essential, and *whilst not necessary* (my italics) teaching qualifications with the former attributes would be most desirable.' Might one suggest a computer could do this job (if anyone knows a suitable programme).

Usually the qualifications asked are as vague as one in the same *Gazette* for a Senior School (sixty girls 15 to 17 years on admission, being trained in 'housecraft, farming and horticulture, together with general education and out-working from a pre-release hostel'): 'The applicant should possess a recognized qualification for work with young people. A knowledge of modern trends in Approved Schools and residential experience would be an advantage.' Presumably a Youth Employment Officer with a pleasing personality would have a reasonably good chance; unfortunately a qualified teacher working in Approved School would appreciate the difficulties ahead and might hesitate to apply. Generally the demands are minimal, University degrees, especially in education or psychology, being of most rare mention, though social science qualifications (which may mean little training in group work) are more in favour. More important, as with all the posts in the schools—many vacant for long periods, to judge by advertising—is the lack of emphasis on training and experience with (a) normal, and (b) disturbed and difficult adolescent girls. A large percentage of the population have failed in the ordinary schools, and in other institutions provided by the Social and educational services. The figures produced in this research show a considerable percentage failed in the kind of régimes supplied in the 1950s; about 30 per cent failed to some extent, while 8·5 per cent failed very badly.

Those whose work is with a classified group of delinquents tend to see the problem with their own slant; those specializing with the more intelligent neurotic delinquent see the answer in terms of deep psychotherapy, and activities suited to 'good' teenage ideals, such as climbing mountains or decorating old peoples' houses; those handling the educationally subnormal delinquent think in terms of calm but very firm lines of discipline, with verbal explanations in sentences suited to the 8-year-old, and repeated practical demonstrations. Among girls there is generally another fairly easy group—the scatter-brained but not so very dim girl who has been socially deprived or untutored probably through parental death, or just through parental inadequacy. Training can be mostly by suggestion or example, if staff can grasp the rather subtle techniques and themselves have integrity.

Those who have worked with the anti-social, warped characters (at their worst requiring the psychopath label) sometimes too think they know how to deal with them—you blow, you bluster, you try not to let them get you down, or if you're too refined to work that way you gently ignore their poisonous attitudes, their distorted toddler-level playing-up.

A doubtful advantage of the Classifying School experience was that one was made aware of the many types, including some we have not mentioned here. There were girls who should never have been there at all. There were just a very few extremely good girls, whom we had quickly to save from the self-depreciation that a Court appearance had inflicted. A few others were borderline problems and should have been salvaged without such extreme measures. But also there was the odd psychotic or pre-psychotic girl, or the very severely subnormal; these confused the whole machinery and were confused by it. Along with the seriously psychopathic girls they took up individual staff time and made a mockery of paper organization. Because lay staff so often had to deal with crises demanding drug-therapy and mental nursing skills within a specialist Adolescent Unit, it was difficult to see the job itself in perspective, and people with tremendous personal resources gave up in perplexity or exhaustion. What was done without the physical conditions considered necessary in hospital is, in retrospect, awe inspiring, especially by the Head-mistress during the main research period (1952–4).

Even the more straightforward groups are likely to be a match for maladjusted adolescents or educationally subnormal adolescents in boarding schools, for delinquents are not too welcome there. To appoint Headmistresses and staff with fewer qualifications than in those schools is therefore not very sensible; if there are reasons why Approved Schools should not come under the control of local education authorities, or some central controlling authority, the right appointment of staff is not one of them.

When we come to the very seriously disturbed nucleus, those 8 per cent with 'poor' success ratings in the 500 sample, and a good many more who were on the downward slope (not to mention most of the fifty girls eliminated before the sample was studied), we must face the fact that they cannot be cured under the conditions that existed in the Girls' Approved Schools as studied in this research. If new and startling methods have been introduced I have not heard of them.* One does still hear of girls admitted to Adolescent Units who are too psychopathic for there, of girls admitted to prison who are too neurotic for there.

It might seem to the reader that the simple and obvious thing was to select the 'most failing' group in this research, and state the prevailing factors in their lives. In fact the research has already highlighted the prevailing factors, and the types of personality (depressed, cheerful, apathetic, etc.) who tended to do better or worse. Some of the classical theories (such as the damage of early maternal separation) have been endorsed, and extended to include (for our girls) paternal deprivation in the latency years as well, perhaps, as rejection by father in later years. Often the damage on doubtful constitutions seemed to have been irreparable before the girls came to Approved School. The challenge, then, if we expect cure, lies far back in the line of Welfare Services, with Child Guidance and Family Guidance Clinics, with local authority Health, Education and Children's Departments, and with all good neighbours everywhere.

* This had gone to the publisher's before the appearance of the Government White Paper 'Children in Trouble' (1968), Cmnd 3601, H.M.S.O., and before the announcement in June 1968 by the Home Secretary of new centres for treating severely disturbed boys and girls from Approved Schools.

Appendix

SIGNIFICANT CORRELATIONS

I. Factors Correlated with success 2 to 3 years after licence—see Table 62 (p. 271).
II. Factors correlated with success after 12 to 17 months at Training School—see Table 58 (p. 259).
III. Factors Correlated with Conduct at Classifying School (Table 8).

Factor	Table*	P value	Comment
Success 12 to 17 months at training school	58	·001	
Success 2 to 3 years on licence	62	·001	
Age first left home	39	·001	Left 0 to 8 years more childish behaviour
Matrices grade	52	·001	Lowest 2 grades more childish
Binet I.Q.	51	·001	I.Q. 84 and below—more childish. Not subversive
Economic status of parents	22	·01	
Relationships in home	44	·05	Barely significant
Material condition of home	21	·05	Barely significant, but those from extremely uncomfortable homes more cooperative
Adults with mainly	30	·1–·05	Those with mother absent tended more to childish outbursts. With father absent tended to be more aggressive

Not Significant: Passalong Scores; Matrices Scatter; Home Area; Major/Minor Detrimental Situations.
* *Tables usually regrouped for statistical purposes.*

IV. Factors Correlated with Age on Committal to A.S. (Table 15).

Factor	Table	P value	Comment
Age on 1st known Court appearance	p. 86	·001	
Age at 1st known delinquency	p. 91	·001	
Success at time of 3rd report from T.S.		·05	Barely significant. 14's and older 16's doing rather better

Not Significant: Success at T.S.; Major/Minor Detrimental Situations.
279

V. Factors Correlated with Residence following Break in Home (i.e. Adults normally lived with).

Factor	Table	P value	Comment
Success 12 to 17 months at T.S.	58	·05	Barely significant
Conduct at C.S.	8	·1 to ·05	Barely significant

Note: In each case where both parents absent the tendency was to do distinctly worse. Did rather better if mother absent than if father absent.

Not Significant: Demand for attention; Later success; Age at first delinquency; Mood at C.S.

VI. Factors Correlated with Material Condition of Home (Table 21).

Factor	Table	P value	Comment
Binet I.Q.	51	·001 ⎱	'Dullest' groups from least
Matrices score	52	·01 ⎰	comfortable homes
Relationships in home	44	·001	Extremely uncomfortable—child slackly disciplined
Size of family	—	·001	Extremely uncomfortable linked with very large family
Scholastic attainment in Reading	—	·001 ⎱	Attainment of girls from more comfortable homes tended to be higher
Attainment in number	—	·01 ⎰	
Conduct at C.S.	8	·05	Barely significant, but girls from extremely uncomfortable homes tended to be more cooperative
Chief misbehaviour before committal	49	·05	Stealing rather more linked with comfortable homes. Truancy rather more linked with uncomfortable homes
1st known Court appearance	—	·1 to ·05	Barely significant

Not Significant: Success at Training School; Success on Licence; Major/Minor Detrimental Situations.

Appendix

VII. Factors Correlated with Economic Status of Parents (Table 22).

Factor	Table	P Value	Comment
Binet I.Q.	51	·001	
Matrices grade	52	·001	
Scholastic attainment in Reading	—	·001	
Attainment in number	—	·001	
Size of family	—	·001	
Conduct at Classifying School	8	·01	Better off girls more in subversive group. Dependent (economically) either more straight or more openly uncooperative
No Major/Minor detrimental situations	37	·01	Troubles piled up for girls of unskilled and dependent families
Mood at Classifying School	7	·05	Barely significant. Girls from better homes (economically) tend to be more resentful or more anxious
Success at Classifying School	58	·1 to ·05	Barely significant, but dependent (economically) tended to do better

Not Significant: Success on Licence; Age when first left Home.

VIII. Factors Correlated with Place in Family

Factor	Table	P value	Comment
Binet vocabulary	—	·02	Significantly more 1st children than later were above average for age in vocabulary
Binet I.Q.	51	·2 to ·1	Not significant but still slight tendency for 1st, 2nd, 3rd to be higher

Not Significant: Matrices Grade; Demand for Attention.

281

Appendix

IX. Factors Correlated with Size of Family (Table 35).

Factor	Table	P value	Comment
Material condition of home	21	·001	As above
Delinquency in family	43	·001	More delinquents in families of 6 to 11
Economic status of home	22	·001	As above
Scholastic attainment in			
(a) Reading	—	·01	As expected
(b) Number	—	·2	—larger families poorer readers. Not significant for arithmetical ability

X. Factors Correlated to No. of Different 'Home' Environments (Table 29).

Not Significant Correlation.

XI. Factors Related to Time in Training School pre-licence (Table 57a).

Factor	Table	P value	Comment
Success 2 to 3 years after licence	71	·01	Very long training linked with extreme failure

XII. Number of Major/Minor Detrimental Situations (Table 37).

Factor	Table	P value	Comment
Relationships in home	44	·01	Those with accumulation of detrimental situations were more unhappy and rejected at home
Success 2 to 3 years on licence	62	·01 ⎫	Those with *NO* major or minor detrimental situations *tended* to do badly, and
Success 12 to 17 months on licence	58	·05 ⎬	definitely worse as time went on
Offence for which committed	16	·05	Barely significant. Tendency to be in beyond control group if *many* detrimental situations

XIII. Factors Related to Delinquency in the Home (Table 43).
See Table IX.

XIV. Factors Related to Age when First Left Home (Table 39).
See III and II.

282

XV. *Factors Related to Conduct at Work* (pre-Committal).*

Factor	Table	P value	Comment
Relationship with Day Schools	45	·001	
Concentration and persistence at C.S.	—	·01	All in expected directions
School sent to	60	·01	
Mood at C.S.	7	·01	
Success 2 to 3 years on licence	62	·02	

* *Not number of jobs, as on p. 197. See p. 198.*

XVI. *Factors Related to Home Relationships (Table 44).*

Factor	Table	P value	Comment
Binet I.Q.	51	·001	Tendency for the duller girls to have been slackly disciplined and the brighter to have been rejected
Material condition of home	21	·001	
Age first left home	39	·001	More felt rejected if left home 0 to 4 years. More felt neglected if left 5 to 8 years
No. major/minor detrimental situations	37	·01	Girls with no major or minor were happier, less rejected
Conduct at C.S.	8	·05	The rejected were more subversive or openly uncooperative

XVII. *Factors Related with Relationships with Day Schools.*
See XV, and I and II.

XVIII. *Factors Related to Binet I.Q.*
See III, VI, VII and XVI.

XIX. *Factors Related to Passalong Test Scores.*
See II.

XX. *Factors Related to Matrices Grades.*
See III, VI and VII.

XXI. Factors Related to Matrices Scatter ('Shaw' Criterion).

Factor	P value	Comment
Prevalent mood	·05	Barely significant
Success at T.S.	·1 to ·05	but interesting
Success 2 to 3 yrs on licence	·1 to ·05	(See text).

XXII. Group Participation, Contribution to Group, Identification with Contemporaries, Expression of Feelings, Mood at C.S.
Character Strength—See Tables 58, 60, 62.

XXIII. Factors Related to Training School to which sent.
See Table 60.

NOTES

Chapter I

1. *Reformatory Schools for the Children of the Perishing and Dangerous Classes and for Juvenile Offenders*, Mary Carpenter (1851), Gilpin.
2. *Seventh and Eighth Reports of the Work of the Children's Department* (1955 and 1961), H.M.S.O.
3. *The Report of the Committee on Maladjusted Children* (The Underwood Report) (1955), H.M.S.O.
4. *Throw Away Thy Rod*, David Wills (1960), Gollancz.
5. *The Sexual Behaviour of Young People*, Michael Schofield (1965), Longmans.
6. *Society of Woman—A Study of a Women's Prison*, Rose Giallombardo (1966), Wiley, N.Y.

Chapter II

1. *Schools for Young Offenders*, Gordon Rose (1966), Tavistock Publications.
2. Van der Slice—*Journal of Criminal Law and Criminology*, Vol. XXVII (1936–7).
3. *Women in Prison*, Ann Smith (1962), Stevens.
4. John Howard (1784), *The State of the Prisons*.
5. Griffiths (1884).
6. *Memoirs*, Elizabeth Fry, Vol. 1. (1847), Gilpin.
7. *Reformatory Schools for the Children of the Perishing and Dangerous Classes and for Juvenile Offenders*, Mary Carpenter (1851).
8. *Report of the Departmental Committee on the treatment of Young Offenders* (1927), H.M.S.O.

Chapter III

1. *Approved School Boys*, John Gittins (1952), H.M.S.O.

Chapter VI

1. *The Psychopath*, William McCord and Joan McCord (1964), Van Nostrand.
2. *Report of the Committee on Children and Young Persons* (The Ingleby Report) (1960), H.M.S.O.

Chapter VII

1. *Manual of Child Psychology*, Carmichael (1946), Wiley, New York.
2. *Brit. J. Educ. Psych.* (June 1966), Vol. 26, Part II, pp. 202–9.
3. *Crime and Personality*, Eysenck (1964), Routledge & Kegan Paul.
4. *Approved School Boys*, John Gittins (1952), H.M.S.O.

5. *Delinquency and Human Nature*, D. H. Stott (1950), Carnegie.
6. *Wayward Youth*, Aichorn (1925), Imago.
7. *The Psychoanalytical Approach to Juvenile Delinquency*, Freidlander (1947), Routledge & Kegan Paul.

Chapter VIII (a)

1. 'Sex Differences in the Life Problems and Interests of Adolescents', Symonds, *School and Society*, No. 43 (1936), pp. 751-2, New York.
2. *L'Uomo Delinquente*, Lombroso (1895), Turin.
3. *Personality*, Allport (1937), Constable.
4. *The Young Delinquent*, Burt (1925), University of London Press.
5. 'A review of some studies of delinquents and delinquency', Healy (1925), *Arch. Neurol. Psychiat.*, 14, Chicago, pp. 25-30.
6. *Varieties in Human Physique*, Sheldon (1940), New York.
7. *Varieties of Delinquent Youth*, Sheldon (1949), New York.
8. *Unravelling Delinquency*, S. and E. Glueck (1950), New York.
9. *Psychiatric Examination of Borstal Lads*, Gibbens (1963), Maudsley Monographs.
10. 'Physique and Temperament', Epps and Parnell, *Brit. J. Med. Psych.*, No. 25 (1952), pp. 249-55.
11. *Approved School Boys*, Gittins (1952), H.M.S.O.

Chapter VIII (b)

1. *Pentonville—A Sociological Study of an English Prison*, Terence and Pauline Morris (1963), Routledge & Kegan Paul.

Chapter VIII (c)

1. *Approved School Boys*, Gittins (1952), H.M.S.O.
2. *Unravelling Delinquency*, S. and E. Glueck (1950), New York.
3. *Brit. J. Educ. Psych.* (June 1955), Vol. 25, Part II, pp. 123-8.
4. *The Normal Child and some of his Abnormalities*, Valentine (1956), Penguin Books.
5. *Psychiatric Examination of the School Child*, M. Barton-Hall (1947), Arnold.
6. Ogle (1871): quoted by Hécaen (below).
7. *Left-handedness*, W. M. Clark (1957), University of London Press.
8. *Left-handedness*, Hécaen and de Ajuriaguerra (1964), New York.
9. Ballard: quoted by Blœdé, 'Les gauchers. Étude du comportement de la pathologie et de la conduite à tenir', Thesis, Lyon, (1946), p. 72. Quoted by Hécaen (above).
10. Pringle, M. L. Kellmer, 'Adverse Conditions in Maladjusted Children', *Brit. J. Educ. Psych.* (1961), Vol. 31, 183-93.

Chapter IX

1. *Seventh Report on the Work of the Children's Department* (1955), H.M.S.O.
2. *Report of the Committee on Children and Young Persons* (1960), H.M.S.O.

3. *Social Science and Social Pathology*, Barbara Wootton (1959), Allen & Unwin.
4. *Youth: The Years from 10 to 16*, Gesell, Ilg, Ames (1956), N.Y.

Chapter X

1. *500 Delinquent Women*, S. and E. Glueck (1934, Reprinted 1965), New York.
2. *The Criminal Area*, Morris (1958), Routledge & Kegan Paul.
3. *Juvenile Delinquency in an English Middletown*, Mannheim (1948), Routledge & Kegan Paul.
4. *The Social Background of Delinquency*, Jephcott & Carter (1954), University of Nottingham.
5. *Delinquency and Child Neglect*, Harriet Wilson (1962), Allen & Unwin.
6. *Psychiatric Studies of Borstal Lads*, Gibbens (1963), Maudsley Monograph.

Chapter XI

1. Epps, 'A Preliminary Survey of 300 Female Delinquents in Borstal Institutions', *British Journal of Delinquency*, Vol. I (1951), No. 3, pp. 187–97.
2. Epps, 'A Further Survey of Female Delinquents undergoing Borstal Training', *British Journal of Delinquency*, Vol. IV (1954), No. 4, pp. 265–71.
3. Stephanos, *Studies in Psychology* (1966). Edited by Banks, pp. 173–203. 'Boys in Detention Centres'.
4. *The Young Delinquent*, Burt (1925), University of London Press.
5. *Young Offenders*, Carr-Saunders, Mannheim & Rhodes (1942), Cambridge University Press.
6. *Unravelling Delinquency*, S. and E. Glueck (1950), New York.
7. *Juvenile Delinquents in a Psychiatric Clinic*, Litauer (1957), I.S.T.D. Publication.
8. *Approved School Boys*, Gittins (1952), H.M.S.O.
9. *500 Delinquent Women*, S. and E. Glueck (1934. Reprinted 1965), New York.
10. *Throw Away Thy Rod*, David Wills (1960), Gollancz.
11. *Psychiatric Studies of Borstal Lads*, Gibbens (1963), Maudsley Monograph.
12. *Maternal Care and Mental Health*, Bowlby (1951), W.H.O.
13. *Delinquent Girls in Court*, Tappan (1949), McGraw Hill.
14. *In Place of Parents*, Trasler (1960), Routledge & Kegan Paul.
15. *Delinquent and Neurotic Children*, Ivy Bennett (1960), Tavistock Publications.
16. *Delinquency and Child Neglect*, Harriet Wilson (1962), Allen & Unwin.
17. 'Adverse Conditions in Maladjusted Children', M. L. Kellmer Pringle (1961), *Brit. J. Educ. Psych.* Vol. 31, pp. 183–93.

Chapter XII

1. *500 Delinquent Women*, S. and E. Glueck (1934. Reprinted 1965), New York.
2. *Psychiatric Aspects of Juvenile Delinquency*, Bovet (1951), W.H.O.

Chapter XIII

1. *Brit. J. of Delinquency*, Vol. 1, No. 3, Epps (1951).
2. *500 Delinquent Women*, S. & E. Glueck (1934. Reprinted 1965), New York.
3. *Juvenile Delinquents in a Psychiatric Clinic*, Litauer (1957), I.S.T.D. Publications.
4. *Brit. J. Delinq.* Vol. 5, No. 1, (July 1954), Lees & Newson, 'Sibship Position and Juvenile Delinquency'.
5. *Unravelling Delinquency*, S. & E. Glueck (1950), New York.
6. *Juvenile Delinquency in an English Middletown*, Mannheim (1948), Routledge & Kegan Paul.

Chapter XIV

1. *The Explanation of Criminality*, Trasler (1962), Routledge & Kegan Paul.
2. *The Social Background of Delinquency*, Sprott, Jephcott & Carter (1954), University of Nottingham.
3. *Growing Up in the City*, Mays (1954), Liverpool University Press.
4. *The Young Delinquent in the Social Setting*, Ferguson (1952), Oxford University Press.
5. *The Criminal Area*, Morris (1958), Routledge, Kegan Paul.
6. *500 Borstal Boys*, Rose (1954), Blackwell.

Chapter XV

1. *Child Care and Mental Health*, Bowlby (1951), W.H.O.
2. *Organisation of Behaviour*, Hebb (1949), New York.
3. *In Place of Parents*, Trasler (1960), Routledge & Kegan Paul.

Chapter XVI

1. *Approved School Boys*, Gittins (1952), H.M.S.O.
2. *500 Delinquent Women*, S. & E. Glueck (1934. Reprinted 1965), New York.
3. *15-18*, (1960), Central Advisory Council for Education.
4. *The Sexual Behaviour of Young People*, Michael Schofield (1965), Longmans.

Chapter XVII

1. *Delinquent and Neurotic Children*, Bennett (1960), Tavistock Publications.
2. *The Psychopath*, W. & J. McCord (1956), New York.
3. *Report of the Committee on Maladjusted Children* (1955), H.M.S.O.

Chapter XVIII
1. *The Sexual Behaviour of Young People.* Michael Schofield (1965), Longmans.
2. *Cider with Rosie,* Lee (1959), Hogarth Press.

Chapter XIX
1. *Measuring Intelligence,* Terman-Merrill (1937), Harrap.
2. *Approved School Boys,* Gittins (1952), H.M.S.O.
3. *The Young Delinquent,* Burt (1925), University of London Press.
4. *Juvenile Delinquents in a Psychiatric Clinic,* Litauer (1957), I.S.T.D. Publications.
5. *Low Intelligence and Delinquency,* Mary Woodward (1955), I.S.T.D. Publications.
6. 'Age & Intelligence of a Group of Juvenile Delinquents', Mann (1939), *J. Abnorm. Soc. Psych.,* Vol. 34, pp. 351-60.
7. *Problems of Child Delinquency,* Merrill (1947), Harrap.
8. *Guide to Using Progressive Matrices,* Raven (1938), H. K. Lewis, London.
9. Epps. *Brit. J. Delinq.,* Vol. 1, No. 3, 1951, Epps.
10. 'Standardisation of Progressive Matrices', Raven, *Brit. J. Med. Psych.,* Part 1, 99, pp. 187-150 (1941).
11. 'The Validity and Interchangeability of Terman-Merrill and Matrices Test Data', D. Walton., *Brit. J. Psych.,* Vol. 25, Part III, Nov. 1955.
12. *The Porteus Maze Test Manual,* Porteus (1952), Harrap.
13. *Crime and Personality,* Eysenck (1964), Routledge & Kegan Paul.
14. *Psychiatric Examination of Borstal Lads,* Gibbens (1963), Oxford University Press.
15. *Porteus Maze Tests: 50 years after,* Porteus (1965), Harrap.
16. *Personnel Selection in the British Forces,* Vernon & Parry (1949), University of London.
17. *Personality,* Allport (1937), Constable.
18. *Performance Tests of Intelligence,* Drever & Collins (1928), Oliver & Boyd.
19. *Intelligence Concrete & Abstract,* W. P. Alexander (1935), Cambridge University Press.
20. *Manual to Thematic Apperception Test,* Murray (1943) Harvard University Press
21. *Explorations in Personality* Murray (1938) New York.
22. 'The Measurement of Personality in Children', Himmelweit & Petrie, *Brit. Educ. Psych.,* Vol. 21 (1951), pp. 9-29.
23. *Psychodynamics,* Rorschach (1942), Bern.
24. Richardson, *The Rorschach Newsletter,* Vol. VIII, No. 2, Dec. 1963.
25. *Adolescent Rorschach Responses,* Ames, Metraux, Walker (1959), N.Y.
26. Schubert, *The Rorschach Newsletter,* Vol. XI, June 1966.
27. *Society and the Criminal,* East W. Norwood (1949), H.M.S.O.
28. *Saving Children from Delinquency,* Stott, D. H. (1952), University of London Press.
29. *Unravelling Juvenile Delinquency,* Glueck, S. E. (1950), Harvard University Press.

INDEX OF PERSONS

SUBJECT INDEX

Index

For Product Safety Concerns and Information please contact our EU
representative GPSR@taylorandfrancis.com
Taylor & Francis Verlag GmbH, Kaufingerstraße 24, 80331 München, Germany